The Alcohol Report

Edited by

Martin Plant and Douglas Cameron

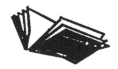

FREE ASSOCIATION BOOKS / LONDON / NEW YORK

Published in 2000 by
Free Association Books
57 Warren Street, London W1T 5NR

A CIP record for this book is available from the British Library

ISBN 1 85343 525 2 hbk

ISBN 1 85343 524 4 pbk

Designed and produced by Chase Publishing Services
Printed in the European Union by TJ International, Padstow

The Alcohol Report

Contents

List of Tables, Figures and Boxes

Tables

FIGURES

BOXES

Notes on Contributors

Colin Bennie RMN. Manager, Community Alcohol and Drug Service, Forth Valley Primary Care NHS Trust, UK.

David Campbell RMN. Community Alcohol and Drug Service, Forth Valley Primary Care NHS Trust, UK.

Douglas Cameron MD. Senior Lecturer (Clinical) in Substance Abuse, Department of Psychiatry, University of Leicester, UK.

Ian Davidson RMN. Research Nurse, Alcohol and Health Research Centre, Edinburgh, UK.

Henk Garretsen PhD. Professor/Director, Addiction Research Institute (IVO) Rotterdam, The Netherlands.

Eileen Goddard BA. Principal Researcher, Office for National Statistics, London, UK.

Kathryn Graham PhD. Senior Scientist/Head of Social Factors and Prevention Initiatives, Centre for Addiction and Mental Health, London, Ontario, Canada.

Nick Heather PhD. Professor/Director, Centre for Drug and Alcohol Studies, Newcastle Upon Tyne, UK.

Ron McKechnie MSc. Consultant Clinical Psychologist, Department of Psychological Services and Research, Dumfries, UK.

Iain McKinney RMN. Charge Nurse, Community Alcohol and Drug Service, Forth Valley Primary Care NHS Trust, UK.

Martin Plant PhD. Director, Alcohol and Health Research Centre, Edinburgh, UK.

Moira Plant PhD. Senior Scientist/Deputy Director, Alcohol and Health Research Centre, Edinburgh, UK.

Bruce Ritson MD. Lead Clinician, Substance Misuse Directorate, Royal Edinburgh Hospital Lothian Primary Care NHS Trust.

Eric Single PhD. Professor, University of Toronto, Ontario, Canada.

Diwakar Sukul PhD. Director, Kamkus Centre for Multidimensional Healthcare and Holistic Dentistry, London, UK.

Anthony Thorley MA, MB, FRC Psych. Consultant Psychiatrist in the Addictions, Bath and Western Wiltshire Specialist Drug and Alcohol Service, Bath, UK.

Christine Thornton CQSW. Research Fellow, Alcohol and Health Research Centre, Edinburgh, UK.

Christopher Thurman MBE. Until recently Director, Economics and Statistics, Brewers and Licensed Retailers Association, London, UK.

Linda Wright PhD. Freelance health promotion consultant, Great Ayton, Yorkshire, UK.

Preface

This book sets out to provide a balanced and informative review of some of the key topics likely to interest those with a serious concern with evidence about drinking patterns and levels of alcohol-related problems. Such people include medical practitioners, nurses, psychologists, social workers, counsellors and those who work in specialist and non-specialist statutory and voluntary agencies providing help and support for those with drinking problems and their families. In addition, it is hoped that the text will be helpful to a wide range of people whose work is likely to bring them into contact with drinking and 'problem drinking'. The latter include the police, social workers, prison staff, people working in the beverage alcohol industry and in the distribution and sale of alcohol, together with students, civil servants and politicians. In short, it is hoped that *The Alcohol Report* will provide an informative and balanced source of user-friendly, dependable information about some of the key issues related to alcohol.

The contributors to this book represent several different disciplines. These include economics, health promotion, nursing, psychiatry, psychology, social work, sociology and statistics. The contributors do not necessarily share a common philosophy or perspective. This book does not aim to provide any type of 'ideological consensus'. It was written by people with their own individual viewpoints. Each of the contributors has special interests in and expertise related to the topics about which they have written.

This book includes a bibliography of the main references found to be helpful in the compilation of this text. It is hoped that this will assist those seeking further information.

The views expressed in this book are solely those of the contributors. Any errors are the responsibility of the editors.

Acknowledgements

The editors are grateful to many people for assistance in the writing of this book. Particular thanks go to Mr Steve Chalmers and Mrs Janet Docherty of the Alcohol and Health Research Centre (A&HRC) and to Ms Emma Plant of the University of British Columbia, Vancouver. Thanks are also due to members of staff at Alcohol Concern, the Health Education Board for Scotland, the Home Office, the Medical Council on Alcoholism, the Scottish Council on Alcohol, the Scottish Executive and the Office for National Statistics.

The A&HRC is an independent charity. The work of the research team has been supported by the beverage alcohol industry, government departments, charities, research councils, the World Health Organization, the European Union, the police, local authorities, health boards and NHS trusts. The A&HRC has recently received core support from Allied Domecq, the PF Charitable Trust and the North British Distillery Company Limited.

1
Drinking and Problem Drinking

Douglas Cameron and Martin Plant

We started this book with the intention of updating *Drinking and Problem Drinking* (Plant 1982), but it soon became clear that that was not possible, and that a different book was required, for it is notable how far our thinking has moved in that short time. We could no longer even sustain that original title, for embedded in it was the notion of dichotomy, that in some ways there are either two sets of behaviours, one set being socially, psychologically or medically problem-free and the other not so; neither would we now maintain that there are 'simply' two kinds of people: those whose drinking is problem-free and those whose drinking is not. It is not like that. Drinking episodes which are defined as problematic in one context may be defined as totally acceptable, even desirable, in another. To talk of problematic intoxication without talking of the intent or purpose behind that intoxication is a road to nowhere.

We acknowledge that alcohol consumption has long been a hugely popular form of human behaviour; that alcoholic beverages are used as an accompaniment to social activity in most countries of the world. People generally consume beverage alcohol because they enjoy its effects and because its consumption receives strong social support, or at least has widespread social acceptance. Alcohol is often an integral component of marking special occasions, such as births, marriages, anniversaries, festivals or funerals. It is also incorporated into some religious rituals. Alcohol consumption is clearly useful to humankind.

That consumption is influenced by a host of factors. These include the personality, relationships, life stage and life experiences of the individual, the setting in which drinking occurs, and the chemistry of the mind-altering substance called ethyl alcohol. This theme is addressed in more detail in Chapter 3.

But since the earliest records of beverage alcohol production and consumption, there have been references to drunkenness or to undesirable consequences associated with inappropriate drinking. Throughout history there have been innumerable attempts to define and to curb the 'excessive' or 'problematic' consumption of alcohol. Excessive or problematic consumption has been variously characterised as a social problem, a sign of weakness of will, immorality, skills or self-esteem deficit, or as sickness. The portrayal of problems related to alcohol has taken up considerable effort and such problems have been defined in different ways in different places and at different times (Trotter 1813, Beecher 1826, Musto 1997).

During recent decades, there has been an explosion of 'scientific' information about alcohol consumption and its consequences, both positive and negative. Indeed, there is even now a substantial body of evidence suggesting that low-level alcohol consumption may be beneficial in health terms. That evidence was not even acknowledged 20 years ago. That is discussed further in the next chapter, dealing with the effects of alcohol. It is hoped that the following chapters provide a useful, if inevitably highly selective, guide to some of this vast literature. Research has examined almost every conceivable aspect of alcohol use. The resulting information has now made it possible to provide a fuller and also probably a more balanced, but more complicated, overview of issues related to drinking and its associated costs and benefits than before. Some of the literature about alcohol and its problems has tried to indicate that there might be a fairly clear-cut distinction between those who consume alcohol without problems and those whose drinking involves some form of adverse effect. In these days of the Human Genome Project, bodily differences to explain that distinction are pursued.

The earlier book *Drinking and Problem Drinking* made mention in Chapter 1 of the founding fathers of Alcoholics Anonymous, and about our emerging reservations of the disease concept of 'Alcoholism' as promulgated by Alcoholics Anonymous (AA). Here, 20 years later, we acknowledge that the dichotomous belief that there are two races of drinkers, so-called 'normal drinkers' and 'alcoholics' or sufferers from the 'alcohol dependence syndrome', remains one of the most widespread and widely promulgated ways of portraying alcohol problems. This defines 'alcoholism' as an incurable, permanent condition with the corollary that an 'alcoholic' should never attempt to drink again: total abstinence is the only viable option (Alcoholics Anonymous 1955, Robinson 1979). In fact, while AA has certainly helped a huge number of people to overcome their problems with alcohol, the distinction between problem-free drinking and problematic drinking is much more blurred than suggested by the AA view, and indeed such a view may well be counterproductive.

It is clear from available evidence that people drink in different ways at different times in their lives. Some of the complexities of these changes are discussed in Chapter 2. For many, initiation to alcoholic beverages may be followed by several years of periodic heavy drinking, sometimes involving a number of adverse consequences. This is a common pattern among those who are young and single, as noted in chapters 4 and 6. It is also clear that there is typically very little continuity between drinking early in life and drinking later on (Plant et al. 1985, Fillmore 1987, 1988). Many of those who drink heavily and often with some adverse consequences while they are young, or not so young, simply drink less at a later phase in their lives. Several of the contributors to this book highlight the fact that the consequences of drinking are related to the pattern and context of consumption. This is emphasised by Thurman in Chapter 5 (section A), and in Chapter 6 which summarises some of the evidence related to trends and patterns in alcohol problems. Chapter 6 and Chapter 5 (section B) outline the economic, social and medical ill-effects of heavy and inappropriate drinking, while Chapters 1 and 5 (section B) also acknowledge evidence that moderate alcohol consumption has positive health effects.

Later chapters consider a number of major areas that could all be classified as 'responses to alcohol problems': Chapter 7 discusses harm minimisation and examines evidence of past success in this field.

It is also clear that many of those who do see themselves as experiencing 'alcohol problems' and are prompted to seek some form of help, manage to overcome such problems with or without giving up drinking. Moreover, it appears that such an improvement may occur following no formal specialist support, or via support from quite different types of agency. This is elaborated by Nick Heather in section A of Chapter 8. Cameron (1995) has emphasised that an important role of treatment services for problem drinkers is to provide help and support at times when they require it, and only for as long as they require it. Such individuals often manage to 'do well' for long periods in between episodes of seeking help. A number of different therapeutic responses to alcohol problems now exist, with quite different methods and philosophies. Sections B and C of Chapter 8 describe two examples of these, home detoxification and a range of approaches that are commonly known as 'complementary/alternative' therapies.

Chapter 9, by Linda Wright, examines in detail the issue of evidence-based alcohol education for young people. This has important implications for health promotion; not only for the young, but also for older people.

So, we need to ask why it is socially useful still to dichotomise the drinking populace, why it may serve the interests of some to believe in a 'them' and 'us' view of the world. It may be no more complex than about blame, guilt amelioration and maintenance of social norms. More fruitful is the notion of construing people who at least sometimes consume beverage alcohol as being on a 'drinking career' (Plant 1979). Such people (most of us) probably experience some alcohol-associated problems at some time in our lives, however trivial, but not at others. Moreover, as elaborated elsewhere in this book, most of those who do drink generally do so without lasting problems. Most episodes of alcohol consumption are moderate and enjoyable.

It has been emphasised in the Preface that this is not a 'consensus book'. The contributors represent varied backgrounds and have distinctive individual views on many issues. Accordingly, this book does not set out to present or impose a single 'party line' or philosophy. Alcohol issues stimulate many debates and this is healthy. It is hoped that this book will provide readers with a useful source of information and that most will find something that is thought-provoking, as well as new, in the following pages.

2
Alcohol and its Effects
A: General Effects

Bruce Ritson and Anthony Thorley

INTRODUCTION

Alcohol has been aptly called 'our favourite drug' (Royal College of Psychiatrists 1986). Humanity and alcohol have always had an intertwined relationship and it will always be so, although humans were, and are, certainly not unique in experiencing the effects of alcohol. Animals, birds and insects all encounter alcohol in the natural setting and become intoxicated. Elephants have been observed crashing about after having eaten rotten fruit; humming birds become less controlled in their flight due to drinking fermenting nectar from flowers. All beekeepers know of the phenomenon of the drunken bee or wasp who has had an overdose of fermented honey. For men and women, alcohol continues to be, perhaps along with tobacco, the most potent and controversial substance that we have in our society.

The Production of Alcohol

Of course, humanity was very much predated by alcohol itself. Chemically written as C_2H_5OH, this extraordinary and fascinating molecule made up of carbon, hydrogen and oxygen, known as ethyl alcohol or ethanol, is the only one of a family of naturally occurring alcohols which men and women can reasonably tolerate in their bodies. Almost all the other alcohols – lighter ones, such as methanol, a wood oil as in methylated spirits; and the heavier alcohols, collectively known as fusel oil – are all highly toxic to people and are generally avoided. Habitual meths drinkers can become blind as a consequence of the direct damage of methanol.

Ethanol is a naturally occurring substance and is made by living bacteria and single-celled organisms. The most important of these is the simple yeast and, in combination with sugar, water and air in warm temperatures, as usually found in a ripe fruit or vegetable, yeast ferments these products to produce ethanol and the bubbling gas, carbon dioxide. As the yeast naturally builds up higher concentrations of ethanol, it becomes more and more intoxicated by its own product. At about 13–15% alcohol in the solution, the yeast is literally poisoned and ceases to ferment. Thus the maximum strength of ethanol possible would be around 15%. This is the percentage of alcohol found in ordinary table wines: no other alcoholic beverage can be made stronger without adding further pure spirit produced by some process of distillation.

To begin with, it was not possible to produce alcoholic beverages with a strength greater than 15%, but it is thought that at some point in the ninth century AD the Arabs developed the process of distillation. This boils off the ethanol from the sugar and water and, by cooling and condensing the alcohol vapour, the pure spirit can be collected. The Arabs gave this unpalatable and toxic essence or spirit the name '*alkuhl*' or '*al kohl*'. To render it drinkable, alkuhl was diluted to generate a variety of beverages.

The history of the development and diversification of various alcoholic beverages in the last thousand years, and their production by brewing, distilling and skilfully mixing and blending, will not concern us here: much has already been written on the subject. Suffice to say that the early products were based on natural fermentation: ales from barley, beer with hops added, meads from honey, wines from the grape, and so on. The distillation of whisky commenced in Ireland in the twelfth century, and the production of brandy, gins and other spirits was developed and organised into a formal industry in the seventeenth and eighteenth centuries.

Measuring Alcohol

'Proof' spirits

By the eighteenth century, it was fairly clear that some form of regulating the standard strength of a bottle of spirits was required and the practice was developed of 'proving' the solution of water and alcohol against a standard measure of gunpowder. Water was added to the 100% pure spirit drop by drop, until the mixed liquid would no longer allow ignition of a small pile of gunpowder. At the critical point when ignition was prevented, the solution was proved to be at a strength of 57% pure ethanol. This is the strength in the UK represented by 100° or 100 proof. Some malt whiskies can be obtained at 100°, but standard bottles of gin, brandy and whisky have a proof label of 70°; this is 70% of a 57% solution, and gives a 40% strength of ethanol. In general, with UK proofs the percentage of ethanol is, very approximately, half the proof on the label. European and North American proof labels, however, are calculated differently.

The ladder of beverage strengths

The strength of an alcoholic beverage refers simply to the amount of ethanol that is present in the drink. This point is emphasised because it is a common misunderstanding that some drinks are stronger and more damaging than others; for instance, that whisky is more harmful than beer. In fact, as will be made clear below, ethanol itself harms no matter how dilute it is. Thus, half a pint of beer and a single measure of spirits or a glass of wine contain roughly equal quantities of ethanol and are equally damaging. The only difference is that it is possible to get drunk quicker on low-volume, high-concentration beverages like whisky or gin.

The spirits – gin, whisky, and so on – are at the top of the ladder of beverage strengths. Vodkas are often labelled at 65° and are therefore about 37% ethanol. Descending the ladder of beverage strengths, one comes to the fortified wines: sherry, port, madeira, and so on. These are ordinary wines to which some spirit, often brandy, has been added. There is a great deal more to making a good sherry, but the strength of fortified wines is between 18 and 20%. Coming a few more steps down the ladder, one arrives at the table wines and here, because natural fermenting processes are used at their most efficient, the strength is between 11 and 14%. Brewed beverages, such as ciders, beers and lagers, are on the next step down and present strengths between 2.5 and 10%.

Here the reputation of beer and lager strengths develops into a rich mythology. Many real ales, whilst allegedly tasting superb, are relatively weak. Ciders, on the other hand, are usually stronger than the average beer. Lagers literally span the whole lower range from 3% to almost 9%, so, to keep a check on blood alcohol concentration, a drinker would need to know the strength of the alcohol. This information in the UK is now displayed on the beverage label or on the pumps for draught beverages.

It is notable how the range of ethanol concentrations in our commonly used beverages runs from less than 2% in some beer and lemonade shandies to almost 60% in some spirits.

The average measures in the UK of these various beverage groups contain a fairly similar quantity of ethanol. Half a pint of 'average' beer, around 3% strength, contains 10 ml of ethanol. An equivalent amount of ethanol is found in a normal 120 ml glass of 11% table wine, a single one-sixth gill measure of 40% spirits or a small 60 ml glass of 18% sherry or fortified wine. British researchers and health educators in the alcohol field commonly refer to this equivalent measure of ethanol as a *'unit'* (this is not an international standard and countries calculate units differently). Counting units of ethanol, rather than simply drinks, reminds us that it is the alcohol which is doing the harm and brings some order to the confusion of different beverages. However, it is important to remember that the alcohol content of beers and lagers varies enormously so that a pint of beer (568 ml) may contain from 2 to 5 units of alcohol depending on its strength.

The Role of Congeners

There is clearly much more to a beverage than alcohol and water: the fascination and variety of drinks and drinking is provided in the main by the other substances which give a drink its particular look, flavour, smell and taste. The collective name for these substances is *congeners*. They include vegetable products, various chemicals and minute amounts of metal and other constituents derived from the recipe of the beverage and/or the technical apparatus in which it is brewed or distilled.

In some drinks, the relatively toxic alcohols, methanol and fusel oil, are found in minute quantities. These are within safe limits, but enough to give the drink a particular flavour or tang. Congeners are metabolised in different ways from ethanol and are strongly associated with the unpleasant symptoms of hangover. However, in spite of much mythology about various drinks – and apart from hangovers – there is little evidence that congeners cause any significant harm or damage in comparison with the quantity of ethanol consumed.

Alcohol as Food

Many countries value alcohol as food and still refer to its 'alimentary' properties. At the turn of the last century, women were encouraged to drink porter (dark beer like Guinness or stout) for its food value – a tradition immortalised in the slogan, 'Guinness is good for you'. At the present time in the UK alcoholic beverages provide about 6% of our daily requirement of energy, almost twice as much as 30 years ago, but a great deal less than in the mid-eighteenth century when average consumption was very high. As a molecule, C_2H_5OH is similar to water, H_2O, and is remarkable in that it appears to move throughout the body as freely as water itself. Thus ethanol need not be digested but passes more or less completely unchanged into the bloodstream. As a carbohydrate it represents a powerful packet of potential energy and, weight for weight, it produces more energy than the equivalent amount of starch or protein and only a little less than the equivalent amount of fat. Each gram of ethanol produces seven calories worth of energy. Thus drinks have a good many calories packed into them. A 'unit' of ethanol contains about 60 calories and, if the congeners involve a lot of sugar and other products, as in sweet wine or cider, the number of calories in any standard drink may rise to over 250! A standard bottle of 70° whisky contains 1,800 calories, and a pint of average beer 180 calories: anyone watching their weight will know the importance of keeping an eye on their alcohol consumption. Incidentally, it is worth remembering that low-calorie lagers are not usually weaker in terms of ethanol strengths, but sometimes lie in the rather strong range. Heavy drinkers often eat little but put on weight. Ten cans of strong lager may contain a total of 2,500 calories, enough for a man doing a heavy manual job. Any addition from merely eating food will just be put on as excess fat.

Although alcohol contains calories and is rapidly turned into energy and fat, beverages do not contain sufficient proteins and vitamins to keep the body at a stable level of function and health. Alcoholic beverages are poor foods and reliance upon them as a sole source of food leads to vitamin deficiency diseases and wasting of high-protein tissues like muscle.

Absorption and Metabolism of Ethanol

Almost all ethanol from beverages passes unchanged into the bloodstream. Some 95% is then burned up or, more technically, oxidised by enzyme action mainly in the liver; the remaining 5% leaves the body unchanged in the sweat, urine and breath; this later fraction being used as the basis for the 'breath test'. There are many factors affecting the rate and efficiency of uptake of alcohol into the blood and further factors which affect how rapidly it is oxidised and excreted from the body. All these factors in part influence how much an individual has a 'head for alcohol' or how much tolerance develops, and it is therefore worth examining a few of them in detail.

Beverage strength

The rate of alcohol uptake into the blood depends on beverage strength. Optimal strengths are between 15 and 30% pure ethanol – so beware of sherry on an empty stomach. Low-strength drinks like beers and lager do not have a sufficiently high concentration gradient to diffuse through the stomach wall to gain speedy entry into the wall blood vessels and therefore absorption is slow. Undiluted high-strength drinks, like whisky or brandy, irritate the stomach lining and, in response, it secretes a copious film of protective mucus which delays absorption. The stomach also reacts to strong drinks by reflexively closing its powerful exit valve, the pyloric sphincter, and so holds up the alcohol with any food in the stomach. Most alcohol is not actually absorbed through the stomach wall, but through the wall of the first two feet of intestine leading from the stomach, the duodenum and ileum. Hence strong drinks, retained in the stomach by exit valve spasm, prevented from absorption by mucus and soaked into ingested food, would tend to have a delayed absorption and therefore to give the drinker a false impression of ability to take more than previously thought. However, all the delayed ethanol eventually gets through into the blood and the drinker may then be surprised at his or her rapid intoxication!

Biological differences between men and women

The absorption of ethanol molecules across the walls of cells in the intestine and then through the walls of blood vessels in the intestine itself all involve complex chemical processes assisted by enzymes. Each of these enzyme stages in the transport from gut to blood is subject to individual variation. Thus, hypothetically, an individual could be genetically endowed either with a highly efficient transport system or with rather sluggish enzymes that only absorb ethanol slowly. Thus some people could be born with a capacity to absorb ethanol more efficiently than others: there is much anecdotal evidence to support this view.

There is evidence that women in general tend to absorb alcohol faster than men, reach higher peak blood alcohol concentrations and excrete the alcohol more speedily. Whereas men achieve fairly constant peak blood alcohol concentrations following standard amounts of ethanol, women show particularly rapid absorption and high peak blood alcohol concentrations in the premenstrual and ovulatory phases of their monthly cycle. Conversely, there is also some evidence that women using oral contraceptives absorb and metabolise alcohol more slowly and evenly (M.L. Plant 1997).

These differences between men and women are accentuated by weight. Women on average weigh 15% less than men of the same age, but, more significantly, young women have 50% of their total body weight in the form of water as compared with 60% in young men. As the ethanol is ultimately concentrated in this 'pool' of body water and women have less than men, both on this count and on the weight factor they will show higher blood alcohol concentrations from standard measures of ethanol. This increased sensitivity to alcohol may ultimately be reflected in the pattern of a woman's drinking. If she is wary of rapid and embarrassing intoxication, a woman may keep her drinking more controlled, intermittent, and therefore develop a 'head for alcohol', or tolerance, more slowly than a man. In addition, she may develop a different pattern of drinking in one part of her monthly cycle as compared with another. The important issue of drinking during pregnancy is considered in detail in section B of this chapter.

The oxidation of ethanol

In the blood vessels that drain the intestines and stomach known as the portal system, the alcohol is carried, together with digested food, straight to the liver. In the liver cells, ethanol is broken down and oxidised (or burned for energy) by means of an enzyme called alcohol dehydrogenase. As far as is known, this enzyme occurs in no other part of the body and exists for no other purpose than breaking down ethanol. It therefore stands as evolutionary testimony to the long-standing relationship between humanity and alcohol.

1.   Ethyl Alcohol ⎯⎯⎯⎯⎯⎯⎯⎯⎯⎯⎯⎯⎯⎯→ Acetaldehyde

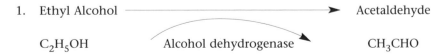

C_2H_5OH Alcohol dehydrogenase CH_3CHO

Ethanol is converted by this enzyme to the more toxic chemical, acetaldehyde. Raised blood levels of acetaldehyde can cause increased blood pressure, a faster heart rate, flushing, nausea, breathing disturbance and a number of other unpleasant side-effects. Some of these symptoms are not unlike those found in excessive intoxication or hangover, and this has led some researchers to hazard a guess that it may be more *acetaldehyde* which causes the difficulties rather than its immediate chemical predecessor, ethanol.

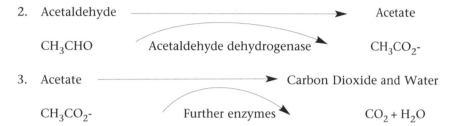

2. Acetaldehyde ⟶ Acetate

    CH$_3$CHO   Acetaldehyde dehydrogenase   CH$_3$CO$_2$-

3. Acetate ⟶ Carbon Dioxide and Water

    CH$_3$CO$_2$-   Further enzymes   CO$_2$ + H$_2$O

The enzyme which rapidly removes the toxic acetaldehyde and converts it to acetic acid is acetaldehyde dehydrogenase, and this occurs not only in the liver but all over the body. This reaction occurs very rapidly and is followed by a further fast conversion by other enzyme systems, of acetic acid to carbon dioxide and water, with a major release of energy. Normally, acetaldehyde dehydrogenase rapidly destroys all acetaldehyde so that it only exerts its toxic influence momentarily, and most people probably feel no effects from it. But what if individuals who get drunk quickly have a tendency to a slower breakdown of acetaldehyde? Is this the key to alcohol problems? Unfortunately, most researchers are very sure it is not as simple as this and that there is no clear evidence that problem drinkers have any significant and consistent defect of alcohol or acetaldehyde dehydrogenase enzymes. However, there are two interesting related features which hinge on this alcohol and acetaldehyde breakdown metabolism.

Alcohol and lactic acid

Alcohol metabolism leads to an increase in an organic acid found naturally in milk, called lactic acid. Usually, both in milk and in the healthy body, levels of lactic acid are harmless, and in fact the substance is an essential component of normal energy-producing metabolism. However, higher levels are found in the blood of heavy drinkers and high levels are also associated with uncomfortable experiences of anxiety, panic attacks and possibly the development of pathological fears, known as phobias. Many heavy drinkers suffer from anxiety, have panic attacks and develop or enhance phobias such as a fear of going out or being in social situations.

Alcohol is used to calm down and control anxiety, but, in high doses, ethanol does seem to increase anxiety. Here is a truly vicious circle: alcohol reduces anxiety only to create further anxiety. Is lactic acid one of the factors behind this interesting paradox?

Alcohol and uric acid

Another acid which is increased in the blood of heavy drinkers is uric acid, and high levels of uric acid are associated with the painful condition of gout. Here, crystals of uric acid salts (urates) are deposited in skin, cartilage and joints, resulting in the extreme pain of a particular kind of arthritis. Heavy drinking may not cause gout, but it may exacerbate it in the predisposed individual. The association between gout and the heavy port-drinking university don or eighteenth-century gentleman (or both) has been recognised for many years.

Alcohol and fat

As ethanol is oxidised and converted to water and carbon dioxide, fat is produced in the blood at a rapid rate. The precise relationship between ethanol metabolism and fat metabolism is complex and will not be pursued here. Commonly, the high levels of fat in the blood are deposited as fat in the liver (fatty liver), fat in muscle and heart tissue (fatty heart muscle) and fat just everywhere (for example, as a 'beer belly').

The effect of alcohol on nerve cells

Cell biologists and biochemists have established that the cell wall is made up of complex fat molecules enclosing the cell both inside and out, like the tufted pile of a double sided carpet. This skin of fat molecules is sufficiently stable to hold substances apart on either side of the cell wall, but, in certain circumstances, they become fluid enough to let certain molecules, for instance sugars and food substances, pass through the wall. Ethanol, outside the cell wall, directly alters its stability so that the wall becomes more fluid, and the functioning of the transport system of essential packets of chemicals used in metabolic processes and, in particular, in transmitting nerve signals, is adversely affected. Consequently, alcohol outside a cell causes a complex disruption of cell function and coordination, and this may best translate itself into the signs and symptoms of more general lack of coordination due to intoxication.

The effect is most marked when we consider the impact of ethanol on the junctions (synapses) which separate one nerve cell from another. Although there is some evidence that alcohol temporarily stimulates nerve signal transmission, this effect is transient and usually insignificant when compared with a general depression of nerve transmission. When nerve transmission rates are slowed down by alcohol, any signal, for instance from pricking fingers with a pin, takes longer to reach the brain and one may not draw one's finger back quickly enough to avoid an unpleasant cut. In much the same way, reaction times are slowed, as is the ability to perform fast, coordinated movements. This has an all-important impact on skills such as driving or operating machinery.

Cellular mechanisms of physical dependence

It is easy to forget that alcohol is a drug that has a profound and wide-ranging effect on the biological integrity of the brain, a characteristic which distinguishes it from many other beverages and foods.

Ethanol, as a chemical, is also particular in that it is potentially 'addictive' (dependence producing) and can produce physical dependence after long periods of high-dose use. Somehow, therefore, chemicals which produce physiological dependence, for instance morphine, barbiturates, nicotine and alcohol, all differ fundamentally from chemicals that do not, for example, peppermint or rhubarb, but which may commonly be associated with some degree or other of psychological dependence. It appears that alcohol and similar addictive chemicals interact in some as yet ill-understood way with the brain's cellular biochemistry and function to become specifically integrated into the normal metabolism, and become, in part, essential for that metabolism to continue without disturbance. The body has therefore made a fundamental adjustment to the presence of ethanol, which becomes, in effect, a paradoxical vital substance, essential for relatively stable functioning. There is a great deal more to alcohol dependence than physical dependence, as will be discussed later in this section, but are there any clues as to what the biochemical nature of physical dependence is?

Although the effects of alcohol on the fatty membranes surrounding the cell walls are important, it is now thought that other major effects of alcohol on the chemistry of the brain are even more important. These effects are very complex and are thought to impact on the pleasure centres of the brain. Key centres of the brain, such as the nucleus accumbens, the basal ganglia and the frontal cortex, are circuits which when activated seem to drive addictive appetites (Nutt 1999). A more general account of brain function can be found in Greenfield (1997, Chapter 3). Our understanding of these brain mechanisms is developing very rapidly at present, principally because of new investigative brain imaging techniques. Alcohol increases the level of Dopamine, Serotonin and Gamma Amino Batyric Acid (GABA), and along with other receptors these have an important part in the activity of the brain. Others have suggested that alcohol has an impact on the brain's own opiate receptor system, including the endorphins. We therefore have an extremely complex system with the effects of small doses, differing from those of larger doses and short-term use, having a very different impact from longer-term use when adaptation will have occurred. There are also important genetic differences in the way in which individuals respond to alcohol at a cellular level. Thus the brain cells adapt to living in an alcoholic environment so that higher doses of alcohol need to be taken before achieving the effects which would have been attained at much lower levels previously – this is the phenomenon of tolerance. The drinker experiences this as 'having a good head for drink'. Far from being an indication of strength or resolution, it is simply evidence that alcohol is beginning to take hold of the individual. In addition to this physical development of tolerance, there is of course a psychological element whereby the drinker gets used to the effects of intoxication and is somewhat more adept at disguising or handling this. No biochemist believes that an explanation of physical dependence could possibly be as simple as this, and all chemical explanations in the final analysis owe more to poetry than precision.

The breakdown and excretion of ethanol

As ethanol in the blood circulates round and round the body, most of it has to pass through the liver repeatedly, to be converted to acetaldehyde in a continuous flow of gradual dilution. The liver manages to maintain its breakdown of alcohol at a fairly constant rate, in spite of the concentration of alcohol in the blood. The rate of breakdown is equivalent to 15 mg of ethanol per 100 ml of blood per hour, or, conveniently, one unit per hour. It is worth remembering, therefore, that however much you have drunk, at whatever rate, your body only burns up the ethanol at a rate of around half a pint of beer or a single measure of spirits per hour.

There is an obvious attraction, therefore, in attempting to discover chemicals which may enhance this breakdown process so as to reduce intoxication more rapidly. It has been found that the sugar fructose can speed up alcohol oxidation, but only when used at levels which induce sickness and vomiting in most people. Consequently, fructose is not a practical chemical to use and, so far, no other practical alternative has been discovered.

One direct action of the alcohol in the blood is that it acts as a diuretic, directly stimulating the excretion rate of the kidneys and the formation of urine. Hence remaining levels of blood alcohol are rapidly excreted, together with large quantities of water, leading to a degree of dehydration. Many drinkers have experienced the effects of dehydration after a bout of intoxication.

To summarise, what does all this metabolic and physiological evidence mean? It certainly does not explain everything about alcohol and alcohol problems, as psychological, social and cultural factors have a more powerful overriding effect. It does, however, provide clues about some basic biological processes upon which one can build a partial understanding of drinking behaviour.

Hence intoxication and lack of coordination are partly explained by alcohol-disturbed cell membranes. Differences between men and women appear to have some sound basis in physiology. Tolerance, the adaptive ability to manage higher and higher consumption without massive deterioration in function, may be *functional*, a general and psychologically enhanced ability to behave normally; *and*/or it may be *cellular*, a specific adaptation in the cell membranes and metabolism to cope with increasing blood alcohol concentrations. Tolerance will also include changes in absorption, oxidation, breakdown, storage and elimination, and is thus a highly complex process.

DRINKING BEHAVIOUR, CONSEQUENCES, HARM AND PROBLEMS

It is convenient to identify three elements of drinking behaviour that may have harmful consequences for the drinker. As emphasised elsewhere in this book, pattern of consumption is a major influence on the consequences of drinking.

Intoxication will be considered first. *Excessive regular consumption* is very frequent or daily drinking beyond a 'safe' (or low risk) level, which often does not produce intoxication or dependence, but does, nevertheless, generate a range of consequences and harm, especially in the medical area. *Dependence* may generate few consequences and problems, as compared with the other two elements of drinking behaviour, but it requires special consideration because of the importance attached to it by many workers in the 'alcohol problems field'.

It must also be apparent that these elements of drinking behaviour, occurring separately or in combination, may be inconsequential or acceptable, or they may be consequential and generate harm. The individual may not recognise or accept the harm as a problem, or conversely may identify consequences and harm where the professional worker does not recognise them.

Intoxication and its Consequences

Becoming 'drunk' is a very individual process and is only loosely correlated with specific blood alcohol concentrations. Thus some individuals become verbose, humorous and loose tongued, whilst others become more passive and morose. The personality of the drinker certainly comes into play and traits may be enhanced, exaggerated, distorted or become virtually unrecognisable. The varieties of drunkenness have been recognised for a long time:

'Nor haue we one or two kinde of drunkards onely, but eight kindes. The first is Ape drunke, and he leapes, and sings, and hollowes, and daunceth for the heauens: the second is Lion drunke, and he flings the pots about the house, calls his Hostesse whore, breakes the glasse windowes with his dagger, and is apt to quarrell with any man that speaks to him: the third is Swine drunke, heuy, lumpish and sleepie, and cries for a little more drinke, and a fewe more cloathes: the fourth is Sheepe drunke, wise in his own conceipt, when he cannot bring foorth a right word, the fifth is Mawdlen drunke, when a fellowe will weepe for kindness in the midst of his Ale, and kisse you, saying; By God Captaine, I loue thee, goe they waies thou dost not thinke so often of me as I do of thee, I would (it is pleased GOD) I could not loue thee so well as I doo, and then he puts his finger in his eie, and cries: the sixth is Martin drunke, when a man is drunke and drinkes himselfe sober ere he stirre: the seventh is Goate drunke, when in his drunkennes he hath no mind but on Lechery: the eith is Foxe drunke, when he is craftie drunke, as many of the Dutch men bee, will never bargaine but when they are drunke. All these *species* and more, I haue seen practised in one Company at one sitting, when I haue been permitted to remaine sober amongst them, onely to note their seuerall humours. (He that plies any one of them harde, it will make him to write admirable verses, and to haue a deepe casting head, though he were neuer so verie a Dunce before.)' (Thomas Nash (1592) *Pierce Penilesse: His Supplication to the Diuell*)

The plasticity of drunken behaviour or comportment may be further altered by emotional, social and cultural factors. There is a good deal of social learning in drunken behaviour. Young children know how to act drunk long before they ever are drunk. Young men and women show their drunken behaviour very differently. Most individuals perceive they are drunk before being recognised as being such. There are over 50 words in the English language alone for being drunk, and most of them are commonly used. To judge from this, drunkenness is one of the richest areas of common experience, pleasures and problems, and yet it is widely accepted that being drunk and incapacitated in Glasgow, in working-class Scotland, means something very different from being drunk in Godalming in middle-class England, or for that matter in France or Italy.

Stages of intoxication
In spite of all the plasticity in drunken behaviour, authorities would agree that physiological dysfunction occurs for most people at blood alcohol concentrations (BACs) in excess of 30 mg per 100 ml blood, the equivalent

of drinking a pint of beer or two glasses of wine or spirits. Intoxication at this level is technical, rather than socially recognised, as it is for many drivers who drink and drive with BACs in excess of 80 mg%. Generally speaking, each unit of ethanol per hour increases the BAC by 15 mg% with general and commonly experienced consequences as shown in Table 2.1.

Table 2.1: Stages of intoxication

Blood alcohol concentration (mg per 100 ml blood)	Approximate effects for average tolerance
20	Enhanced sense of well-being; reaction times reduced
40	Mild disinhibition; reduced driving ability at speed
60	Mild impairment of judgement and decision-making
80	Physical coordination diminished; UK legal driving limit
100	Deterioration in social and physical control
150	Observable intoxication; amnesic episodes possible
350	Incontinence; sleepiness
500+	Coma, breathing difficulties and death

The 'Breathalyser' is only one technical application of a legal threshold of intoxication. Many drivers count as legally intoxicated, but are socially acceptable (outside a car) in their behaviour. Regulations related to the 1974 Health and Safety at Work Act may cause employers and unions in the future to agree upon other technical levels of intoxication linked into disciplinary procedures and alcohol policies in order to safeguard employees with regard to alcohol-related accidents (Hutcheson et al. 1995).

As someone drinks and becomes drunk, there is no direct experience of the temporary stimulation effect upon nerve transmission. The overriding physiological depressant effect becomes increasingly apparent and is usually anticipated, consciously, by the seasoned drinker. Thus, when stopping for a 'quick one' in the pub, the rapid consumption of a single drink may very much derive its effects in the first 20 minutes from psychological factors, rather than directly from the physiological impact of alcohol. The relaxation and the bonhomie rely more on bar atmosphere and habit than on beverage alcohol. Confirmation of this initial anticipatory psychological stage has been provided by experiments with subjects unaware that they were

drinking non-alcoholic beverages and yet feeling the same degree of relaxation and well-being as if they were consuming alcohol.

Further drinking produces a physiological effect superimposed on the
psychological reaction and the two become inextricably interrelated. The
drinker knows he or she is going to feel more distanced from stimuli, external
and internal. If these are painful, for instance anxiety about work or financial
problems, the drinker will value such distancing as pleasurable. Attitudes or
behaviours that may be unacceptable to express may be shown without any
thought for the consequences. Thus alcohol can facilitate the expression of
normally repressed desires, for example to harm or insult others. Public
houses are also places where wild ideas can be ventilated or extreme behaviours exhibited and relatively tolerated. Dissociation therefore facilitates
role-playing and hedonistic expression, as well as more threatening behaviour. To the extent that mild intoxication aids relaxation and leisure, it may
be a considerable benefit to society in acting as an acceptable safety valve for
more fundamental frustrations. The drunken man in the pub (the behaviour
is unlikely if he is on his own) can take on the world – and win!

To state that ethanol merely disinhibits the higher centres is probably too
simplistic. Some individuals become extrovert and funny and temporarily
can make delightful companions. Others exhibit sensitive irritation and are
verbally sarcastic and unpleasant. Yet others show a maudlin sadness which
borders on the suicidal. The variety of drunken behaviour is much wider
than usually admitted or represented in the music hall caricature. Ethanol
does not *cause* aggression by any direct and consistent physiological effect,
but dissociation may potentiate its expression in those predisposed by
personality or inclination.

'Alcoholic blackouts' or amnesic episodes

Rapid drinking leading to intoxication and blood alcohol concentrations in
excess of 150 mg% is associated with periods of impaired or totally absent
memory. These memory blanks may last several hours and are commonly
known as 'alcoholic blackouts': they are medically referred to as amnesic
episodes. Such episodes can be very disturbing to the drinker, particularly if
nothing is remembered of part of the night before until the morning after.
Drinkers cannot recollect how they went from pub to pub, how they got
home, with whom they spent the night or whom they insulted or promised
a favour. Occasionally, when an individual is drunk, there is difficulty in
remembering details of events, although, when pressed, a hazy recollection
is possible. This is a more common experience and is to be distinguished
from a true amnesic episode.

It is important to emphasise that this memory impairment occurs in
normal drinkers who get intoxicated rapidly, that it does not itself imply a

drinking problem and, especially amongst young men celebrating at, for example, engagement parties or sporting triumphs, that it is relatively common. In several general population surveys, over 15% of those interviewed reported an amnesic episode in the previous twelve months. However, if it occurs frequently, this consequence of intoxication may constitute a drinking problem in its own right.

The mechanism of these amnesic episodes is not understood. It is a disturbance of memory recording rather than memory recall or playback: in many cases there is no recall possible for the amnesic period as no memory was laid down. The law does not accept amnesia as a defence with regard to an offence carried out during an amnesic episode, any more than intoxication itself is an acceptable defence. Many individuals during their period of amnesia are relatively coordinated, clear-minded and able to distinguish between their actions as right or wrong, and to appreciate the consequences.

Coma and death

At high blood alcohol concentrations, above 350 mg%, the individual becomes more and more uncoordinated until unable to stand. Muscles controlling bladder and bowels may be affected so that the drinker becomes incontinent or involuntarily defecates. Further depressant activity in the central nervous system and brain induces sleep: when the individual is unconscious and unrousable, this is referred to as coma. Continuing increases in alcohol concentration finally interfere with the area of the brain (medulla) which controls involuntary mechanisms such as breathing and the beating of the heart. Breathing becomes irregular, and the heart may develop arrhythmias. Unless the situation is rapidly reversed, death will ensue. In other circumstances the drinker may vomit while unconscious, inhale this into his or her lungs and drown in his or her own vomit.

Hangover

For those who have survived a night of intoxication, the only consequence (or problem) the following morning may be a hangover. Although a hangover is characterised to some extent by depressed mood, headache, dehydration, nausea and hypersensitivity to outside stimuli such as noise, its variety is considerable. In one survey, people reported that hangovers lasted from 45 minutes up to 2.5 days, and that for some it began, not in the head, but in the knees! It may not be possible fully to explain hangover, but some of its features are produced by the wide variety of toxic congeners, described earlier, which are added to drinks for taste and aroma. In combination with the dehydration caused directly by ethanol itself, the congeners may be responsible for the headache or mood change. Some drinks or mixtures contain more congeners than others and therefore produce a more painful hangover. Vodka, for example, has very few congeners, whereas brandy, port or rich red wine have many: evidence is strong that mixing drinks is more likely to produce hangovers. The simple 'hangover scale' shown in Figure 2.1 suggests what to avoid. Clinical experience suggests that many young people who go on to develop drinking problems have never significantly suffered from hangovers, and therefore hangovers may have an important protective effect on most people in moderating their drinking.

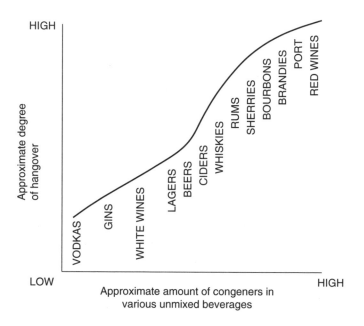

Figure 2.1: A simple guide to hangovers

Medical problems

As can be seen from Box 2.1, most of the medical problems arising from intoxication are accidents and emergencies, secondary to the lack of coordination, or due to acute toxic effects of ethanol on various organs.

The biggest single factor is alcohol-related road traffic accidents. In the UK, one in seven road deaths is the result of a drink-drive related accident. Other accidents occur at home and in the workplace. Overdose of alcohol leading to coma and death, as described above, is referred to as *acute alcoholic poisoning*. Alcohol also interferes with the production of insulin in the pancreas and, occasionally, with sugar metabolism more directly, to produce symptoms of diabetes or diabetic coma. This is a quite common hospital presentation of infants who have opened the domestic drinks cupboard and sampled the contents for themselves. In some individuals, recurrent intoxi-

---

Box 2.1: Harm due to intoxication

Medical problems

Acute alcohol poisoning or overdose	Pancreatitis
	Trauma
Amnesic episodes	Head injury
Drug overdose	Accidents
Suicidal behaviour	Epilepsy
Acute gastritis	Hangover
Diabetic symptoms	Fetal alcohol syndrome

Social problems

Social isolation	Sexual problems
Aggressive behaviour	Domestic accidents
Passive behaviour	Industrial accidents
Domestic violence	Absenteeism
Child abuse	Poor time-keeping
Child neglect	

Legal problems

Driving offences	Criminal damage to property
Drunkenness offences	Fraud
Theft	Deception
Shop-lifting	Assault
Taking and driving a vehicle	Homicide

---

cation can cause the very serious condition of inflammation of the pancreas, known as acute pancreatitis. More commonly, many drinkers will develop inflammation of the stomach lining (acute gastritis), experienced as pain or indigestion, and there may be some bleeding from the red raw tissue. In some predisposed individuals intoxication can precipitate the major seizures of epilepsy, as well as more minor forms of seizure.

Interaction of ethanol and drugs, both illicit (for example, cannabis, ecstasy (MDMA), heroin, crack/cocaine and amphetamines) and medically prescribed, is a very important and complex area. Good advice, when in any kind of doubt, is not to combine alcohol with any medication until formal advice from a doctor or pharmacist has been taken. As indicated above, alcohol itself can be the cause of an overdose. Alcohol is commonly used together with other drugs in suicide attempts and risk-taking suicidal behaviour (parasuicide) by disturbed and unhappy people.

Social and legal problems

The social and legal problems related to intoxication and drunken behaviour speak for themselves and are much easier to understand. It is noteworthy how much of the work of the social worker, probation officer and police officer is taken up with the effects of a range of unacceptable drunken behaviours; also how circumstances, social class and social expectation of intoxication-related behaviour all come into play. Thus in some social settings domestic violence and injuries to children related to drinking are commonplace, whereas in other social settings they are relatively rare or strongly proscribed and consequently well-hidden. To make an impact on intoxication-related social and legal problems, it becomes necessary for professional workers not simply to tackle consumption alone but to use treatment strategies which seek specifically to minimise the harm they produce.

Regular Excessive Consumption and its Consequences

For many years it has not been possible to define with any confidence exactly what constitutes 'heavy drinking'. 'Heavy' for one person is light for another, and heavy by cultural standards may not be heavy by medical standards. However, in the last ten years it has become clear from a number of international studies that a man of average weight who drinks on a regular daily basis more than ten units (80g) of ethanol, equivalent to five pints of average beer, has an increased likelihood of future alcohol-related illnesses, social problems and legal offences. For some of the reasons described above, women's threshold of regular excessive consumption is lower than men's, being set at about six units a day, or three pints of average beer. Neither of these daily consumption levels has much significance in terms of harm (other than possibly through intoxication) if drunk on one occasion. However, if this consumption is regularly exceeded, daily or more than four days a week, there are good biological reasons why the average body cannot cope, and fairly logical reasons why most of the medical harm occurs.

It is evident that the body can only process a certain amount of alcohol per day. Consider the liver, the organ that has to do so much of the metabolic work: it appears that a healthy liver can only process and oxidise 80g of alcohol for a man and as little as 40g for a woman, in a 24-hour period. Even these levels may cause some fatty liver and minor damage in some people, but for those who drink beyond these levels on a regular basis, their livers cannot cope with the excess and consequently there is damage. At a very rough estimate, it takes approximately 72 hours for the slightly damaged liver to return to normal. However, if the body is subjected to another damaging dose the day after, and another the following day, and so on, the liver and other damaged organs have no chance to recover and the damage accumulates. It is this accumulation which is the really significant outcome of regular excessive consumption, as compared with a single drinking episode with or without intoxication. The body does, however, make some basic adjustments to a daily perfusion of damaging alcohol. Tolerance is one of the adjustments already described that affects behavioural functioning, but this also applies to biological functions of various organs. Tolerance is not enough, however, and many organs in the body are unable to avoid incurring harm. As alcohol gets everywhere in the body, it follows that damage due to regular excessive consumption is going to be very widespread; in fact, there is no organ or tissue that is not affected.

It is this damage, often from relatively innocent regular drinking, which provides much alcohol-related illness in hospital beds. In the UK approximately 25% of general hospital beds amongst men are occupied by patients with alcohol-related illnesses. Accordingly, the preventive significance of communicating sensible drinking in the context of regular excessive consumption to both clients and the general public cannot be over-emphasised.

The widespread damage and the mass of disorders and symptoms shown in Box 2.2 comprise a most confusing area, and one ripe for its own mythology. In fact, there is a good deal of logical common sense about the trail of damage which ensues as alcohol passes around the body. The following account of medical harm due to regular excessive consumption may therefore insult those readers with a medical or biological background by its necessary simplification, but, it is hoped that it will give non-medical readers sufficient illumination to make them more confident as practitioners and health educators.

Box 2.2: Harm due to excessive drinking

Medical problems

Cancers of the mouth throat and gullet	Testicular atrophy Anaemia	Alcoholic hepatitis Liver cirrhosis
Gastritis	Chronic myopathy Cardiomyopathy	Liver cancer Distributed fat metabolism
Stomach haemorrhage	Peripheral neuritis	Gout
Pancreatitis	Wernicke's encephalopathy	
Diabetes	Korsakoff's psychosis	Fetal alcohol syndrome
Vitamin deficiency	Brain damage	Epilepsy
Fatty liver	Depression	Feminisation
Anxiety	Sexual impotence	Phobic illnesses

Social problems

Financial debt	Marital problems	Absenteeism
Homelessness	Sexual problems	Employment problems
Family problems		

Legal problems

Theft	Deception	Drink driving
Fraud	Vagrancy	

Medical problems

Digestive system

Alcohol that is swallowed passes through the mouth, throat and gullet (oesophagus) and damages the inner skin lining of all these organs; as with all such chronic tissue damage, some of the damaged cells can become cancerous. It can therefore be stated with confidence that alcohol consumption is associated with cancer of the mouth, throat and oesophagus and that regular excessive drinkers run greater risk of suffering these cancers. The higher the dose of alcohol, the greater the risk of cancer. Furthermore, heavy drinkers are also often heavy smokers, and this increases the risk of cancer (Anderson et al. 1993). In the US, where smoking and drinking levels are similar to those in the UK, tobacco consumption causes 30% of all cancer deaths, but alcohol causes 3% of cancer deaths and, next to tobacco, is the most significant identifiable carcinogenic factor. Tobacco and alcohol may therefore be the two factors most accessible in terms of prevention of cancer in general.

Liver
Beyond the duodenum, in the next two feet or so of the small intestine or ileum, most of the food, vitamins and alcohol are absorbed and transported to the liver. Inflammation of the intestine wall due to regular excess drinking can interfere with efficient absorption of vitamins and iron, contributing to *vitamin deficiency* and various types of anaemia. As most of the alcohol goes first to the liver, it bears the brunt of the attack. As described earlier, it first becomes infiltrated with fat, the condition of *fatty liver* and, after a period of several weeks or months of regular excessive consumption, an inflammation may set in called *alcoholic hepatitis* (this is not to be confused with infectious hepatitis, which is not due to alcohol but to various infective agents). *Fatty liver* and some early hepatitis will cause the liver to expand in size and perhaps be tender, but for many people two or three months' abstinence or much reduced drinking will allow the fat to be reabsorbed and the hepatitis to settle. These liver conditions are therefore reversible when regular excessive consumption ceases.

Amongst those people who develop *alcoholic hepatitis,* the reversibility on ceasing to drink is less predictable. If the individual goes on drinking regularly, the chronic inflammation proceeds to damage the liver irreversibly: the damaged liver tissue is called *liver cirrhosis.* The chances of getting cirrhosis depend on how long a person has been drinking and at what daily rate of consumption. Usually over four years' heavy drinking is required, at a daily consumption of around 20 units (10 pints of beer or two-thirds of a bottle of 70° spirits), virtually no one had cirrhosis after three years of drinking, 8% had cirrhosis after eight years of drinking, 21% had cirrhosis after 13 years, and 51% had cirrhosis after 22 years of drinking. Cirrhosis can be caused by other agents, and a familial tendency may indicate genetic factors which may increase vulnerability or act as a protection for the individual. Nevertheless, the death rate from liver cirrhosis is for problem drinkers about ten times the average in the UK.

As noted in Chapter 6, both cirrhosis deaths and alcohol-related mortality in the UK have continued to rise, and the greatest increase in cirrhosis deaths has been among men (Medical Council on Alcoholism 2000).

There is also emerging evidence that women under 40 are particularly likely to develop hepatitis leading to cirrhosis at much lower daily consumption levels and after shorter periods of drinking heavily. Thus the predictions given above may have to be radically revised for women. The reasons behind this propensity of women to develop hepatitis and cirrhosis appear to be biological, possibly hormonal, as well as an ill-understood and complex immunological response which is currently the subject of world-wide research.

When the liver is damaged by cirrhosis, it responds by utilising a high regenerative capacity, growing new liver tissue to replace the dead cirrhotic tissue. As the dead tissue is not significantly absorbed, the chronically damaged liver, logically, grows larger in volume and this, along with *fatty liver*, is the main reason why the livers of regular excessive consumers are often enlarged. However, as heavy drinkers get older they are less and less able to grow new liver tissue, and eventually the liver is unable to do its metabolic work in separating out vital substances from poisons and other products which are not required. This is the clinical condition of *liver failure*, which is extremely difficult to treat and may even require liver transplant.

The enlarged, engorged, inflamed liver places an increased strain and back pressure on the blood in the portal vessels which pass from the intestines and stomach to the liver. Therefore, as blood cannot pass easily through the damaged liver back to the heart, so the condition of *portal hypertension* arises. In order to bypass the liver, the blood seeks to make short-cut connections with alternative veins leading to the heart and causes localised varicose veins. Where these occur at the base of the gullet, they are referred to as *oesophageal varices*. As the varices sometimes balloon out into the inner wall of the oesophagus, it is clear they may become eroded or damaged by passing food or drink. Sometimes a varix ruptures in this way and the resultant bleeding is a major and often fatal emergency.

Finally, the alcohol-damaged liver, after many years of harm from regular excessive drinking, may develop a primary cancer called a *hepatoma*. This condition is relatively rare in the UK, but is common in high-alcohol-consumption countries like France. Primary liver cancer is a serious condition and is often rapidly fatal.

Heart
After leaving the liver, with its massive variety of damage, the blood reaches the heart and is pumped around the lungs to collect oxygen from the air; freshly oxygenated, it returns to the heart. Excessive regular alcohol

consumption is associated with a number of diseases of the heart and blood circulation system. The heart muscle becomes infiltrated with fat and this may lead to permanently damaged heart muscle, known as *alcoholic cardiomyopathy*. This condition can predispose individuals to heart attacks and premature death and almost certainly contributes to the higher level of heart attacks amongst heavy drinkers.

Brain and nervous systems
The freshly oxygenated arterial blood is now pumped by the heart all over the rest of the body: the alcohol will return to the heart in the veins to be pumped round and round until all the alcohol is eliminated. The first and most sensitive organ to receive fresh arterial blood is the *brain,* and it now appears certain that the brain is damaged directly by alcohol and may take months, if not years, to recover fully. Long-term regular excessive consumption, for five years or more, can lead to the brain being so damaged that it shrinks in size: new X-ray and scanning techniques have allowed doctors to measure this effect. The functional effects of this brain damage are probably more serious than previously realised. Many problem drinkers complain of difficulties in concentration, adverse effects on problem-solving abilities and abstract thinking, and memory impairment, but even some who do not have these complaints identifiable at a clinical level still have X-ray evidence of *brain shrinkage.* There has been a suggestion by some researchers that such *minimal brain damage* might predispose the drinker to functional difficulties in controlling his or her drinking.

After a few months' abstinence (a minimum of three is usually recommended), many of these psychological dysfunctions and handicaps will have melted away. Although the brain regenerates tissue very poorly, this is compensated for by the brain making more efficient use of its reserve function. There is, however, evidence in individuals who go on drinking excessively that the brain can become permanently damaged: it manifests its dysfunction in the serious condition of *alcoholic dementia.* This is similar to senile dementia in the elderly and may, in life-long heavy drinkers, be a contributory factor to the clinical picture of this common, distressing and irreversible condition. It is possible, therefore, that drinkers could avoid some of the later psychological hazards of regular excessive drinking by reducing their daily consumption earlier in their lives.

There are several serious brain pathologies which are related to regular excessive consumption of ethanol, together with vitamin deficiency. Two of these, *Wernicke's encephalopathy* and *Korsakoff's psychosis*, are linked and lead to serious disturbances of balance, vision, thinking and perception. To some extent these conditions can be avoided by adequate vitamin intake, and vitamins are used in the treatment of the acute onset of these conditions.

Both require skilful psychiatric and medical management in a hospital setting.

Alcohol passing out from the arterial blood system into the rest of the body damages almost every tissue it meets. Nerves are damaged and, along with vitamin deficiency, this may lead to pain, abnormal tingling and loss of sensation in fingers and toes known as *peripheral neuritis*. Muscles are damaged, work less efficiently, become painful and may show wasting in the condition known as *alcoholic myopathy*.

Other systems

Alcohol also affects the levels of sex hormones; certainly in men, but probably, although this is less well-understood, in women also. In men this leads to shrinkage of the testicles (*testicular atrophy*), with loss of sexual drive, impotence and loss of male sexual characteristics. Some men go on to develop breast tissue (*gynaecomastia*) and other features of *feminisation*. Many regular excessive drinkers suffer from sexual and marital difficulties and, in part, this may have a physiological basis.

As intoxication can lead to acute pancreatitis and diabetic symptoms, so regular excessive consumption can lead to more established pancreatic disease and some degree of *diabetes*. The damage of *chronic pancreatitis* is sensitive to even minute quantities of alcohol and a metabolic crisis can easily be precipitated after a few drinks. Pancreatitis, therefore, becomes a definite indication for advising complete abstinence.

Depression and anxiety

Alcohol is clearly a potentially very harmful substance: some readers may already be experiencing anxiety and depression simply on contemplation of the physical damage alone! Chronic excessive consumption causes emotional and mental illness, although less commonly than imagined by many members of the general public. It has already been noted that alcohol causes *increased anxiety* in some individuals and that this may generate *panic attacks* or *phobic illnesses*, which might require psychiatric treatment in their own right.

It is often reported that most problem drinkers are depressed, but this is not entirely correct. It is more accurate to say that over 90% of problem drinkers are deeply unhappy, but a relatively small number, possibly less than 5%, have the significant clinical illness of *depression*. Notwithstanding the relative absence of formal psychiatric illness in problem drinkers, many individuals have a variety of personal difficulties and emotional problems, and alcohol use may have enhanced and exaggerated profound problems of appropriate personal and social functioning. This area of dysfunction becomes most significant for the therapist concerned with treatment and rehabilitation.

Social and legal problems

It is clear that this vast potential of medical damage and pathology will spill over as illness to generate more specific social and legal problems. Illness leads to unemployment and this leads to reduced income. If scarce financial resources are still being spent on alcohol by a regular excessive consumer, there will be resultant financial problems like debt, non-payment of bills leading to disconnection of power supplies, rent arrears, and so on. The spouse of such a drinker is likely to present with these global financial problems at the local Social Services office, but the essential cause will be the problem drinker's regular excessive consumption. The harmful consequences for children and the quality of family life are obvious.

Another common difficulty may be the effect on sexual relations and marital life due to the reduction of sex drive produced by this pattern of drinking. The wife of a male problem drinker might present at a local general practice or Social Services office complaining of a deteriorating marital relationship, and many men clearly use alcohol as a way of avoiding the full responsibility of dealing with their own sexual inadequacies. In addition, women sometimes value their husbands' regular drinking and intoxication as a way of avoiding their own sexual difficulties. Although alcohol is occasionally referred to as an effective contraceptive, it is not to be recommended.

Chronic financial problems may lead some individuals into crime, such as theft, fraud and deception, as a way of obtaining funds to service their regular heavy consumption.

Alcohol dependence and its consequences

For many people, it is dependence on alcohol that is the issue at the centre of problem drinking. They might say, 'If it could only be explained why it is that some people can't give up drinking easily, or why they lose control over their drinking, then surely it would be a giant step towards "solving" alcohol problems.' By now it should be apparent that dependence is not the most significant or damaging problem as far as alcohol is concerned, but is nonetheless of great importance. It is most important not to overemphasise the role of dependence – many serious alcohol-related problems can occur amongst drinkers who never become dependent.

As has been described in Chapter 1, the concept of 'alcoholism' as a disease has, for many alcohol workers and clinicians, been superseded by a more complex view of problem drinking.

Dependence in general

All people are dependent – on each other, on special relationships, on sunlight, on their pay packets and pensions, on the media, on status, on their roles in various settings, and so on. The degree and significance of this normal non-problematic dependence is established by the emotional reaction when one is deprived of a dependent activity; for example, loss of status, or having one's pay stopped. If some degree of sadness, anxiety or loss is then experienced, then some degree of dependence has been demonstrated. The experience is similar to a minor bereavement or grief reaction. Many individuals who have been dependent on alcohol talk about abstaining as being comparable to having lost a close friend, and partners of problem drinkers frequently describe alcohol as a rival for their affections.

Alcohol dependence syndrome

Alcohol dependence syndrome is a clinical description of a cluster of experiences reported by many drinkers who are dependent on alcohol. It provides a useful framework for understanding the problem and from which to help some patients or clients. The main features are a narrowing of the drinking repertoire, increased tolerance to alcohol, increased salience of drinking, withdrawal symptoms, a subjective awareness of a compulsion to drink and relief or avoidance of physical symptoms by further drinking. More controversially some would add the phenomenon of reinstatement after abstinence, whereby a drink even after a prolonged period of abstinence precipitates a recurrence of the syndrome with all its damaging consequences (Edwards and Gross 1976).

Dependence in many respects is a psychological phenomenon which exists in many forms, ranging from personal to cultural. Dependence can be on the substance or indeed its effects. Frequently it is also based on an association with particular objects, a specific glass or a personal pewter mug, or with a social role such as being a 'heavy drinker', being 'sociable', and so on, or a particular activity such as going into a pub and buying rounds of drinks. There is also the reinforcing effect of the distinctive sub-cultural aspects such as drinking with the boys, growing up as a man in a heavy-drinking part of the country, or the atmosphere and conviviality. In all forms of dependence on alcohol there is a strong psychological element, and it is often this aspect which is the most challenging in the recovery process. We should never underestimate the strength of habits and their importance in our lives. The habit of drinking can become very deeply ingrained and acquire multiple associations. If we think for a moment about our own habits and the difficulties we have experienced in changing them, it may help in understanding the task faced by the dependent drinker who needs to find a new way of life that excludes, or certainly greatly diminishes, the role of alcohol.

Many people are dependent upon one or two drinks in the evening, and without them the day is not the same. This habit has no particular consequences or problems. Often marriages and relationships are aided in their harmony by this kind of 'normal dependence'. Drinking alcohol can be a rewarding habit and, in the manner of classical conditioning, habits which are rewarding become more and more strongly learned and reinforced. Many of the associated trappings of drinking strengthen this reinforcement and add to the number of cues which allow the drinker to feel drawn towards a further drink, and so the cycle of psychological dependence becomes more and more deeply scored.

Physical dependence

Physical dependence is an inevitable consequence of drinking regularly over time at a very high consumption level. Many authorities would agree that this daily level for a man would be about 16 units, or eight pints of beer or the equivalent (and less for a woman), drunk over a matter of many months or several years. There is no strong evidence that one sort of drink, for example spirits, is any more likely to produce physical dependence than another, for example beer. Like other forms of damage, it is the amount of ethanol itself that matters, not the beverage type. Many researchers report that it takes up to 15 years of regular excessive consumption for a man to become physically dependent and up to 6 years for a woman. There is a huge amount of individual variation in susceptibility to physical dependence – genetic, biological and psychological factors all play a part in this.

It is well-known that it takes only a matter of a few weeks of regular injected heroin use for a drug taker to become physically dependent or addicted. How long does it take with alcohol? Experiments conducted over 30 years ago with prisoners in the USA, and unlikely to be repeated for ethical reasons, exposed subjects to unlimited daily access to alcohol, found that all the men had become physically dependent and showed withdrawal symptoms after only 60 days' drinking. So, whilst the social distinctions between alcohol and illicit drugs remain clear, perhaps the *chemical* gap between alcohol and drugs is not so wide.

The cellular and metabolic explanations for physical dependence and withdrawal symptoms were considered earlier. How does this metabolic insight help us to understand the dependent drinker? It appears that most physically dependent drinkers develop for themselves a critical blood alcohol concentration below which withdrawal symptoms are manifest, as the alcohol level falls. The typical drinker has been topping up all day, staying above his or her critical level and not experiencing withdrawal. Now he or she falls asleep, intoxicated, at midnight and, whilst asleep, continues to burn off alcohol at the rate of about 1 unit per hour, until the level falls below the critical point. Sweating and excessive perspiration are often the first symptoms to emerge, so that the drinker awakes in the early morning bathed in sweat, and then becomes aware that his or her hands and feet are quivering and tremulous. Nausea and vomiting may occur, together with anxiety and extreme agitation. Often the excessive drinker feels profoundly depressed and at that time may consider life not to be worth living.

The naive drinker may not connect this uncomfortable scenario with the need to take another drink. The experienced physically dependent drinker is, however, well-prepared. This individual has a drink ready by the bedside and takes a few mouthfuls, say 1 unit, of alcohol. Twenty minutes later all the unpleasant symptoms – tremors, nausea, agitation and black mood – have virtually melted away and there is no significant intoxication. However, an hour or so later, that drink has also been burned up and withdrawal symptoms will begin to creep back again. Some drinkers, to use the terms of alcohol dependence syndrome, go on to drink to relieve withdrawal symptoms (relief drinking) and others drink to anticipate or avoid them (avoidance drinking). Some business people with easy access to a bottle of whisky and business lunches, for instance, have become masters of titrating drinks throughout the working day so as to control the physical dependence symptoms, but never become markedly drunk or intoxicated. Thus, paradoxically, for some drinkers even physical dependence is not, as they perceive it, a particular problem.

It is worth noting that the four or five diagnostic features of physical dependence – tremors, sweating, nausea, anxiety, and so on – do not all start abruptly one morning. Heavy drinkers who are becoming physically dependent usually drift very gradually into the symptoms over a period of weeks: perhaps some slight tremor at first, or a little sweating, followed later by tremors, then some nausea and retching. Sometimes it is difficult to distinguish the drift into physical dependence from the effects of regular severe hangovers, but most drinkers soon recognise that something is essentially changed about their normal response to alcohol.

Many individuals, particularly young men and women at a time in their lives when they are drinking heavily, drift in this way into physical dependence. In some heavy-drinking parts of the UK, as many as one adult in twenty may report having had the 'shakes' during the previous twelve months. Most physical dependence goes undetected by medical and other helping agencies, as the drinkers appreciate that something has changed about their response to drinking. Consequently, and often without any specific plan or conscious desire, they slowly cut down their daily drink consumption, day by day, until the shakes in the morning and other unpleasant symptoms have faded away. This natural process of self-regulated alcohol withdrawal, or, more technically, detoxification, is going on in bedrooms, on building sites, in board rooms and on park benches every day of the year, and is usually entirely without significant consequence or mishap. Almost all alcohol-dependent individuals will have 'detoxified' themselves in this way, sometimes on many occasions, before seeking help.

In summary, dependence is a universal phenomenon existing in many forms, all of which rest firmly on psychological principles and the experience of sadness and loss. Consequences and problems from such general dependence may be much greater for some drinkers than for others who are also physically dependent. Physical dependence, although qualitatively different, amplifies the basic psychological pattern of loss. The implication of this loss reaction, however powerful, is that the drinker will anticipate ceasing to drink with great anxiety and will tend not to be able to stop drinking when he or she may need to. At a therapeutic level, there is no such thing as 'getting rid of dependence', as it is normal and implicit, but the problematic consequences related to drinking can be avoided by channelling dependence needs more constructively in a series of therapeutic interventions which help the client or patient to help him- or herself. As will be seen below, there are really very few medical problems specifically caused by dependence itself, as most are more directly related to intoxication and regular excessive drinking, but dependence may have helped to generate these problematic drinking patterns. (For an interesting critique of the concept of dependence see Davies (1992a).)

Medical problems arising from dependence

The major medical problems related to physical dependence are the severe or complicated manifestations of alcohol withdrawal symptoms (Box 2.3). Although, as made clear above, these symptoms are usually transient and without hazard, occasionally some two to three days after the last drink an individual may develop very severe withdrawal symptoms, including *delirium tremens*. The latter is not simply the 'shakes' with some additional agitation, but a serious condition characterised by disorientation and confusion; vivid visual and, more rarely, auditory hallucinations; severe tremor and agitation; fever and sweating; possible epileptic seizures; and other evidence of a severe debilitating illness. This is a major medical and psychiatric emergency and hospital referral is essential for specialist treatment and care. With adequate medical treatment the crisis is usually over within a week, but further hospital support may be needed for some time. The hospital admission may be life-saving, but it will be less than adequate in avoiding future episodes of delirium tremens unless the problem drinker is put immediately into contact with a competent agency, which can enable him or her to sort out the underlying drinking problem and make lifestyle changes.

Elements of this syndrome may occur in a more isolated and less severe form. Visual hallucinations, traditionally in the form of monsters, animals, insects or even the famed pink elephants, may be experienced with great

Box 2.3: Harm due to alcohol dependence

Medical problems

Anxiety	Delirium tremens
Depression	Withdrawal epilepsy
Hallucinations	Multiple drug-taking
Paranoid states	Alcoholic psychosis

Social and legal problems

Stigma	Costs and social consequences of maintaining the habit

agitation, especially when the light is off and the room is dark. The 'horrors', as this experience is sometimes referred to by drinkers, tend to be less intense or absent altogether when the light is on and the sensory system is flooded with an input of external stimulation. Physically dependent drinkers are often only able to sleep with the light on because of the risk of the 'horrors'. Sometimes the visual hallucinations of withdrawal are accompanied by disturbing auditory hallucinations, but usually this profound disturbance clears up as the patient passes through alcohol withdrawal. Occasionally the hallucinations continue for some weeks in the absence of drinking, or even more rarely commence during a period of sustained abstinence. In addition, there may be much prickly and unreasonable suspicion by the drinker of people and the world around him, a form of *paranoid reaction*. These serious and rare disturbed psychiatric conditions are known as *alcoholic hallucinosis* and/or *alcoholic psychosis,* and occasionally may require expert psychiatric diagnostic skills to distinguish them from similar elements found in schizophrenic illnesses. *Epileptic seizures* can also occur in relation to alcohol withdrawal and are a risk when anyone physically dependent ceases drinking abruptly and does not have medically supervised tranquillising medication. Another much more common problem related to alcohol dependence, especially amongst young people, is the tendency to become involved with other dependence-producing or potentially problematic drugs and solvents, to develop the picture of *multiple drug use.* When in doubt about the presence or absence of any of these serious conditions, it is essential to consult a doctor or an experienced and trained alcohol counsellor.

Social and legal problems other than those of stigma, financial hardship and general rejection do not arise from dependence itself, except of course through the manifestation of intoxication and regular excessive consumption.

The Benefits of Alcohol

The benefits of alcohol also need to be acknowledged. Alcohol drinking is without doubt one of the most important factors in maintaining social cohesion and wider social stability. At a personal level, appropriate drinking brings marvellous opportunity for fun, recreation, good company and good conversation. Some of the greatest literature, music, poetry and scientific and philosophical concepts have been created or developed out of a setting of not a little intoxication.

There is increasing medical evidence that to drink modestly, up to a unit a day (or a glass of wine a day), may confer a longer life, with less heart disease and circulatory problems, as compared with those who do not drink at all (Macdonald 1999). These benefits are only evident amongst older men and post-menopausal women, and it is misleading to assume that they necessarily act in the same way for all age groups. In France, the medicinal properties of various wines taken in modest quantities have been represented in several books by influential medical men, in a manner reminiscent of claims for the subtle health-giving properties of spa mineral waters. Much remains to be learned from this area of benefit. In a final analysis, it may therefore be true to say that a little beverage alcohol does much good and is possibly better for many people than total abstention.

B: Drinking During Pregnancy

Moira Plant

INTRODUCTION

This chapter now moves on from a general consideration of alcohol and its effects to a more detailed review of one particular topic, the effects of maternal drinking during pregnancy. There have been a number of advances in the field of drinking in pregnancy since the first reports were published in the 1960s by Lemoine and his colleagues in France (Lemoine et al. 1968) and later Jones and his colleagues in the US (Jones and Smith 1973). The term 'Fetal Alcohol Syndrome' was first described when the latter group of American dysmorphologists became aware of a common set of features found in a number of infants from different racial groups. One of the few common factors amongst the mothers of these children was the fact that they were all very heavy drinkers. Indeed, in the paper published by Jones and Smith to alert physicians to the syndrome, the description of these mothers was 'chronic alcoholics during pregnancy' (1973: 1267). The other factor common to all the mothers in the original group was that they were all poor women, part of the welfare system in the US, which almost by definition means that the degree of social deprivation experienced by these women was high, compared to the general population. Although descriptions of babies damaged by their mothers' drinking have been in the literature, both scientific and fictional, for many years (Warner and Rosett 1975, Plant 1985, Plant et al. 1999), there was little consistency in the descriptions given.

The question of alcohol being a factor in spontaneous abortion is still unclear. Much of the original research was conducted for reasons other than alcohol consumption and therefore the alcohol consumption information was often poorly collected. However, while some studies found an association (Harlap et al. 1979, Kolata 1981 and Windham et al. 1992), others did not (Halmesmäki et al. 1989, Walpole et al. 1989, Parazzini et al. 1994).

Diagnostic Paradigms

The patterns of malformations noted by Jones and Smith (1973) and named the Fetal Alcohol Syndrome (FAS) fell into three groups:

1. Pre- and postnatal growth deficiency: the babies were short in length, light in weight and had a smaller than normal head circumference when born. This growth deficiency did not improve as the children grew older with continued growth below the 10th percentile for gestational age.
2. Morphological anomalies, including a rather distinctive set of facial features such as a short upturned nose, receding chin and forehead, asymmetrical ears and short palpebral fissures, giving the appearance of a broad nasal bridge.
3. Central nervous system involvement, with severe learning difficulties and later cognitive and behavioural problems. Around 50% of children with FAS have IQs below 70.

However, a further aspect was included in the original description – that the mother had to have an 'identifiable' drinking problem. This latter aspect quickly began to be ignored in the ensuing few years. A further diagnosis emerged, that of Fetal Alcohol Effects (FAE). Initially this was the diagnosis, '*possible* fetal alcohol effects', babies found to have individual features of FAS. As noted by Abel:

> The 'possible' was subsequently dropped and, like fetal alcohol syndrome, the term *fetal alcohol effects* (FAE) took on a life of its own (Aase 1994). (Abel 1998: 8)

Fetal Alcohol Effects as a diagnosis then began to be misused as a way of explaining any abnormality for which an explanation could not be found. The position at this point in relation to FAE is that the two original researchers, Lemoine and Jones, have both commented on the problem with this diagnosis and have recommended that the term be avoided (Lemoine 1994, Aase et al. 1995).

The most recent development in relation to diagnostic paradigms took place in 1996 when the United States Institute of Medicine (IoM) (1996) developed an updated categorisation which put maternal drinking clearly in the frame in a way that could not be ignored or excluded. FAS was divided into three categories:

1. FAS with confirmed maternal alcohol exposure.
2. FAS without confirmed alcohol exposure.
3. Partial FAS with confirmed alcohol exposure.

A further, fourth, category, defined as 'alcohol-related birth defects' (ARBD) was included and a final, fifth, category, 'alcohol-related neuro-developmental disorders' (ARND) highlighted aspects such as impairment of fine motor skills as well as behavioural problems in older children.

LEVEL AND PATTERN OF MATERNAL DRINKING

Over the past two decades a major question for debate has been, how much alcohol does it take to show harm in the fetus? Often the level of consumption has been seen as the most important aspect; however, it has become clear, in this area of alcohol research as in many others that the pattern of consumption often defines the type of problem. The debate has recently focused on this area and it has become clear that much of the initial work clouded the issue of pattern of consumption because of the way in which the alcohol information was analysed. An example of this is that a pregnant woman was asked how much she had drunk the previous week. This amount was then divided by the number of days in a week. Therefore, we have studies stating that alcohol-related deficits can be found in women who drink 'an average' of 14g a day (approx 1.5 UK 'units' or 'standard drinks' a day). However if the work is examined closely, the drinking pattern was not that of 1.5 for 7 days, but 5 or 6 drinks on 2 days. Thus the dose of alcohol tended to be concentrated in a short period of time. It is becoming clearer that this higher dose pattern is the one most often, if not solely, found in alcohol-related birth defects. FAS has only been found in women whose drinking can be classified as heavy, problematic or alcoholic.

Maternal Characteristics

A number of factors have been found to be associated with FAS, the main factors being:

- Socio-economic status. This factor relates to the degree of poverty found in this group. It also includes poor nutritional status, access and use of antenatal care and poor general health.
- Past obstetric history. Clearly, problems in the past obstetric history increase the risk of subsequent problems (Cavallo et al. 1995). Another aspect of this is the possibility that the women may be older and may therefore have a longer drinking history.
- Poly drug use. The topic of poly drug use/multiple drug use has been cited earlier in this chapter. The association between heavy drinking and smoking has been established for many years. The majority of pregnant women in the UK and in other countries use over-the-counter preparations. Use of illicit drugs such as cannabis is now also common. The possible synergistic effects of alcohol and these other substances still need to be monitored.

Paternal Characteristics

In the majority of cases of FAS, it is evident that paternal drinking is usually heavy (Abel 1991). Anomalies associated with paternal heavy drinking include cardiac anomalies (Savitz et al. 1991), problems in the immune system (Gottesfield and Abel 1991) and reduced birth weight (Sokol et al. 1993, Windham et al. 1995).

Development

The development of the fetus has been described above. After birth the child with FAS frequently has difficulties with feeding, sleeps poorly, is hypersensitive to sounds, and suffers from hyperactivity. Another distressing factor for both baby and mother is that these babies will often cry when touched. Thus, one of the major ways a mother comforts her child, by cuddling, is therefore not possible.

Poor coordination, another common feature, causes these children to appear clumsy. As they grow older, different difficulties appear. Quite extreme mood changes may develop along with frequent attention-seeking behaviour, heightened anxiety, aggressive behaviour and a low tolerance for frustration (Abel 1998).

As children with FAS reach school age they are already having difficulty in communicating with other children; in general they communicate better with adults. Speech difficulties may relate to motor dysfunctioning but are also related to physical anomalies such as anomalies of the jaw and palate (Becker et al. 1990). A further difficulty may arise if hearing has also been affected.

In relation to learning abilities, children with FAS or other alcohol-related birth defects score below average on reading and comprehension and will often have problems with arithmetic. Writing development is also delayed. These children also encounter difficulties in socialisation. As noted by Morse (1993), these children do not seem to learn from their mistakes; they tend to be extreme in their behaviour and may therefore be aggressive with other children, or conversely are unable to stand up to being bullied and withdraw into themselves. A particularly worrying aspect for parents is the tendency of FAS children to 'make up stories'. According to Morse this may be related more to the problems of poor memory. The child may be trying to fill the gaps in memory rather than actually meaning to be dishonest. However, as can be seen from this list of problematic behaviours, school life for these children, their parents, teachers and fellow students can be extremely difficult and frustrating (Davis 1994, McCreight 1997).

IDENTIFICATION AND TREATMENT

As noted by M.L. Plant (1997): 'There are now a number of studies on identifying pregnant women problem drinkers (Streissguth et al. 1977, Hinderliter and Zelenak 1993, Russell et al. 1994) and treating the pregnant woman with a drinking problem (Rosett et al. 1983, Finkelstein 1993, 1994, Finnegan 1994, Stevens and Arbiter 1995).' However, the majority of studies do not give clear, detailed descriptions of just how to treat a pregnant problem drinker in relation to such aspects as withdrawal regimes. What is clear is the need for supportive, non-judgemental attitudes, and acceptance that many women in this situation lead quite chaotic lives and will often not attend appointments on time. It would be useful if support staff could find ways of accepting this situation and working with the women rather than trying to get the women to adhere to the hospital structure and rules. Although this may be frustrating for the staff, the number of women in this situation will be small and therefore the amount of disruption weighed against the benefits to the baby are clear. Many women in this situation are frightened and feel guilty and ashamed. They will judge themselves more severely than anybody else will. They need help, not condemnation.

3
Drinking at Cross Purposes

Ron McKechnie and Douglas Cameron

A CASE HISTORY

Mark is aged 39, married with two children, a boy aged 13 and a girl aged 10. He works in London as a partner in a firm of chartered accountants and lives 50 miles north of London in a small town. His wife, Judy, used to be the office manager in Mark's firm. The couple have lived together for 16 years, and moved to their current home 8 years ago so that the children could go to a 'better' local school than the ones that were near their London flat. Judy also wanted to move nearer her parents. She has been a full-time housewife since the children were born but has helped out in the local playgroup, which is operated by the church of which she is a member but not a particularly regular attender. To the consternation of his in-laws, Mark never goes to church.

Both Judy and Mark are drinkers. They used to have wine with dinner most evenings but Judy has tried to restrict their drinking together to weekends, holidays and special occasions. She has done this because she is concerned about Mark's drinking.

Mark has been a regular drinker since his mid-teens. He used to play rugby for the school and the lads were in the habit of 'having a few jars' after training and after the match on Saturday. He drank heavily when he and his mates went to watch the England team play their international matches at Twickenham (London) and he always went to Dublin for the weekend every other year when England were playing there. He told Judy tales of the drunken sprees that took place in Dublin. Mark gave up playing rugby in his late twenties following a knee injury, and left the rugby club when he and the family moved out of London. Now he goes to the local pub to watch rugby matches on the big TV screen there. Even so, the ritual trip to Dublin is still seen by him as 'a must', and he still gets excited when he talks to Judy about it. Judy has worried about sexual infidelity in Dublin, and has toyed with the idea that he has a 'regular woman' there. Mark denies this.

Mark accepts that he drinks more than Judy, but does not believe it is a problem. He is in the habit of having a few drinks on the commuter train on the way back home from work and says that he has earned it after a hard day's work. He has to leave early in the morning and, as much of the work of the accountancy firm involves bankruptcy and liquidation work, dealing with stressed clients and having to make ruthless decisions, he uses drink to 'wind down'. After a meal at home in the evening, he will sometimes go to the local pub for the last half-hour which in reality means that he is often not home until midnight. Sometimes Judy will go with him, although that means leaving the children unattended. Whether Judy goes depends upon how drunk she perceives Mark to be when he makes the sugges-tion. She will go if she wishes to have a little time with Mark and feels that he will be reasonable company. She will not go if she feels he has already had too much to drink and will not be attending to her. Mark has occasional hangovers but mostly he is able to 'get his head on' sufficiently to go to work, although he has told Judy of occasions when he had to meet clients and was clearly the worse for wear.

One year ago, Judy tried to stop Mark from going to Dublin. It coincided with a function to mark her father's retirement from work in the local council's planning department. Mark went to Dublin, and during her father's retirement party Judy, according to her, 'inexplicably' burst into tears. She told her mother about her problems with Mark. Her mother said that she would not have mentioned it herself, but that she also had been worried for some time. She said that she had found an article in a woman's magazine about alcoholism and it had a question-naire in it. She thought on the basis of the questionnaire that Mark was an alcoholic. Judy got the article from her mother next morning and could not but agree with her. She decided that she would have to take it up with Mark when he came back from his weekend in Dublin. Mark duly arrived home, still somewhat intoxicated, and wanted to tell Judy about how England had 'trounced' Ireland. He gave the kids little Leprachaun glove puppets. He gave Judy a bottle of Irish Whiskey which he knew she liked. Judy burst into tears again. The kids were hurriedly asked to sit in front of the television while 'Mum and Dad talk'. Judy told Mark about the article, the questionnaire, her mum's view and that she thought he should get help. Mark said that he thought she was talking rubbish, that he didn't drink even as much as the mates with whom he had spent the weekend, and that his mother-in-law had never liked him because he was not a churchgoer. He termi-nated the conversation by asking Judy if she wanted to go out for a drink. She refused, so he went to the pub by himself. When he came home, Judy was in bed. He crept in beside her and next morning left the house at his usual time to get the train to work. When he came home in the evening, neither he nor Judy mentioned what had happened the night before …

INTRODUCTION

The development of drinking problems is not like the development of a disease such as tuberculosis. Tuberculosis develops because an unwitting and presumably unwilling human host is invaded by the tubercle bacillus and becomes the site of its proliferation, accompanied by various responses of the body to that proliferation. This produces signs and symptoms of the disease. The disease is the problem that creates those signs and symptoms. In the world of alcohol use, the signs and symptoms *are* the problem, as noted in the previous chapter. The ingestion of alcohol is undertaken knowingly and wilfully. The behaviours generated following that ingestion are also wilful.

That is not to say that all of the consequences of alcohol ingestion are intended. Most drinkers do not deliberately damage their livers or their brains with alcohol. They drink because they want to, and the liver damage is an unintended consequence of that pattern of drinking. Nor is it to say that some people are not more vulnerable to the effects, physical, psychological and social, of a particular pattern of alcohol use. It is to say that the key focus is on behaviours and the impact of those behaviours upon those around the person displaying those behaviours. Essentially, alcohol problems are socially created, defined and maintained. They are defined at three levels: at the level of the intimate interpersonal, at the level of the person's social matrix and at the level of society as a whole. As illustrated by Figure 3.1, this can be conceptualised as three concentric circles.

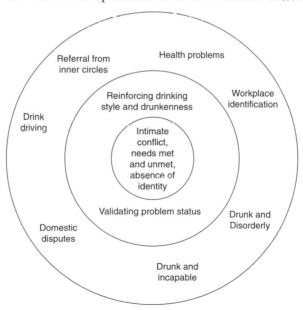

Figure 3.1: Three levels of alcohol problems

Each of these levels has an impact upon the process of problem creation, identification, and interacts with the other levels. Some of the factors in each level are listed in Box 3.1.

Box 3.1: Three levels of alcohol problems

Level 3
Health problems
Opportunistic screening
Workplace identification
Identification by police:
Drunk and incapable/disorderly
Domestic disputes
Drink driving

Level 2
Validating:
Reinforcement by peers of personal identity and 'world view'
Reinforcement by peers of acceptability of drinking style
Reinforcement by peers of acceptability of drunkenness
Reinforcement by peers of problem-free status
Validating positive effects of drinking

Invalidating:
Implicating problem status
Scapegoating of drinking as the cause of problems in relationship
Validating position of partner as a 'drunk'
Supporting removal
Highlighting problems, personal effects preoccupied or 'uncontrolled' drinking

Level 1
Intimate conflicts:
Needs met/unmet
Autonomy
Absence of identity
Dependence/independence
Expectation

Drinking behaviour that is most likely to attract the problem label tends to be generated at level 1. It is there that the behaviour of an individual is under its most intimate scrutiny, and there that judgements about the acceptability or unacceptability of the behaviour are constantly being made and adjusted.

The role and place of drinking and drunkenness for an individual are learned, and learned in part from the family of origin. What behaviours and attitudes are acceptable to this person with whom I live; what baggage from the families of origin is acceptable and what is not? Rules of drinking behaviour are established at the time of new family formation. Is 'he' still 'allowed' to go out with 'the boys' and get 'ratted' after the football? Can 'she' still go out after work with the 'girls' on Friday night after work? There is no right and wrong about these rules. It is just that members of every newly formed relationship have to work them out for themselves. There may be considerable conflict involved.

There is also the issue of what behaviours are shared in these domestic relationships. Does the new couple go out drinking together, do they drink alone or together at home? What are the rules about intoxicated aggression, verbal or physical, and about hangovers? How much must the behaviour remain 'within limits', upon tramlines? How wide are those tramlines? Are they infinitely wide: does one partner have a 'stand by your man' attitude? – he will be tolerated and accepted regardless of his drinking and its consequences? This might be true, and lead to a much lower possibility of problem definition at levels 2 and 3. 'Stand by your woman' is a much less probable position.

Drinking behaviours are not fixed: are there occasions when slightly unusual drinking purposes are tolerated? Is special occasion celebratory drinking, or holiday drinking, or funeral drinking, accepted as being of a different quality from everyday domestic drinking? These and related issues will be explored in more detail below.

Once drinking behaviour has been deemed to be unacceptable at level 1, that may or not be the end of the matter. It depends upon the degree of permeability of those particular domestic boundaries. If the boundaries are highly impermeable, and the behaviour takes place only in private, level 2 involvement might not occur.

More likely, the 'problem' – for that is what it has now become – will become visible to a larger audience, the social matrix of one or other partner. The level 2 response can be either positive or negative. The drinker's 'mates' might be entirely validating of him or her and his or her behaviour. They might say: 'We all do it, it is just our nature', or: 'You've earned the right to behave like that because ....' Or they might invalidate the complainant: 'You're right, she nags, she's never satisfied.'

The negative response could be from peer support for the person having to 'live with' the person with the drinking problem: 'Why do you put up with this, what does he/she do for you?' or as an entry to level 3, 'He needs help or treatment.'

In level 2, we are dealing with conflicting local societal values and norms, and with attempts to validate locating the problem which has become manifest in level 1 as residing in one or other individual.

The level 3 response is interestingly almost always validating of problem definition. Once 'the problem' has been presented to more formal social agencies – medicine, social work, criminal justice, AA – the *a priori* assumption is that there is indeed a problem, and that the problem rests within the designated individual. Here other people's definitions of what is a problem come into play. The problem may be defined simply in terms of weekly levels of consumption, or upon the presence or likelihood of various allegedly alcohol-related harms: to bodily health, to legal status, to work performance or, in a circular way, to domestic relationships. Of course, the individual presenting for a level 3 response may reject the attribution. This is often called 'denial'.

The level 3 definitions feed back into defining the discourse in levels 2 and 1. 'She says I'm an alcoholic'; 'How much do you drink?'; and, of course, the issue of will: 'Can't stop, won't stop.'

It is within this framework that we will examine in greater detail the processes which take place as an individual's behaviour becomes progressively negated, with the concomitant invalidation of identity and being.

LEVEL 1

The Beginning: Becoming Adult and Drinking's Part in This

To become a problem drinker it is necessary to engage in the activity of drinking. In our society the status of drinker is valued; we shun non-drinkers and remove the right to drinking from those we view as not full citizens (children, the mentally disabled and criminals). To ask why young people drink is to ignore this fact and also the fact that we introduce children to alcohol in a systematic fashion similar to that for other 'adult' beverages like tea and coffee (Davies and Stacey 1972, Jahoda and Cramond 1972, McKechnie et al. 1977).

Mastering the art of drinking is not an easy task and this early introduction is part of a long learning period. As with other skills it is inevitable that the learner drinker will make mistakes, somewhat akin to the learning cyclist. Such early mistakes will be attributed to the stage in the drinker's learning. It is necessary to overdo consumption to find out how much is enough. Hangovers and excessive levels of intoxication are thus essential ingredients in the process of learning to drink and not of themselves thought to be a problem. Seen within the context of new learning, they are perceived with amusement and tolerance.

However, it is not simply quantities that one has to learn. In most societies there are clear rules governing drinking behaviour. These rules embrace the hierarchy of rituals that surround this activity but also prescribe how one behaves when intoxicated. The effects of alcohol are therefore seen not as purely pharmacological, but as social too (see MacAndrew and Edgerton 1969). We learn not only from our bodies' reaction but also from our social groupings and their reactions. After an appropriate period of learning, the repetition of mistakes or the breaking of rules is no longer seen in the context of new learning and begins to be seen in different contexts. The inability to learn from mistakes is a key feature here.

One's mistakes can be seen as due to inexperience, but only for a limited time. After that they may be seen as the exuberance of youth or the excesses of studenthood. Thus the mistakes are tolerated and made meaningful within certain contexts and for a limited period of time. However, the repetition of mistakes is sufficient reason to question the purpose and meaning of the behaviour.

Departing from society's rules brings one's behaviour to the attention of others. The severity of the reaction depends not just on the magnitude of the infringement but on the rigidity and latitude allowed by the audience. We know that different societies have different ranges of tolerance of different aspects of drinking problems, and some are more ready to label problems than others. What we are drawing attention to here is not simply labelling but the idea of the problem existing in the eye of the beholder and not necessarily anywhere else. It also stresses the interactive nature of the kind of problems we are discussing.

We have argued elsewhere that one's drinking can go wrong for a variety of reasons to do with the skilled nature of drinking, especially in the domains of dose, purpose and context (Cameron 2000, McKechnie forth coming). It will be argued that the audience questioning someone's purposes or the meaning of that person's drinking is the first step towards the possibility of their becoming labelled a problem drinker.

Whilst one is embarking on the process of learning to be a drinker, this is simply one small part of a larger project: the development of one's identity. Harre (1979) talks of the identity project as the achievement of being known as the kind of person one is. Within the theory of the social construction of emotions it is held that the display of emotion is also part of that identity project (Harre 1986). We are in fact declaring to the world: 'I am the kind of person who gets upset, angry or happy when such and such happens.' Implicit in it is also a statement of values. So this is a moral enterprise as well as a social one. Being a drinker is part of the identity with which we adorn ourselves. There are, of course, many varieties of drinkers, so we can adorn ourselves with different cloaks. Our identity as a drinker is an essential part of our overall identity, especially in societies that value drinking or abstinence – and there are few that do neither.

On Becoming a Problem Drinker: The Difference between the Likely Candidate for Problem Status and Others

We have known for many years that children brought up in the homes of 'alcoholics' and abstainers are more likely to get into difficulty with their drinking than those brought up in families where neither of these characteristics is present (McCord and McCord 1960). There is a continuing argument, probably unresolvable, regarding the relative contribution of nature and nurture to this phenomenon, but it is clear that faulty learning is of great importance.

We also know that children who are not introduced to drinking according to the culturally prescribed fashion are also likely to be the heaviest drinkers in adolescence and therefore more likely to attract attention at this time. Similarly, those whose introduction to alcohol is delayed also seem more prone to problem status in adult life (Ullman 1962).

So there are basic pointers to do with the drinking or non-drinking environment in which one grows up and to do with the process of learning to drink that increase the risk of later vulnerability.

As if that were not enough, there are other factors, to do with neglect and responding to childhood needs, which exist in many families but are especial features of 'alcoholic families', which interfere with the development of identity and the development of personal agency (Steinglass et al. 1987). These appear to heighten the development of later alcohol problems. At a simple level, children who learn that their needs will be ignored or not seen, have to learn to look after their own needs and cope with this kind of neglect. In some studies it has emerged that it is not poverty as such that heightens the risks, but other aspects of deprivation (Vaillant 1983, Hanninen and Koski-Jannes 1999).

The Attention

We have noted above that we all make mistakes when drinking. This is true, not just when learning but also later in our drinking careers. In one population survey a large minority report 'overshooting', the phenomenon of reaching a higher level of intoxication that one reports as the most desirable and the one aimed at on that occasion (McKechnie 1989). The significance of mistakes alters as we progress. Repeated mistakes of the same type will only be tolerated so far. Then they will be sanctioned. If the sanctions do not succeed in altering them, the mistakes will come to be reconstrued. Explanations in terms of experimentation or youthfulness are no longer adequate to the observer. The repetition demands a search in terms of other meanings and these meanings, are likely to be less positive and more sinister.

From this point the drinker will be judged externally, for the observer can no longer see any benefit accruing to the drinker. They have to look elsewhere for explanation. There is a shift away from understanding in terms of the person and his or her agency towards notions of damaged will or bodily addiction. The person's explanations or justifications will no longer be taken seriously, since 'We have heard it all before!'

The assumption is that such persons are no longer in control of themselves. Yet as a corollary of this, no one can do anything for them unless they decide to do it for themselves. Alcoholics Anonymous (AA) advises that we ignore their behaviour and get on with our own lives. In effect we are to ignore them. Their behaviour is not to be construed as having meaning in human or relational terms. Whilst this is intended to apply to their drinking behaviour, it all too easily generalises to other domains and the person soon finds that their role in the family is also affected and they virtually become displaced persons, beyond the normal arena of family relationships and arrangements (Drewery and Rae 1969). Undermining of the person has begun in a serious fashion.

Alcohol plays an important part here, but not the one usually prescribed. Such dislocation from the family is usually seen as the result of the person's drinking; however, it is possible that this process has begun much earlier. The universal and increasing popularity of alcohol even among cultures which have previously shunned alcohol has been explained in terms of alcohol's inherent signalling system. By that we refer not only to the presence of a glass in the hand but also to the inevitable lack of muscle coordination that follows from consumption even at low doses. Perhaps noteworthy here is the tightening of the upper lip (from which the term 'getting tight' derives) which is apparent long before any slurring of speech. The usefulness of this signalling system is that it communicates publicly that the person has been drinking, and is in alcohol intoxication mode. With this information we can then decide how seriously to take this person. As there is in our culture a tendency not to take too seriously things said when the speaker is under the influence, we have all that is necessary to begin the process of undermining the status and 'personhood' of the drinker. This process is probably well underway long before we begin to look at alternative explanations.

Different social groups have different levels of tolerance to problems arising from drinking and different levels of readiness to attribute them to alcohol. An extreme example might be a young orthodox Muslim or Mormon for whom the consumption of any alcohol at all would lead to the risk of being perceived as having a drinking problem. The risk is due to his or her preparedness to break with conventional values and not to the amount of alcohol he or she may have consumed. But we are addressing here something more subtle: the breaking of drinking rules within a drinking culture.

It was not that Mark, in our case study, was drinking at all that has caused Judy to designate him as a problem drinker. It was about the purpose and place of drinking in his life compared to its place in hers. For instance, for her, the party to mark the retirement of her father *should have* been a more important place for Mark to be than the biennial Dublin visit with his mates. After all, her father would retire only once. Mark could have been at the retirement party and possibly consumed just as much as he did that evening in Dublin. So it was not the consumption of a certain quantity of alcohol that was the problem either. It was about the relative importance that Mark attributed to a couple of events. One of them was a family event which would not be repeated. The other was a 'boys only' ritual which had occurred before and no doubt would occur again. Mark chose the latter. He had not left behind that particular piece of youthful spree drinking: it remained part of his identity project, to the exclusion of being a dutiful son-in-law party attender. His absence became part of the process by which his 'problem' became visible at level 2.

The scene is now set for a dominance battle. If Judy attempts to control Mark's behaviour, as she has done already regarding his drinking, any further attempts are likely to be seen as focusing on his drinking rather than his freedoms. A common response to this is to protest: 'I will not be controlled in this fashion.' So Mark continues to drink and to exercise his freedoms. His freedoms or the lack of them are never addressed as a problem. It is important for Mark to preserve some semblance of himself as a man who is not under his wife's thumb. Mark may already have brought some problems into his relationship with his in-laws. We know he thinks his mother-in-law doesn't like him. It is possible that he already did not have a great image of himself and, as Steffenhagen and Burns (1987) have noted, low levels of self-esteem are the cause, not the result, of deviant behaviour.

There is a vast literature on relapse within drinking problems based upon the original work of G. Alan Marlatt (Marlatt and Gordon 1985). This alludes to the phenomenon of resuming old drinking habits. The literature encourages drinkers to identify the triggers for resumed drinking as a way of predicting risky situations and engaging in appropriate incompatible behaviours. This body of literature could equally be read as showing how problem drinking comes about in the first place, rather than simply how and when it comes to be reinstated. Thus all the relapse triggers can be seen as creators of the problem in the first place. Most of the triggers that people mention are inevitably to do with social situations (for example, Fichter et al. 1997). We should not be surprised by this when we think of the vast literature that exists on the personality characteristics of the partners of alcoholics which predict good outcome. This must lead us to the view that partners and family are not just innocent by-standers but are intimately involved in the creation, development and maintenance of problems. This is the view essentially taken by the systems theorists Finlay (1978) and Steinglass et al. (1987).

LEVEL 2

Level 2 is the world of family, friends and neighbours. The people at this level have varying views about the nature of drinking and of drinking problems, informed by personal experience, by what they have observed in others and by what they have gleaned from the 'professionals' who inhabit level 3. Each member of this community will have their own symptom checklist for what constitutes an alcohol problem. Of course, they will not have this as an explicit corpus of knowledge, but they will 'know' when someone is breaking the rules of drinking in their culture. They will readily make judgements that somebody is or is not an 'alcoholic' or problem drinker. They will know that, for instance, *early morning drinking*, or *drinking every day*, or *missing work because of hangovers*, is what alcoholics do.

So, contingent upon the beliefs of those consulted, the level 2 response can be either 'Yes, *he has* or *you have* an alcohol problem', or, 'No, *what is being done is normative.*' That is, there is a validation or invalidation of the phenomena under scrutiny.

One example of how members of a community define their problem drinkers is provided by Mulford (1977). He examined the community labelling process in Iowa, USA, and found four phenomena demonstrated by drinkers which made it likely that they would be labelled problem drinkers:

1. trouble due to drinking
2. personal effects drinking
3. preoccupied drinking
4. uncontrolled drinking.

According to Mulford, these phenomena were cumulative and non-sequential. That is, if you showed one of them, you might be labelled an 'alcoholic'. But if you showed two, the odds of being labelled an alcoholic went up; even more so if you demonstrated three. His perception was that if a person in Iowa showed all four, he or she would almost certainly be labelled an 'alcoholic'.

In our case study, Mark has displayed 1, 2 and possibly 4 on Mulford's list. Mulford's criteria are, however, rather coarse. We are concerned with rather more intimate detail. In the real world, the behaviours are not so clearly exclusively about alcohol. It was Mark's non-appearance at a certain place that was the problem, not his appearance in an intoxicated state. That non-appearance was linked to the possibility of him being intoxicated in Dublin, but the people in Mark's level 2 had no data other than hearsay to go on. But that was enough for them to create an image, a mantle, which it was agreed fitted.

Loss of Personhood

We have alluded to this phenomenon earlier and it is now time to consider it in greater detail. The process of loss of personhood is insidious, beginning very early in a drinker's career and almost without notice. This is one of the reasons why it has gone largely unreported in the literature. Yet it may be of sufficient seriousness for drinkers to feel they are second-class citizens, and it may be one of the reasons why in the eyes of some authorities they are not worth spending money on.

We have mentioned the beginnings of the process in relation to no longer seeing social meaning in the behaviour of the drinker or recognising that the drinker is not engaged in a communal activity: they are doing their own thing, albeit with others. However, the seeds are probably sown much earlier in some of our reactions to drinking, which apply to all drinkers and not just those who are candidates for problem status.

As noted above, ingesting alcohol results in the communication of signals that indicate that the person is now in an intoxicated state. This system may account for the popularity of alcohol. However, it also allows us, having noticed the intoxicated signal, to react in such a way as to revise the level of seriousness with which we take the behaviour exhibited. We can ignore what is said on the basis that 'It was just the drink talking', and not hold the problem drinkers responsible because they wouldn't have done whatever it was they did had they not been drinking. Initially this applies to utterances during the intoxicated period and happens to us all to some extent. However, it is then only a small step to begin also to disregard what is said when the drinkers are sober, particularly when 'drinker' or 'drunk' becomes an integral part of the definition of self.

In a similar vein, we can ignore anything said or done if we suspect that the drinker will have no recollection of it the next day. This often suits both participants in the exchange. *'He's a lovely man when sober but he says the most terrible things when he's drunk and doesn't remember.'* This allows the observer to continue to hold a positive picture of the drinker without questioning the validity of the 'terrible things'.

Drinkers are therefore confronted with a system which initially does not take their utterances seriously when they are drunk but later proceeds not to take them seriously at any time, as if they have lost the right to a voice within the system.

Those who experience a series of consistent changes when drinking are frequently referred to as undergoing a Jekyll and Hyde transformation. In other words, they are behaving like someone else rather than expressing another side of themselves. Again, this view can suit both participants. In much of our work with couples who report these phenomena, when asked if the things said were true or needed to be said, they often replied in the affirmative. In these instances the drinking has 'enabled' the drinkers to say something that they would have found difficult to say when sober yet which they felt needed to be said. The defence of being intoxicated is the excuse that allows both parties to avoid looking at a difficulty in their relationship.

These consistent changes in a person when 'under the influence' must be seen as manifestations of part of the person and not as some alien presence. Such changes do not come from the bottle but from the personality of the drinkers functioning in one of their environments. This is not to argue that 'the drunk man always speaks the truth', it is to argue that they are as capable of doing so as the rest of us, but that they also speak as much rubbish. The fact that the speaker may have been drinking does not in itself invalidate what has been said. Some other criteria for rejection would have to exist.

It is useful to note that the Jekyll and Hyde explanation is usually only invoked when there is a negative appraisal of the behaviour and is not used when 'drunken changes for the better' are prominent.

In disputes where one party has been drinking, the moral high-ground is taken by the significant other *who in the process defines reality.* Any disagreement with that definition of reality is then construed as denial. Again, the drinker's point of view is invalidated.

We judge normal behaviour by the standard of an ideal other. In Western society that ideal other is thought to be a fully functioning independent individual capable of self-control. He or she is a sentient agent. When people behave out of the ordinary we have to make sense of that. Since our ideal contains the notion of self-control, we frequently invoke a lack of self-control in our understandings of others' behaviour. As a society we generate disorders based on the notion of flawed control (Gaines 1992). Having concluded that the person is no longer in control of him- or herself we are totally justified in not taking him or her seriously. That person is no longer a full citizen and therefore not entitled to the same rights and privileges as others.

Even if we conclude that he or she is sick (that is, having the disease alcoholism) the person is undermined because he or she is no longer expected to be functioning normally. *'What else do you expect from a sick person?'* This allows condemnation and caring at the same time.

LEVEL 3

Enter the Professionals

We define a level 3 response as one which involves professional agents or alcohol-specific charitable or self-help personnel. It is the involvement of people other than family and friends. The involvement may occur as a direct result of wishes and actions of the problem drinkers or their families and friends. But it may occur inadvertently. Drinkers may, for example, 'be presented' by an employer, as a result of some health screening procedure, as a result of some unrelated contravention of the law, or as a result of an accident. Something happens that places drinkers and their drinking under professional scrutiny. Signs and symptoms are elicited, and almost always the problem drinker status is validated. What is usually elicited these days is evidence of 'alcohol dependence' and/or alcohol-related disability.

As noted in the previous chapter, the 'common elements' of dependence on alcohol are:

1. narrowing of the drinking repertoire
2. salience of drink-seeking behaviour
3. increased tolerance to alcohol
4. repeated withdrawal symptoms
5. subjective awareness of compulsion to drink
6. relief or avoidance of withdrawal symptoms by further drinking
7. reinstatement after abstinence. (Edwards and Gross 1976)

This list is increasingly being claimed to be a real and meaningful nosological entity, and has become central to such works as the *Diagnostic and Statistical Manual* (*DSM*) and the *International Classification of Diseases* (*ICD*). Yet it contains a number of phenomena with no real claim to be evidence of pathological status and which are, at best, value judgements.

Alcohol-related disabilities are even more of a rag-bag of phenomena:

1. social disabilities, such as 'the failure of the individual to perform adequately in any role expected of him or her (spouse, parent or employee, for instance)'. This includes problems in the family, at work, and the committing of crime, including drinking and driving
2. psychological disabilities, such as nervousness and moodiness, personality problems, memory blackouts, alcohol withdrawal states
3. physical disabilities, such as gastrointestinal tract and liver damage, heart disease and hypertension, damage to brain and nervous system, accidents and trauma, adverse effects on sexual function and effects on the fetus. (Royal College of Psychiatrists 1986)

The prevalence of these phenomena in the general population is well documented (Kristenson and Hood 1984). It is widely accepted that their prevalence seems to go up and down contingent upon the overall level of alcohol consumption in the country: the more awash with alcohol a community is, the higher is the prevalence of these problems, although more recent data on drinking patterns suggests that intake per drinking session may be a better predictor of disability than overall consumption (Rehm et al. 1996).

It is notable that over the past 30 years professionals in all the caring disciplines are being informed over and over again by the alcohol experts that they are failing to recognise substantial numbers of people on their caseloads where alcohol use is 'the real, or underlying cause of their problems' (for example, Walsh 1995).

What this means is that in any drinking community a number of alcohol-related problems are widespread and professionals are exhorted and trained to recognise them as alcohol-related in individuals who present to them. They are then taught to try and intervene in the presenter's drinking career by advocating reduction or cessation of consumption of alcohol. Thus the level 3 response to a presenter is most likely to concur with the invalidating views at level 2. It is a one-way street.

This is not to say that there are no people whose drinking has damaged their health. Of course there are. Nor is it to say that there are no people who, to any balanced observer, would benefit from reduction or cessation of their alcohol consumption. Of course there are. It is to say that professionals tend not to focus on the purpose of an individual's drinking. So invalidation of personhood may well be part of the process of assessment: 'This person is alcohol dependent, or an alcoholic', meaning that his or her drinking can be explained in terms of a pathological process and that no other explanation need be posited.

It is thus not surprising that many people who are referred to professionals either fail to show up or refute the label they believe they are having attached to them. Some time ago, we reported the sequence of thinking that non-attenders (to a psychiatrist) go through:

1. 'Treatment involves mental hospitals and consultant psychiatrists. They are for people who are "mental", "lunatics", "not right in the head".'
2. 'I am being referred because of my drinking.'
3. 'This means I am being considered "mental" because of my drinking and "mental" people who drink are called "alcoholics".'
4. 'Am I an "alcoholic"?'
5. '"Alcoholics" are people who ... [hide bottles, neglect their responsibilities, have no control, keep falling over, drink all day, drink more than others, and so on].'
6. 'I am not like that. Therefore I am not an "alcoholic". Therefore I do not need treatment, so I will not attend.'

These people did not attend for interview; they negotiated for themselves an explicit though vague definition of an 'alcoholic' which placed them at a distance from the label, and temporarily modified their drinking to reinforce their notion of not being an 'alcoholic' (Cameron 1983).

What of those who do manage to pass through a professional's consulting room door? If they do not accept the professional's judgement, they are deemed to be wrong. They have been variously termed 'in denial', 'unmotivated' or 'pre-contemplators', depending upon in which of the last few decades they were referred for help. The tricks used to convince them of the error of their ways and perceptions become ever more sophisticated, involving such techniques as motivational interviewing, workplace interventions and good old-fashioned compulsion, particularly if there has been some contact with the criminal justice system.

It is perhaps worth noting that the so-called prevalence of alcohol problems is based upon the rates of presentation to professional agents, but the assumption is made that those presenting to professionals represent only a minority (usually claimed to be in the range 10–20%) of those with such problems.

To extend our case study, Mark would now reach the professionals and they know best. Since Mark reports that he has found it difficult in the past to abstain, he has been persuaded that this is what he should at least try, albeit for a short period of time. To assist him in this he could be offered a drug that is supposed to have the effect of reducing craving. His problem is now internalised to his body, which is viewed as having altered in some sense. His duty in this is to faithfully take the medicine or it may have been arranged that his wife has the responsibility of making sure that he takes it. The other widely used specific pharmacological alternative would be to prescribe Disulfiram which, rather than reducing craving, leads to very unpleasant side-effects if alcohol is consumed. All other ('psychosocial') treatments or interventions would be aimed at Mark as a person: towards his will, his motivation or his sense of agency. The view is promulgated that he is either biochemically challenged or wanting in the personality department.

The success of community reinforcement programmes and family therapy for alcohol problems is due not so much to increasing the problem drinkers' sense of agency as to repositioning them within their immediate social group as people whose behaviour is to be attended to and whose needs have to be listened to. They are reincorporated as persons. This is also seen in so-called spontaneous recovery where the trigger to recovery is a new relationship in which the previously invalidated person feels valued.

In conclusion, this chapter has highlighted something which some will find disturbing. It is that the most intimate observer of someone's drinking is at least an equal partner in generating the problem. It is his or her perception of what is or is not a problem that is critical. In our case study, Judy, with the encouragement of her mother, focused on Mark's drinking as the sole and sufficient cause of their interpersonal difficulties. This made his drinking a problem. She could have focused in on his long hours at work, his disinterest in church, her feelings of neglect, or his absenting himself from family events and rituals.

All these aspects were clearly problems for her, too, but she did not call them problems. Why one aspect of someone's behaviour gets placed into the category of problematic by the intimate observer is, of course, a result of many things. The visibility of the problem behaviour plays an important part not just in this case for Judy, but also as it is the main thing which is obvious to Mark's mother-in-law. This visibility means that the drinking takes precedence over the more hidden, but possibly more important, dimensions of the relationship. This depends on many factors, including the upbringing of the observer, his or her beliefs, prejudices and self-image, and the likelihood that he or she will be supported. In short, the observer's own identity. When we look at what might lead to a change in Mark's behaviour, Judy is as crucial as she was in the creation and maintenance of the problem. The likelihood of Mark becoming abstinent or 'improved' is going to depend to a large extent on Judy's personality and resources as well as Mark's, and on the continuing dance they engage in regarding what they want from each other and their marriage.

It is the mismatch between the two identity projects which is at the core of why somebody develops a drinking problem. This is what creates drinking at cross purposes.

4
Drinking Patterns

Eileen Goddard, Martin Plant, Moira Plant, Ian Davidson and Henk Garretsen

Beverage alcohol has been in use for at least 7,000 years (McGovern et al. 1996). Drinking patterns have changed markedly throughout history. They also vary markedly between different social, cultural and national groups of people. Alcohol is both legal and widely enjoyed in most societies. Even so, its consumption has often been controversial and there have been periods, such as the eighteenth-century British 'Gin Epidemic' and the Prohibition era in the US, when alcohol consumption has been the subject of intense debate and disagreement (Musto 1997, M.L. Plant 1997).

Information about alcohol consumption patterns is currently available from several sources. These include 'official statistics' related to the production, sale and purchase of alcohol. These figures often relate to alcohol taxation, which is discussed further in Chapter 5. In some countries 'official' information about alcohol consumption is extremely limited or non-existent. Most of the detailed information available relates to developed countries. Even so, some information does exist in relation to developing nations. A considerable body of such information has recently been reviewed by Grant (1998). In some countries and regions, alcohol consumption is illegal. Elsewhere, in places such as India, Norway and in some parts of the former USSR, a considerable proportion of the alcohol consumed is illicitly produced and not covered in official statistics. Another invaluable body of information about drinking habits has been generated by surveys of self-reported alcohol consumption. Again, most of the studies of this type have been conducted in developed countries. Survey coverage is generally patchy and uneven. Many studies have collected only limited amounts of information and there is great variation in survey methods. Self-reports of drinking are not necessarily accurate and, as noted by Midanik (1982a, 1982b), may be seriously distorted by poor coverage, bias, under-reporting and over-reporting. The possible limitations of surveys are discussed in more detail later in this chapter.

Since the Second World War, per capita alcohol consumption in many countries has varied considerably. In the UK, for example, consumption rose until 1979, then levelled off (Brewers and Licensed Retailers Association 1998). A number of authors have maintained that the drinking habits of several sections of the British population changed little over much of this period (May 1992, Plant and Plant 1992). More recently, however, it has been suggested that drinking patterns have undergone changes and that there might have been a shift in the position of the sexes in relation to several alcohol-related variables (M.L. Plant 1997).

INTERNATIONAL ALCOHOL CONSUMPTION LEVELS

Neither levels nor trends of national per capita alcohol consumption have been uniform. This perplexing variation is illustrated in relation to 43 countries in Table 4.1.

Table 4.1: Per capita alcohol consumption in 43 countries (1970–96) (litres of pure alcohol)

Country	1970	1975	1980	1985	1990	1993	1994	1995	1996
Europe									
Austria	10.3	11.0	11.0	11.3	11.9	11.6	11.2	11.2	11.0
Belgium and									
Luxembourg*	9.0	10.6	10.9	10.6	11.1	10.5	10.3	10.1	9.1
Bulgaria	6.7	8.2	8.7	8.8	9.4	6.0	6.3	5.6	6.2
Croatia						9.9	11.3	11.5	11.6
Czech Republic						12.3	12.5	11.7	11.9
Denmark	6.8	8.8	9.3	10.3	9.8	9.9	10.0	10.1	10.1
Finland	4.3	5.9	6.1	6.3	7.8	6.8	6.6	6.4	6.3
France	17.2	17.0	15.6	13.8	12.6	12.3	11.8	11.9	12.1
Germany**	12.0	13.1	13.3	12.5	11.7	11.8	11.5	11.2	10.8
Greece						7.5	7.5	7.4	7.2	7.7
Hungary	9.9	11.0	12.9	12.6	12.1	10.7	10.7	11.0	10.1
Ireland	5.9	7.8	7.4	6.6	7.3	7.3	7.1	7.2	7.5
Italy	16.0	14.9	13.9	12.5	9.5	8.0	8.2	8.0	7.7
Netherlands	5.5	8.6	8.6	8.3	8.1	7.8	7.9	7.9	8.1
Norway	3.6	4.3	4.6	4.1	4.1	3.8	3.8	3.9	4.0
Poland	5.1	6.9	8.4	6.7	6.7	6.0	6.2	6.0	6.0
Portugal	9.8	13.1	10.8	12.9	11.7	11.4	10.3	10.4	10.8
Romania	5.8	7.3	7.6	7.4	8.5	8.6	8.7	9.0	9.9
Russian Federation						5.5	5.3	5.2	5.2
Slovak Republic						7.3	8.4	9.2	8.5
Slovenia						8.1	7.8	7.7	6.7
Spain	12.0	13.9	13.5	11.8	10.8	9.7	9.7	9.6	9.4
Sweden	5.8	6.3	5.6	5.3	5.8	6.0	6.1	5.7	5.2
Switzerland	10.8	10.7	11.1	11.5	11.4	10.2	9.8	9.5	9.4
United Kingdom	5.3	6.8	7.3	7.2	7.6	7.1	7.3	7.0	7.2
Ukraine						4.3	2.8	2.1	1.4

Table 4.1: (*cont ...*)

Country	1970	1975	1980	1985	1990	1993	1994	1995	1996
Africa									
South Africa	3.0	3.6	3.8	4.2	5.1	4.6	4.8	4.8	5.1
Asia									
China						3.2	3.3	3.5	3.7
Japan***	4.8	5.4	5.6	6.1	6.5	6.8	6.8	6.8	6.7
S. Korea****						1.2	1.4	1.5	1.5	1.5
Philippines			4.0	3.7					
Australasia									
Australia	7.8	9.2	9.4	9.2	8.4	7.8	7.9	7.7	7.8
New Zealand	6.3	7.8	8.2	8.0	7.9	7.4	7.4	7.2	7.0
North America									
Canada	6.4	8.3	8.7	8.0	7.3	6.2	6.1	6.1	6.1
US	7.0	7.7	8.1	7.8	7.4	6.6	6.6	6.6	6.6
Central & South America									
Argentina	11.5	8.8	7.6	7.7	6.8	6.8	7.0		
Brazil*****	0.7	1.0	1.3	1.4	2.5	2.0	2.2	2.8	3.0
Chile*****	5.6	5.4	6.4	5.5	4.5	3.6	3.2	3.3	3.1
Colombia****	1.4	1.4	1.8	2.3	2.5	2.4	2.4	2.1	2.2
Cuba	0.8	1.1	1.2	1.3	1.5	0.9	0.7	0.6	0.7
Mexico****	1.9	2.0	2.5	2.5	2.7	2.7	2.7	2.5	2.5
Peru*****	1.0	1.5	1.6	1.6	1.4	1.6	1.5	1.7	1.8
Venezuela*****	2.6	2.5	3.8	3.1	3.4	3.8	3.6	3.8	3.2

Notes: *Luxembourg has not been listed separately, since cross-border trading reportedly leads to inaccuracies.
**Prior to 1991 figures only refer to Federal Republic of Germany.
***Including sake.
****Beer only.
*****Beer and wine only.
Source: BLRA (1998: 81).

Per capita alcohol consumption, as noted by Thurman in Section A of Chapter 5, though useful, does not give much insight into drinking patterns. There are, for instance, big differences between the north and south of Europe. In the south, quite often wine accompanies a meal and the consumption of alcohol is distributed throughout the day, so that the level of inebriation is not high. Social norms have traditionally not approved of intoxication. In the north (Finland, Norway and Sweden, for example) alcohol (beer and spirits) is 'looked upon as something with which to get drunk at festival get-togethers, where being intoxicated is considered a normal condition' (Hauge 1999).

As Table 4.1 shows, international trends in per capita alcohol consumption have been far from uniform. Levels in countries such as Austria, Australia, Belgium and Luxembourg, Canada, Greece, Peru, Poland, the UK and the US have not varied much over the period 1970–96. In contrast, per capita consumption has increased considerably in countries such as Denmark, Japan, Romania and South Africa. Conversely, there have been marked falls in alcohol consumption levels in Argentina, Chile, Italy, France and Spain. In Italy, for example, per capita alcohol consumption has declined from 16 litres in 1970 to only 7.7 litres in 1996, a fall of over 50%. As reported recently by Rossi and Tempesta (1999b), Italian drinking habits have undergone a major transformation, moving towards those more commonly associated with Northern Europe or North America. This change has involved a move away from frequent drinking with meals to less frequent drinking, not necessarily linked with meals. The overall proportion of abstainers has not changed much, though this has increased amongst young people (Osservatorio Permanente Sui Giovani e L'Alcool 1998). In Western Europe there has been a reduction in the differences in per capita alcohol consumption. This may reflect a process of 'Europeanisation'. In Eastern Europe, trends have been quite different and, as indicated in Chapter 6, rates of problems, such as liver cirrhosis, have increased substantially in some Eastern countries. It has also been stressed by several authors that per capita alcohol consumption in some countries is probably much higher than indicated in Table 4.1. Vroublevsky and Harwin, commenting on the situation in Russia, have noted:

> Between 1990 and 1995, per capita alcohol consumption more than doubled. According to a recent report from the Russian Presidential Commission on Women, Family and Demography, average per capita consumption has now reached 13 litres per year, 5 litres more than the level the World Health Organization considers dangerous. (1998: 207)

CHILDREN AND ALCOHOL

It is widely accepted that men are generally more likely than women to consume beverage alcohol, that male drinkers consume more alcohol and experience higher rates of alcohol-related problems than their female counterparts. Many authors have commented upon the existence of traditional double standards in public attitudes to alcohol consumption by either sex. These are reflected in the disapproval of drinking by women, and the use by 'respectable' women of drinking locales such as public bars (Cavan 1966, Camberwell Council on Alcoholism 1980, M.L. Plant 1997, Thom 1999).

Evidence suggests that these types of attitudes towards drinking begin to develop at a very early age. Research has shown that even amongst young children in England and Scotland, this type of sexism is evident, with a greater disapproval of alcohol consumption by adult females than by males. Children as young as four years of age often appear able to differentiate between alcoholic and non-alcoholic drinks. Children are clearly influenced by the use of alcohol by those with whom they have contact, in particular, their parents, older siblings and other people in their lives. In some societies, such as France and Italy, it has long been considered normal to allow young children to taste strictly monitored samples of wine or other alcoholic drinks. The legal minimum age of alcohol consumption in the UK is five years, so it is possible for British parents, should they wish to do so, to follow a similar mode of introducing their children to drinking in a regulated context. Many children have parents and other contacts who provide an example of generally moderate, harm-free drinking. Some children, however, do not have such good role models, but are exposed to heavy and problematic drinking. Some may have little or no close personal experience with alcohol consumption, because their parents do not drink at all for religious or other reasons. Youthful exposure to adult heavy drinking may have profound and possibly harmful consequences. Some children have their lives badly damaged by such experiences (Plant et al. 1989).

Periodic 'moral panics' have focused attention on alleged heavy or problematic drinking by children or other young people. Some of these concerns are justified, while others have been exaggerated or unfounded. A recent example of such a media panic is the controversy over the production, marketing and sale of so-called 'alcopops' (alcoholic lemonades and colas). These alcoholic beverages, characterised by sweet flavours and often packaged in a way likely to attract younger drinkers, were widely condemned as being likely to blur the boundaries between alcoholic and non-alcoholic drinks and to appeal to children. In fact there has been little evidence to suggest that alcopops have had much impact on youthful alcohol consumption. Young heavier drinkers appear to prefer cheaper forms of alcoholic beverage, such as cider. Most of those who consume alcopops appear not to be children or even younger teenagers (MacCall 1998).

Young children in Britain have been shown to have rather negative, moralising, attitudes towards drinking (Jahoda and Cramond 1972, Fossey 1994). This negativity appears to be reversed once young people pass through puberty and enter their teenage years.

TEENAGERS AND ALCOHOL

Teenagers and young adults in drinking cultures appear to be generally enthusiastic about alcohol consumption. Indeed, many authors have reported that such young people commonly regard drinking as a hallmark of maturity, sociability and attractiveness (Davies and Stacey 1972, Plant and Plant 1992). Teenagers are legally able to drink at least under some circumstances in most industrial countries. A notable exception is the US, where the legal minimum age of alcohol purchase or consumption is 21 (Hingson et al. 1997). May (1992), reviewing the drinking patterns of British adolescents, concluded that relatively little had changed in the previous 20 years. He also noted that some media reports related to the alleged excesses of youthful drinking had been unfounded. However, evidence does now suggest that a change has occurred in the alcohol consumption patterns of British teenagers. In fact, there is evidence of increased heavy drinking amongst teenagers and young adults in several countries – in Rotterdam in The Netherlands, a significant sharp rise was evident for the age group 16–24 (Garretsen et al. 2000).

During 1995 a major international survey was carried out to investigate the drinking, smoking and illicit drug-using habits of 15–16-years-olds (Hibbell et al. 1997). A total of 26 European countries participated in this exercise. This study, 'the European School, Survey Project on Alcohol and Other Drugs', is known simply as 'ESPAD'. The participating countries were: Croatia, Cyprus, the Czech Republic, Denmark, Estonia, the Faroe Islands, Finland, Hungary, Iceland, Ireland, Italy, Latvia, Lithuania, Malta, Norway, Poland, Portugal, the Slovak Republic, Slovenia, Sweden, Turkey, the Ukraine and the four component parts of the UK. This study was significant because it collected information from thousands of teenagers using a common questionnaire. As a result, a substantial body of comparable information was gathered. This survey indicated that UK teenagers reported the highest levels of illicit drug use amongst school children of any of the countries surveyed. Moreover, levels of alcohol consumption and intoxication amongst UK teenagers were also high by international standards. Other countries in which a similar pattern was evident included Denmark and Finland (Hibell et al. 1997). Similar striking international differences in the drinking patterns of young people have also recently been reported by Currie et al. (2000).

The ESPAD study showed that levels of illicit drug use were higher amongst UK teenagers than amongst those in any of the 22 other participating countries. The great majority of the 7,722 UK teenagers surveyed had at some time consumed alcoholic beverages. A total of 94% of girls and boys had done so. In addition, 11% of girls and 15.4% of boys had reported consuming alcohol on at least 9 occasions in the previous 30 days. Considerable proportions, 78.5% of girls and 77.3% of boys, had also experienced intoxication. The survey indicated that there were some differences between the drinking experiences of those in different parts of the UK. The highest proportion of girls who had never had a drink (15%) was in Northern Ireland. The highest proportions of boys who had never done so were in England and Northern Ireland (6%). Consistent with these findings, the lowest proportion of teenage girls who had been intoxicated or who had consumed alcohol 9 or more times in the previous 30 days or who had consumed 5 drinks in a row over the same period were in Northern Ireland. Amongst boys, the lowest proportion of those who had been intoxicated were in England and Northern Ireland (76.5% and 78.4% respectively). The lowest proportions of those who had consumed alcohol on 9 or more occasions in the past 30 days were in Scotland and Northern Ireland (9.6%). The lowest proportion who had consumed 5 or more drinks in a row in the previous 30 days was in England (50.6%), while the highest was in Wales (48%) (Miller and Plant 1996).

The high rate of non-drinking in Northern Ireland was consistent with the results of an earlier study by Loretto (1994). High levels of non-drinking amongst UK youth have also been noted amongst those living in the Western Isles of Scotland. A survey in this area indicated that there was a marked polarisation in teenage drinking habits, with high proportions of both abstainers and heavy drinkers (Anderson and Plant 1996).

The ESPAD exercise was repeated during 1999. This time even more countries took part. The UK survey elicited information from a sample of 2,641 students in 223 state and private schools. The findings of this study have already been described in detail elsewhere (Plant and Miller 2000, Miller and Plant 2000a, 2000b) Overall, alcohol consumption amongst 15- and 16-year-olds had changed little between 1995 and 1999. Again, the great majority, 94% of girls and boys, had at some time consumed alcohol. In addition, 74% of girls and 78% of boys reported having experienced intoxication. There were again notable differences between teenagers in different parts of the UK. The highest proportion of abstainers amongst girls (11%) and boys (9%) was in Northern Ireland. English and Welsh boys and girls were more likely than those in Scotland or Northern Ireland to have had more than 9 drinking occasions in the past 30 days.

Older teenagers – those aged 16–19 – are covered on surveys of the adult population, but a different method is used to obtain information about young people's drinking. The first government survey of drinking among young teenagers (secondary school children aged 11–15) was carried out in 1984 (Marsh et al. 1986). Since 1988, information has been obtained biennially from surveys (primarily of smoking behaviour) carried out for the Department of Health and the Scottish Office (now the Scottish Executive)

(Goddard and Higgins 1999a, 1999b). These surveys are carried out at school, where sampled pupils are gathered together in a classroom where they fill in a self-completion questionnaire under the supervision of an interviewer, but with no teacher present. They are asked general questions about drinking, and more detailed information is asked about what they drank in the previous week. On the whole, children appear to answer questions about drinking honestly, although one or two in each survey may exaggerate the amount they drink, this is usually easy to detect and they can then be excluded from the analysis.

The surveys show that the overwhelming majority of children aged 11–15 drink little or nothing, and most of the remainder drink only modest amounts. Drinking increases sharply with age – there is very little drinking among boys and girls aged 11, but by the time they are aged 15, about half will report having had an alcoholic drink in the last week. The surveys suggest that those who drink small amounts tend to do so at home under the supervision of parents. However, at the other end of the scale, there are small but significant proportions of boys and girls who drink substantial amounts: in 1996, 5% of boys and 3% of girls had drunk 15 or more units in the previous week.

Boys drink on average more than girls, but the difference is proportionately less than among young adults. Among those aged 11–15, boys drink about 1.5 times as much as girls, whereas young men aged 16–24 drink twice as much as young women of the same age.

There was considerable concern following the introduction of 'alcopops' in 1995 that these drinks, which have an alcoholic content (about 5%) similar to many lagers and ciders, would encourage children to drink. The 1996 survey found some evidence to support the suggestion that those who drank 'alcopops' may do so because the taste of alcohol is masked by the addition of fruit juice or cola, but little for the contention that they encourage children to drink who would not otherwise be doing so.

TRENDS IN ALCOHOL CONSUMPTION AMONG YOUNG TEENAGERS

Between 1990 and 1996, the government surveys have shown a marked increase in alcohol consumption among both boys and girls. There has been little change in the proportion of children aged 11–15 who drink at all, but the average amount drunk by those who do drink, and the frequency with which they drink, has risen. In 1990, 22% of those aged 11–15 had drunk alcohol in the previous week, but in 1996, 27% had done so. The average number of units drunk per pupil per week in 1990 was 0.8: in 1996, this had more than doubled to 1.8 units (Goddard 1997a, 1997b).

Table 4.2:* Percentage who drank last week, by sex and age, England 1996

All pupils aged 11–15

Age	Boys	Girls	Total	1996 base (=100%)		
				Boys	Girls	Total
11 years	7	6	7	269	266	535
12 years	12	9	11	296	272	568
13 years	27	22	24	275	277	552
14 years	37	35	36	297	285	582
15 years	50	55	53	295	291	586
Total	27	26	27	1432	1391	2823

Source: Goddard (1997a).

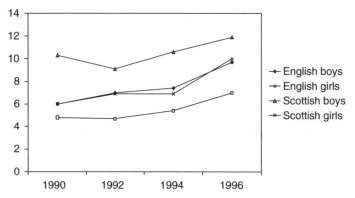

Figure 4.1:* Mean past week's alcohol consumption amongst young teenagers who had drunk in the previous week, England and Scotland, 1990–96

Table 4.3:* Usual drinking frequency, by sex, England 1996

All pupils aged 11-15

Usual drinking frequency	Boys %	Girls %	Total %
Almost every day	2 ⎤	2 ⎤	1 ⎤
About twice a week	8 ⎬ 21	7 ⎬ 18	7 ⎬ 20
About once a week	12 ⎦	10 ⎦	11 ⎦
About once a fortnight	8	10	9
About once a month	8	9	9
Only a few times a year	22	21	21
Never drinks now	4	3	4
Never had a drink	37	39	38
Base (= 100%)	1431	1387	2818

*Source for Table 4.2, figure 4.1 and Table 4.3 is Goddard (1997a).

Table 4.4: Trends in drinking among young teenagers, England 1990–96

All pupils aged 11–15

	1990	1992	1994	1996
Percentage of pupils who drank last week				
Boys	22	24	26	27
Girls	20	17	22	26
Total	21	21	24	27
Average units drunk last week per pupil				
Boys	0.9	1.4	1.5	2.1
Girls	0.7	0.7	1.0	1.5
Total	0.8	1.1	1.3	1.8

Source: Thomas et al. (1998).

It should be noted, however, that trends in consumption among a narrow age group such as this are likely to be indicative more of changing fashions among successive cohorts of children than of longer-term trends in consumption.

Comparison of these substantial data sets between 1990 and 1996 showed that mean previous week's consumption levels had risen amongst most sub-groups. The mean alcohol consumption of girls who had consumed alcohol in the previous week rose by 12.5%, from 4.8 to 5.4 units. The corresponding rise amongst boys was greater, 23.3%, increasing from 6.0 to 7.4 units. (A unit is equivalent to 7.9 g / 1 cl pure alcohol. This is *roughly* equivalent to half a pint of normal strength beer, stout, lager or cider, a single bar measure of spirits or a single glass of wine.) An additional survey carried out in 1996 supplies some further detail to this picture (Goddard 1997a, 1997b). Over the period 1988–96 the proportion of girls in England who had drunk in the previous week rose from 17% to 26%. In contrast, the corresponding proportion of boys rose relatively little, from 24% to 27% (Goddard 1997a). Scottish results were comparable, since the rise in the proportion of girls who had drunk in the previous week over the period 1990–96 was greater than the rise in the proportion of boys, from 12% to 21% and from 16% to 24%, respectively (Goddard 1997b). Amongst Scottish young people the mean alcohol consumption of those who had consumed alcohol in the previous week rose by 66.6% amongst girls and by only 15.5% amongst boys aged 12–15. Amongst young people in England the mean previous week's alcohol consumption amongst girls rose by 45.8%, and that of boys rose by 61.7%.

Surveys generally confirm that teenage girls drink less than teenage boys. This conclusion has been supported by UK-wide surveys of young people's drinking and by recent studies in other European countries (Miller and Plant 1996, Hibell et al. 1997, M.L. Plant 1997, Currie et al. 2000, Miller and Plant 2000a, 2000b).

TEENAGERS WHO ARE HEAVIER DRINKERS

The UK findings from the ESPAD study showed that teenagers whose house-holds were headed by a single parent, who had few constructive hobbies, who had psychiatric symptoms and aggressive, outgoing lifestyles, were those most likely to drink heavily, to use tobacco and illicit drugs and to be truant from school (Miller 1997, Miller and Plant 1999a). There were few differences between alcohol, tobacco and illicit drug use in rural, suburban and urban areas (Miller and Plant 1999b). These results are consistent with a substantial body of evidence. This indicates that young people who drink heavily are particularly likely to use tobacco and illicit drugs and to engage in a variety of potentially risky or health-damaging behaviours (Jessor and Jessor 1977, Plant and Plant 1992).

The spreading HIV/AIDS pandemic has led to considerable concern about the possiblity that alcohol consumption, through its 'disinhibiting' effects, may lead to unprotected sex (Room and Collins 1983). A number of studies have examined this topic. Several authors concluded that young heavier drinkers were at risk, or believed themselves to be at risk, in relation to unprotected sex (Plant and Plant 1992, Stall and Leigh 1994). In fact evidence on this topic now suggests that the alcohol–sex connection is not so clear-cut as had previously been supposed. It seems that people who are heavier drinkers are more risk-inclined. Even so, it has not been convinc-ingly demonstrated that an individual's chances of engaging in high-risk sex do increase following alcohol consumption. Some people simply take more risks than others, whether they are drinking at the time or not (World Health Organization 1994b).

ADULT DRINKING

Warner (1992) has reported that women in medieval England did drink alcohol, but that they seldom did so in public 'taverns'. The Industrial Revolution did little to enhance the image of the public bar in Britain. The latter was widely regarded as being a disreputable place, often associated with prostitution (Williams and Brake 1982, Plant 1992). During the twen-tieth century, there was a great improvement in the nature and range of facilities available in most public bars in Britain. Licensing arrangements were liberalised and encouragement was given to the provision of meals, entertainment and children's rooms. Even so, women were excluded from some public bars in Britain until the 1970s.

As noted above, alcohol consumption and drinking patterns in Britain have been measured since the 1970s by a variety of government surveys of the general adult population. The first ad hoc surveys were carried out in England and Scotland (Dight 1976, Wilson 1980, Goddard 1986). These studies were conducted mainly to collect information not available up to then about people's drinking, and also, in Scotland, so that the effects of changes in licensing legislation in 1976 could be assessed. Two further ad hoc surveys were carried out in the late 1980s (Goddard 1991) to assess the effects of the 1988 Licensing Act in England. In 1978, the collection of information about drinking was put on a regular footing by the inclusion of a set of questions on the General Household Survey (GHS) (for example, Thomas et al. 1998). These have subsequently been repeated biennially, with some modifications from time to time in the information collected. More recently, questions about drinking have also been included each year on the Health Survey for England (HSE) (Prescott-Clarke and Primatesta 1998), which began in 1991. There have been no major government ad hoc surveys of drinking in the 1990s, although specific topics have been covered occasionally as part of the Office for National Statistics' Omnibus Survey (for example, Goddard 1999).

Information obtained regularly from the GHS and the HSE has the advantage that trends over time can easily be monitored. The disadvantage, however, is that because neither survey is dedicated solely to the collection of information about drinking, the extent of questioning is limited. Both surveys concentrate almost entirely on obtaining information about alcohol consumption, and are not able to explore more widely the circumstances in which people drink, as has been done by the ad hoc surveys.

Estimating Alcohol Consumption

If a measure of alcohol consumption is required which characterises the respondent's drinking in a general way, account has to be taken of the fact that an individual's consumption may vary both from day to day during the week, and from one week to the next. Surveys typically use one of two alternative methods of estimating alcohol consumption: the retrospective seven-day drinking diary, and the quantity–frequency method.

With the retrospective seven-day drinking diary, drinkers are asked about their alcohol consumption over a seven-day period beginning with 'yesterday' (the day before the interview), and back day by day through the preceding week, and are encouraged to remember each occasion on which they had a drink. They are asked detailed information about each of those occasions – typically, the type of drink and how much they had to drink, when the occasion started and finished, and where they were. Thus this approach gives not only information about the previous week's alcohol consumption, but also detailed information about drinking occasions and patterns within that week. The disadvantage is that it is time-consuming, and can only generally be used on a survey dedicated to drinking. Where drinking is just one of a number of topics covered, the quantity–frequency approach, which is quicker to administer, is generally used.

This method provides a measure that averages out behaviour over a period of time, to enable people to be classified into broad groups according to how much they drink. The quantity–frequency measure has been used by the General Household Survey since 1978 and, more recently, by the Health Survey for England and other surveys of which drinking is a component. Respondents are asked how often, during the previous year, they have drunk each of a number of different types of drink, and how much they have usually drunk on any one day.

Both of the above measures give estimates of weekly consumption. The first, the seven-day drinking diary method, may not be typical for a partic- ular respondent, but taking the sample as a whole (or sub-groups), it should give a representative picture of what people drink in an average week. The quantity–frequency method also gives a measure of average weekly consumption, but here the averaging is done at the respondent level. Although individual respondents are not always classified the same on the two measures, they give almost identical proportions of the population drinking different amounts.

Accuracy of Survey Estimates of Alcohol Consumption

As noted above, survey findings may be subject to bias and distortion. Surveys which estimate alcohol consumption are invariably criticised on the grounds that they are bound to severely underestimate it, to the point that doing the survey may not be worth while.

There are a number reasons for this, and although none of them individ- ually are probably large enough to be problematic, they all tend to underestimation rather than the reverse, and in combination the effect is considerable:

- Survey samples of people living in private households by definition exclude those living in institutions and people who have no fixed address – groups which probably contain a higher than average proportion of heavy drinkers.
- Heavy drinkers may be more likely than others to be difficult to contact. For example, young single people are generally under-represented in

survey samples, and their alcohol consumption is substantially higher than average.

- People tend to understate the amount they drink. Deliberate under-reporting is probably quite rare, but unintentional under-reporting is very common indeed. On one level, there is probably a subconscious tendency to underestimate rather than overestimate amounts drunk, and on another, people sometimes genuinely forget occasions on which they had a drink. They also forget how much they had to drink, particularly at social occasions, and if they have had a lot to drink.

- Estimating amounts drunk is particularly difficult for people drinking at home, where drinks are not dispensed in standard quantities, and are probably usually larger than those bought on licensed premises.

- It is also difficult to estimate the proportion of people who do not drink alcohol at all, because surveys differ in the way they try to establish this. Many surveys overestimate the proportion of non-drinkers, because some of those who say in answer to an initial question that they don't drink, either drink very occasionally, or do not realise that some drinks are, in fact, alcoholic. In order to identify them as drinkers, albeit infrequent ones, it is therefore necessary to ask supplementary questions of those who initially say they do not drink. In consequence, surveys that do not do so overestimate the proportion of non-drinkers. The GHS, which asks a supplementary question about very occasional drinking, has over recent years typically identified about twice as many women as men as non-drinkers, and has shown the highest rates of non-drinking among older people. In 1996, 7% of men and 13% of women aged 16 and over said they never drank alcohol, even occasionally: among those aged 65 and over, the proportions were 12% of men and 24% of women.

The Brewers and Licensed Retailers Association (1997) have used Customs and Excise figures to estimate that adults in the UK drank on average 9.4 litres of pure alcohol in 1996. Since one UK 'unit' of alcohol contains approximately 10 ml of pure alcohol, this is 940 units in a year, an average of 18.1 units a week. Surveys typically estimate average weekly consumption as 10–11 units a week, suggesting that they pick up about 60% of alcohol consumed.

Even if this estimate of coverage is roughly correct, the shortfall is not entirely due to under-representation of heavy drinkers and under-reporting of consumption by those who are interviewed. For a variety of reasons, estimates are not defined in such a way that they would give a good estimate of annual consumption – for example, surveys are not likely to reflect alcohol consumption at peak periods such as Christmas, New Year, and when people are on holiday.

DRINKING PATTERNS

On average, men drink much more than women do: as shown above, they are less likely to be abstainers, and those who drink, drink more. In 1996, the GHS showed men as drinking on average 16.0 units a week, compared with 6.3 for women. This is shown in Table 4.5.

Table 4.5: Average weekly alcohol consumption, by sex and household socio-economic group, 1996

Age	Men	Women	Total	Bases (= 100%) Men	Women	Total
Professional	14.6	7.9	11.3	447	432	879
Employers and managers	17.1	7.5	12.3	1650	1672	3322
Intermediate non-manual	17.1	7.2	11.5	700	916	1616
Junior non-manual	14.8	5.7	8.6	475	1014	1489
Skilled manual and own account non-professional	16.0	5.9	11.0	2411	2340	4751
Semi-skilled manual and personal service	15.5	5.3	9.6	985	1330	2315
Unskilled manual	13.4	3.5	7.6	299	434	733
All aged 16 and over	16.0	6.3	10.7	7151	8491	15642

Source: Thomas et al. (1998).

The peak age group for drinking for men is the early twenties, and a year or two earlier for women (albeit at a much lower level than for men): after that, alcohol consumption declines with increasing age. Among those aged 16–24, average weekly alcohol consumption was 20.3 units for men and 9.5 units for women in 1996. Among those aged 65 and over, the averages were 11.0 units for men, and 3.5 for women (Table 4.6).

Table 4.6: Average weekly alcohol consumption, by sex and age, 1996

Age	Men	Women	Total	Bases (= 100%) Men	Women	Total
16–24	20.3	9.5	14.7	881	969	1850
25–44	17.6	7.2	11.9	2628	3182	5810
45–64	15.6	5.9	10.5	2215	2509	4724
65 and over	11.0	3.5	6.8	1445	1836	3281
All aged 16 and over	16.0	6.3	10.7	7169	8496	15665

Source: Thomas et al. (1998).

It is likely that age in itself is not an important determinant of how much people drink, but that it is associated with other factors that are, particularly their living circumstances. In the late teens, consumption is still rising. There are probably several reasons for this. First, those under the age of 18 are below the legal age for buying alcohol: although this does not stop them drinking, it reduces the opportunities for doing so. Furthermore, most of this age group are still living at home with their parents, and some are at school and will have limited money available to spend on drink. Alcohol consumption among men rises in the late teens and early twenties with increasing freedom and disposable income, and then falls when they marry or set up home with a partner. There is a more pronounced fall when they have children, presumably because they have more responsibilities and other calls on their time and money. The pattern is similar for women, but, as noted above, women's consumption peaks a few years earlier. This is probably because, on the whole, women marry or form partnerships with men a few years older than them, so for women, the life events of marriage and childbirth occur earlier (Table 4.7).

Table 4.7: Percentage of adults who drink almost every day, by sex and age

				Bases (= 100%)		
Age	Men	Women	Total	Men	Women	Total
16–24	5	1	3	335	343	678
25–44	10	7	8	864	1113	1977
45–64	15	11	13	862	887	1749
65 and over	23	14	18	489	617	1106
All aged 16 and over	14	9	11	2550	2959	5509

Source: Goddard (1999).

As the children grow up, the consumption of their parents rises slightly, although there is an underlying tendency for consumption to fall as people get older, whatever their marital condition. The groups whose consumption is relatively high compared with others of similar age tend to be those whose circumstances differ from the general pattern – the divorced and separated of both sexes, and widowed men.

As alcohol consumption changes in relation to age and the circumstances associated with different ages, so do other aspects of drinking behaviour. Young people, for example, tend to drink only on one or two days in the week – typically Friday and Saturday – but drink a lot when they do drink.

Older people, however, drink more often, but drink much more modest amounts. Thus, among those aged 65 and over, 23% of men and 14% of women drink every day, compared with only 5% of young men and 1% of young women aged 16–24. The topic of older people is elaborated on later in this chapter.

Regional Variations in Alcohol Consumption

Contrary to popular belief, alcohol consumption is not significantly higher in Scotland than in England – indeed, for women, it is considerably lower. In 1996, men drank an average of 16.1 units in England and 16.2 units in Scotland: for women, the figures were 6.3 units in England and 5.5 in Scotland. Neither is it the case that drinking behaviour is more polarised in Scotland than in England ('polarised' means that there are more heavy drinkers, but also more abstainers). In fact, patterns of consumption in the two countries are similar. Within England, the GHS has tended to show higher consumption in the north than in the south, and that was so for men in 1996, but there was little regional variation among women. This is elaborated on in Table 4.8.

Table 4.8: Average weekly alcohol consumption, by sex and region, 1996

Region	Men	Women	Total	Bases (= 100%) Men	Women	Total
North	19.1	5.9	11.8	432	532	964
Yorkshire and Humberside	16.8	6.6	11.2	606	754	1360
North West	18.4	7.9	12.7	804	933	1737
East Midlands	15.3	5.8	10.2	550	630	1180
West Midlands	16.2	5.9	10.6	664	790	1454
East Anglia	13.7	5.5	9.4	305	330	635
Greater London	14.5	5.6	9.8	770	884	1654
Outer Metropolitan Area	15.4	6.4	10.6	702	811	1513
Outer South East	15.8	6.7	10.9	666	778	1444
South West	15.0	6.1	10.1	646	785	1431
England	16.1	6.3	10.8	6145	7227	13372
Wales	15.0	6.8	10.4	367	476	843
Scotland	16.2	5.5	10.3	657	793	1450
Great Britain	16.0	6.3	10.7	7169	8496	15665

Source: Thomas et al. (1998).

Drinking, Social and Economic Characteristics

The association between drinking and social class or socio-economic group is not as clear as for many other health-related behaviours, such as smoking, where prevalence is much higher among unskilled manual workers than among professionals, and there is a clear gradient across the social classes. In comparison, social class differences in relation to alcohol consumption tend to be in the reverse direction, particularly for women. In 1996, consumption was lowest for both men and women in unskilled manual households. Among men, average weekly units ranged from 13.4 among those in unskilled manual households to 17.1 units for employers and managers and those in intermediate non-manual households. The variation was much greater among women, and the association with socio-economic group considerably clearer: consumption was highest, at 7.9 units, among women in professional households, more than twice as much as that in unskilled manual households, where the average was just 3.5 units.

Associations with other indicators of socio-economic circumstances, such as earnings and economic activity status, tend to be weaker, or largely explained by the association of these characteristics with the age of the respondent.

Trends in Alcohol Consumption

According to the Brewers and Licensed Retailers Association (1997), overall UK per capita alcohol consumption has fluctuated over the last two decades, but has not shown any pronounced trend in one direction. This is illustrated in Figure 4.2 and is further elaborated by Thurman in section A of Chapter 5.

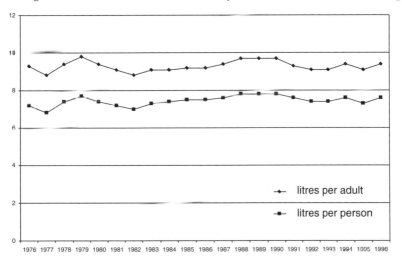

Figure 4.2: UK consumption of alcohol, 1976–96

Survey findings tend to confirm this, although they suggest that patterns of consumption may have changed over that period. The GHS provides the longest series of survey results (having included questions on drinking since 1978), but changes in methodology mean that data have been collected on the current basis only since 1984. Consumption among men has remained fairly stable (although there is some suggestion of an increase among men aged 65 and over). Among women, however, there has been a steady rise over the period. The GHS shows, for example, that in 1986, 10% of women were drinking more than 14 units a week: 10 years later, in 1996, the proportion had risen to 14%. Since women drink much less than men, the effect of the increase in women's consumption on consumption overall has been fairly small. The increase in women's consumption has occurred in all age groups, although it has been most marked among women under the age of 25. This is shown in Table 4.9.

Table 4.9: Trends in alcohol consumption, by sex and age, 1984–96

	1984	1986	1988	1990	1992	1994	1996
Percentage drinking more than 21 units a week							
Men							
18–24	35	39	35	36	38	35	41
25–44	31	32	34	33	31	31	30
45–64	21	23	24	25	25	27	26
65 and over	12	13	13	14	15	17	18
All aged 18 and over	25	27	27	28	27	27	27
Percentage drinking more than 14 units a week							
Women							
18–24	15	19	17	18	18	20	24
25–44	11	13	14	13	14	15	16
45–64	8	8	9	10	11	12	13
65 and over	3	3	4	5	5	7	7
All aged 18 and over	9	10	10	11	11	13	14

Source: Thomas et al. (1998).

Several UK studies conducted in the 1970s indicated that women were approximately twice as likely as men to be abstainers and that women were also much less likely than men to be regular drinkers (Scotland – Dight 1976, Northern Ireland – Harbison and Haire 1980, England and Wales – Wilson 1980).

Information from the GHS shows clearly that the proportion of British women who consumed larger quantities has changed more than that of men over the period 1984–96. First, the proportion of women drinking over 35 units in the past week doubled, from 1% to 2%. The proportion of men consuming over 50 units in the past week remained unchanged at 6%. (Note: these levels have been described as 'high risk' drinking by the Royal College of Psychiatrists (1986).) To express this type of change in a different way, Thomas et al. (1998) have noted that the proportions of those over the age of 18 whose alcohol consumption exceeded the 'sensible'/'low risk' weekly amounts of 14 units for women and 21 units for men had changed, as shown in Figure 4.3.

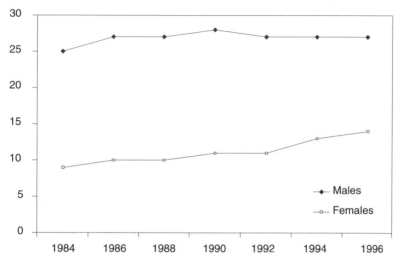

Figure 4.3: Proportions of British adults exceeding 'sensible' weekly alcohol consumption levels, 1984–96

As indicated by this figure, the proportion of males who drank at or above this level has risen only slightly, from 25% to 27%. In contrast, the corresponding proportion of women who did so has risen markedly, from 9% to 14% (Thomas et al. 1998: 186).

OLDER PEOPLE

An increased amount of research is being carried out in the United Kingdom. The General Household Surveys have asked about drinking every two years since 1978 (Bennett et al. 1996). As with all such surveys, they produce figures which under-report consumption when compared with sales and tax returns. They always include older people, and ask about alcohol along with many other areas of interest. Across these years the surveys have consistently reported women drinking less than men, and young and middle-aged people drinking more than older people.

Table 4.10 shows that older people were more likely both to have stopped drinking and to have been life-long abstainers. The number of life-long abstainers points to the possibility that the current generation of older people has always drunk less. It is not surprising that older people, who have by definition lived longer, have had time to develop a reason to stop drinking.

Table 4.10:* People who have stopped drinking and life-long abstainers

| | % Life-long abstainers | | % Stopped drinking | |
	Men	Women	Men	Women
16–24	30	12	5	6
25–44	25	25	26	22
45–64	20	25	31	31
65+	25	39	37	42

Table 4.11 shows the percentages for 1984 and 1994 of those drinking above what were, at the time of the surveys, thought to be low-risk levels (14 units a week for women and 21 units a week for men). Each of the biennial surveys between these years shows a gradual step-wise increase in the drinking of older people. Over the decade there was a rise of 5% for men and 4% for women.

Table 4.11*: Drinking above low-risk levels, 1984 and 1994

| | % Men over 21 units a week | | % Women over 14 units a week | |
Age	1984	1994	1984	1994
18–24	35	35	15	20
25–44	31	30	11	15
45–64	21	27	8	12
65+	12	17	3	7
All Ages	25	27	9	13

Table 4.12 shows the percentages of those drinking over what has been thought of as high-risk levels (50 units a week for men and 35 units a week for women). Here again there has been an increase in the percentage of older people drinking at this level.

Table 4.12:* Drinking above high-risk levels, 1984 and 1994

| | % Men over 50 units a week | | % Women over 35 units a week | |
	1984	1994	1984	1994
18–24	11	11	3	4
25–44	8	7	2	2
45–64	5	6	1	2
65+	2	3	0	1
All Ages	6	6	1	2

*Source for Tables 4.10, 4.11 and 4.12 is Bennett et al. (1996).

Stall (1987) suggested six possible explanations for older people drinking less: morbidity, mortality, biology, cohort effects, excessive drinking as a self-limiting disease, and under-measurement. The first three, simply put, mean that as people get older they either develop illnesses, or even alcohol problems that make drinking less attractive; heavy drinkers die early, removing them from the figures; or biological ageing makes the effects of alcohol less rewarding. All of these are certainly evident to some degree. The idea of cohort effects is that each generation retains a specific pattern of drinking from its early adult life into old age. Those who learnt to drink at times of low consumption are likely to continue this as times change. This has recently been supported by longitudinal study (Levenson and Spiro 1996). This suggests that we can look forward to future generations of older people drinking more. That alcohol problems may be self-limiting is a contentious idea. At least two-thirds of older people who have alcohol problems have long-standing alcohol problems, and a proportion develop alcohol problems late in life (Atkinson 1994). In longitudinal studies many alcohol-dependent people get worse or die (Vaillant and Milofsky 1982). Measuring alcohol consumption amongst older people certainly seems to be fraught with problems (Graham 1986). However, this is true for all age groups. There is no evidence to support the contention that there is a dispro-portionately large and hidden problem amongst older people

Older people generally do not see themselves as being at risk of alcohol-related problems. Focus groups conducted for the Health Education Authority (Baton and Atherton 1995) found that older people perceived alcohol as enjoyable, medicinal and a relaxant; felt they knew how much they could drink, and saw people either as being alcoholics or as not having any problem. Unsurprisingly, given these attitudes, there was found to be resistance amongst older people to education about alcohol and its effects.

Alcohol is a drug: a vasodilator and central nervous system depressant. In common with many drugs used in medicine, the way the body responds to it changes as people age. A lot of research has been conducted to try and determine at what level of drinking risks to health are lowest. The guidance such research gives us is based on assessments of relative risks based on large representative samples. It should be recognised that an individual's response to alcohol is complex. There is no absolutely 'safe' level of drinking as there is no certainty of damage at a particular level of drinking, only a higher or lower probability. Age is an important factor that has an influence on how an individual reacts to alcohol. A full stomach will slow the absorption of alcohol. Foods high in carbohydrates are particularly good at this. This appears to be particularly important for older people. In a fasted state they will experience more subjective and objective intoxication, and take longer to recover than younger people (Beresford and Lucey 1995). Drinking history will influence the presentation of the effects of alcohol. Those that drink heavily for a prolonged period develop tolerance. Their behaviour appears to be less affected by what they drink. It is not that they are immune to the effects of alcohol. Older people appear to have a reduced capacity to develop a tolerance to alcohol (Brower et al. 1994). Health is an important consideration for many older people. In Britain older people carry the greatest burden of both acute and chronic ill health (Bennet et al. 1996). Many of the common disorders of old age can be affected by anything more than moderate amounts of alcohol; for example, hypertension, diabetes, digestive tract problems, Parkinson's disease, dementia (Gomberg 1982). The metabolism of alcohol by the liver does not decline with age (Vestal et al. 1977). However, illness or disease that reduces the functioning of the liver or the gastrointestinal tract will leave the body open to the full toxicity of alcohol. As we get older, lean tissue turns to fat, particularly for men (Tupler et al. 1995). Experiments comparing metabolism and intoxication in young and elderly, men and women revealed that for weight-standardised doses of alcohol, older subjects experienced more subjective and objective intoxication and subsequently took longer to recover. The implication for older drinkers is that they will experience problems at a lower level of consumption than young and middle-aged people (Beresford and Lucey 1995).

In summary, older people, well and ill, are likely to be more greatly affected by alcohol. Slowly, more research is being done to establish the implications for the health of older people. Meanwhile, age differences need to be considered in appreciating studies conducted with young or middle-aged people.

In conclusion, it is evident that different groups of people in different social positions and in different places exhibit considerable variety in relation to their use or non-use of alcohol. It is emphasised that pattern of drinking is a major factor in influencing the consequences of alcohol consumption (Grant and Litvak 1998). This issue is discussed further in Chapter 6.

5
Economic Aspects

A: Alcoholic Drinks: Demand and Supply*

Christopher Thurman

INTRODUCTION

So many articles on the economics of the beverage alcohol industry commence with the structure of the industry set up to meet the demands of the consumer. However, this author has always thought that this is a bit like putting the cart before the horse. If people did not want to drink the different types of alcoholic beverages, there would be no industrial structure to supply those requirements. Nor would there be any agricultural suppliers either – whether it is producing barley for conversion to malt for beer and whisky, or the myriad varieties of grape used in wine. Consequently, this chapter commences with some thoughts on the consumption of these drinks before moving on to considering the industrial structures.

MEASURING CONSUMPTION: THE CONCEPT OF PER CAPITA CONSUMPTION

A Crude Measure

As noted in Chapter 4, per capita alcohol consumption is an important variable, often used to compare alcohol consumption between countries and within countries over a period of time. This concept is used in several figures within this chapter, and consequently it is appropriate to consider the nature of its limitations. It is a very crude measure, and has sometimes been used uncritically in an alcohol policy context.

Quite simply, it can give a quite different picture from what is happening in reality. Overlooking the logic of adding together the volumes consumed of very different drinks, the main problems concern population trends and

---

Author's note – all figures relate to the UK unless stated otherwise. A list of the abbreviations used is given at the end of this part of the 'Economic Aspects' chapter).

changes in population structure, as well as changes in the number of drinkers. While the reality of long-term population change is obvious, short-term changes can also undermine the precision of the measure.

A Typical Per Capita Graph

Figure 5.1 shows UK consumption for the main types of drinks related to *total* population over the twentieth century. It is a classic example of a per capita graph.

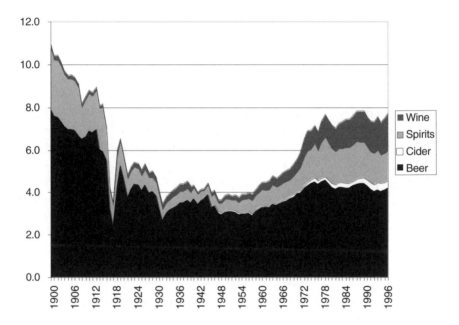

Figure 5.1: Alcohol consumption in the UK, 1900–97

Source: Brewers and Licensed Retailers Association (BLRA).

Changes in Population Structure: Long Term

The drawback of the 'classic' graph is that over a period of time there has been a substantial change in the age structure of the UK population.

Figure 5.2 analyses the UK population over a 90-year period into four age categories. There has been very little change in the number of under-15s and 15–30-year-olds but there have been considerable increases in the numbers above the age of 30. The signs of greater longevity are quite apparent.

In 1901, 33% of the population was below the age of 15, but by 1991 the proportion was 19%. Conversely, the over-65s accounted for only 5% of the population in 1901, rising to 16% by 1991.

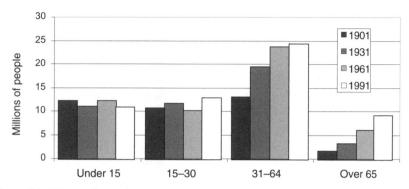

Figure 5.2: UK population by age, 1901, 1931, 1961, 1991

Source: Office for National Statistics (ONS). The data are taken from the UK national population censuses that are carried out every ten years.

The relative decline in importance of the youngest age group has a key implication for the interpretation of consumption trends. In Table 5.1 the 1901 and 1991 figures are taken from the UK Population Census and are divided into the total volume of alcohol consumed. Simply altering the population base to 15-and-over means (not surprisingly) an increase in the consumption-per-head figure, but it is the trend difference which is crucial. The decline in consumption over this 90-year period appears to be 27% when using the total population base. But excluding the under-15s (which is logical in terms of alcohol consumption) means that a more realistic appraisal of the decline in alcohol consumption over this 90-year period is 39%. The key figures are given in Table 5.1.

Table 5.1: UK alcohol consumption, 1901–1991

	Lpa* consumption per head	% of population under 15	Lpa consumption per head of population aged 15+
1901	10.4	32.5	15.4
1991	7.6	19.1	9.4
% decline	27	na	39

Sources: ONS and BLRA.
Note: *Lpa: litres of pure (100%) alcohol.

Figure 5.3 shows this effect graphically.

The conclusion is that using total population as a proxy for adult population can give misleading trends, interpretations and conclusions.

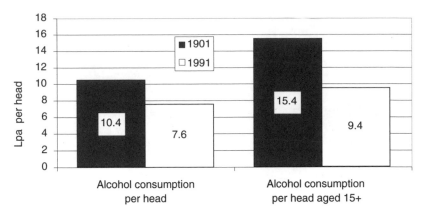

Figure 5.3: The effect of changing population base, 1901 and 1991

Sources: BLRA and ONS.

Changes in Population Structure: Short Term

Short-term population changes are also important, as the following example dealing specifically with the oldest group of people shows. Evidence collected by Public Attitude Surveys (PAS), an independent market research company, shows that the proportion of the population drinking alcohol has grown from 63% in 1988/89 to 67% in 1996/97 (the oldest PAS age group is 50+). Information derived from the General Household Survey (GHS), a survey undertaken by the ONS, shows weekly consumption by the 65-and-over age group to have grown from 5.6 units in 1992 to 6.8 units in 1996. A unit of alcohol is defined in the UK to be half a pint of UK-strength beer, or a small glass of table wine, or a 25 cl glass of spirits. The upward trend in consumption amongst this group is reasonable, but even at this level it is still well below the overall average (see Chapter 4, and also Thomas et al. 1998). Given the forecasts of even greater longevity and knowing that, in general, people of this age have greater prosperity than ever before, then it could be anticipated that these trends might continue. The talk of a 'grey market' (a reference to the consumers' supposed hair colour) is based on sound market information.

The impact upon per capita consumption is obvious and extremely relevant to the interpretation of consumption trends.. The greater volume consumed by this group will clearly increase per capita consumption even if the consumption levels of all other groups remain unchanged: if UK per capita was unchanged overall, then the increased consumption by this group implies a reduction in the consumption of some other group or groups.

At this stage it is useful to look at the recent history of alcohol consumption divided by the 15-and-over population from just before the peak year of 1979 (Table 5.2).

Table 5.2: Alcohol consumption per capita among those aged 15 and over, 1978–97*

Year	Litres of alcohol per head	Year	Litres of alcohol per head
1978	9.4	1988	9.7
1979	9.8	1989	9.7
1980	9.4	1990	9.7
1981	9.1	1991	9.3
1982	8.8	1992	9.1
1983	9.1	1993	9.1
1984	9.1	1994	9.4
1985	9.2	1995	9.1
1986	9.2	1996	9.4
1987	9.4	1997	9.6

Source: BLRA.
Note: *Excludes cross-border shopping and smuggling.

The growth of the 'grey market' leads to the inevitable conclusion that consumption in the other age groups has declined.

Changes in numbers of drinkers

The true denominator in per capita calculations should be the number of drinkers, and this is not easily available over any long time series. A rise in per capita consumption is generally taken to imply that there has been an increase in the level of drinking by the population generally, while a fall in per capita volumes is taken to imply that people have been drinking less. This is not necessarily true, and the following figures show that it is possible for *consumption to fall when the number of regular drinkers increases*. The converse is that per capita consumption could rise when the average volume consumed per person is falling (for example, the effect of the 'grey market'). As noted elsewhere in this book, the pattern of alcohol consumption amongst specific groups of people is an important consideration. Table 5.3 shows how beverage preferences have changed in the UK since 1988. Table 5.4 shows that there have been some changes in the frequency with which people in the UK have consumed certain types of beverage.

Table 5.3: Proportion of people aged 18+ consuming alcohol at least once a month, 1988, 1989, 1996, 1997

	1988 (%)	1989 (%)	1996 (%)	1997 (%)
Any drink	74.1	73.0	76.4	76.8
Beer	49.9	48.9	51.6	51.5
Spirits	35.9	34.9	37.6	38.1
Wine	41.5	40.5	48.5	48.8

Source: PAS.

PAS interview over 20,000 people per year regarding their drinking patterns and these interviews are carried out continuously throughout the year. Without doubt this information provides the most comprehensive insight into the UK drinks market. The investigators ascertain what proportions of the population consume each type of alcoholic drink on at least a monthly basis, from which they can deduce what proportion of the population drink any alcoholic drink at least once a month.

The proportions in Table 5.3 can be converted into numbers of people by using ONS population statistics (Table 5.4).

Table 5.4: Numbers of people drinking at least once a month, 1988, 1989, 1996, 1997

	1988 (Millions)	1989 (Millions)	1996 (Millions)	1997 (Millions)
Total 15-and-over base	46.2	46.5	47.4	47.6
Any drink	34.2	34.0	36.3	36.6
Beer	23.1	22.8	24.9	24.5
Spirits	16.6	16.2	17.8	18.2
Wine	19.2	18.8	23.0	23.2

Sources: ONS and PAS.

The figures upon which the information in Tables 5.3 and 5.4 are based are inclined to 'wobble' from year to year. In order to add a degree of stability/consistency, 1988 has been averaged with 1989 and 1996 with 1997. Table 5.5 compares changes in numbers of regular drinkers against changes in volume.

Table 5.5: Comparison between numbers of regular drinkers and per capita consumption, 1996/97 compared to 1988/89

	Number of regular drinkers	Consumption per head of total population
All alcohol	+6.8%	–2.6%
Beer	+7.0%	–9.4%
Spirits	+9.6%	–20.5%
Wine	+21.7%	+35.9%

Sources: The change in per capita volumes is derived from the data published in table D2 of the 1999 edition of the BLRA *Statistical Handbook*.

By way of comparison it should be noted that the 15-and-over population changed by 2.5% over this period.

Table 5.5 shows that, as noted in Chapters 4 and 6, the relationship between per capita alcohol consumption and the number of regular drinkers is complex. The increase in the number of regular (monthly) drinkers of 6.8% is at complete variance with the downturn in alcohol consumption per head of –2.6%. This fact can only be explained by a fall in the mean quantity consumed by drinkers in general.

An increase in per capita consumption is generally taken to imply an increase in drinking levels within the country. However, for several different reasons this does not necessarily follow. These reasons include the following:

- changing age structure, both long term and short term, such as the relative decline in the proportion of young people in the population
- numbers of people drinking
- people at lower levels drinking more, such as the 'grey market' (another example in the UK is evidence from the PAS survey of a substantial increase in the number of wine drinkers from low-income consumers)

Per capita alcohol consumption is thus a vague and imprecise measure that is clearly confounded by many factors.

DEMAND: TASTE AND TYPES OF DRINKS

The per capita concept adds together different types of drinks on the basis of their alcohol content. However, people drink different beverages according to whether they are thirsty, having a meal, relaxing with friends, and so on. There are many permutations of drink, drinking occasion and drinking venue. The choice of drinks facing the consumer is illustrated in Figures 5.4, 5.5 and 5.6.

Figure 5.4 shows the proportions of the market taken by the different types of beer. But even this is a major simplification. The ale sector includes beers such as stout, mild, light ale and pale ale, as well as bitter. Bitters vary in colour, strength, style of conditioning and taste, as well as having distinct regional variations. Lagers vary equally.

Figure 5. 5 shows a similar analysis for the wine market.

Within each colour of still table wine there are major variations in taste, whether in terms of sweetness (contrast a Sauterne with a Chablis) or robustness (contrast a Shiraz with a Merlot, or a Burgundy with a Bordeaux). The leading types of fortified wine are sherry and port, while sparkling wine includes champagne, other sparkling wines (for example, from the Loire) and semi-sparkling wine.

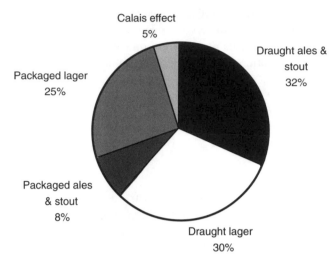

Figure 5.4: Beer sales by different types, 1997

Source: BLRA. The BLRA conducts an annual survey of members' beer sales, plus information regarding sales of imported beer – see tables 14a and 14b of the 1999 edition of the BLRA *Statistical Handbook*. In addition, the BLRA undertakes a regular survey of cross-border shopping and smuggling (details are given later in this section of Chapter 5).

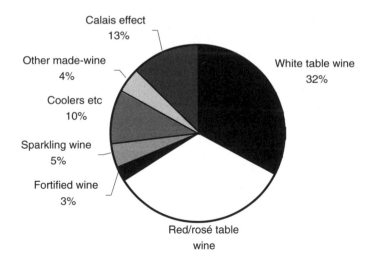

Figure 5.5: Wine sales by different types, 1997

Sources: BLRA, HM Customs and Excise (HMCE) and the Wine and Spirit Association of Great Britain (WSA). The total volume figures are given by HMCE – see table C2 of the 1999 BLRA *Statistical Handbook* – while an analysis by wine type is given in the WSA *Annual Statistical Bulletin*. The BLRA undertakes a survey of cross-border purchases of wine.

The spirits graph is another overview. Scotch whisky includes single malts as well as blends; and the taste of an island malt can be very different from one produced in the Highlands. Other spirits comprise brandy, cognac, whiskey and dark rum, while liqueurs comprise a very wide range of different drinks.

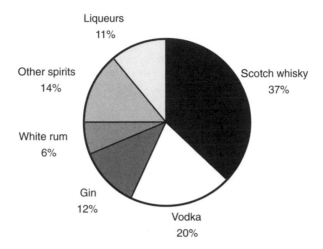

Figure 5.6: Spirit sales by different types, 1997

Sources: HMCE, Gin and Vodka Association (GVA) and WSA. HMCE publishes the total volume of spirits and the volume which is whisky; the GVA and WSA publish statistics on the mix of other spirits in their *Statistical Bulletins* and duty submissions to the Treasury.

In addition, there are drinks such as cider and perry.

With such a wide choice, it is not surprising that there have been major consumer trends. One remarkable change within the UK has been the growth of wine consumption. In 1960, this accounted for 7.8% of alcohol consumption, but by 1997 it had risen to nearly 23%. In 1960, spirits accounted for 16.9% of consumption, rising to a peak of over 24% in 1979 before falling back to 18.5% in 1997. The one drink to lose share consistently over this period has been beer, falling from almost 74% in 1960 to 54% in 1997. This change in taste is clearly demonstrated in Figure 5.7.

Such a taste change is not limited to the UK. Wine consumption has sometimes been growing in other countries where beer was the main drink, while, conversely, beer has been growing in wine-drinking countries. In the case of the UK there are many reasons put forward for this change, such as the very large increase in the numbers of people taking holidays in wine-drinking countries.

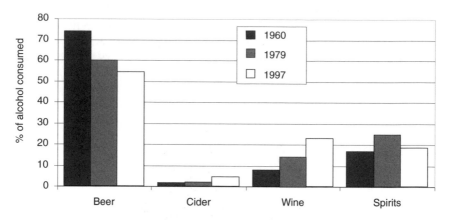

Figure 5.7: Alcohol consumption by type of drink, 1960, 1979, 1997

Notes: 1960 is the base date as this was about the first year in which all the post-war and import controls had been lifted. The purpose of these controls included priority of building materials for housing rather than the renovation of pubs, overseas sales of whisky given preference to UK sales as a means of earning foreign currency, and wine imports subject to control as a means of saving foreign currency. Britain was at the centre of the sterling area. Furthermore, Britain was no longer involved in wars overseas and national conscription had ended. 1997 is the latest available date, while 1979 is a convenient mid-point. It was also the point when beer consumption peaked, and, as shown in Figure 5.1, there has been little change in per capita alcohol consumption since then. Source: BLRA; full details are given in table D3 of its 1999 *Statistical Handbook*.

With beer, there have also been significant taste changes. In 1960, lager accounted for 1% of total consumption; in 1997 it was 58%. Conversely, mild has declined from over 40% to some 2–3%. However, such changes are not new. In the late eighteenth century the large porter breweries developed in London, but by the middle of the nineteenth century the lighter, more sparkling, Burton ales had become popular.

The taste changes over the past 40 years have occurred during periods of different economic performance, of low unemployment and high unemployment, of rapidly rising incomes and falling gross domestic product (GDP – which measures economic activity within a country).

Three conclusions emerge from the above.

- Taste changes have taken place over and above all the normal economic criteria, such as income and price.
- The fact that there are taste changes in other countries suggests some more fundamental changes in cultural attitudes.
- It is the rate of change that has speeded up, not the fact of change itself.

DEMAND: INCOME

It has sometimes been assumed that as income rises, so the consumption of alcohol rises. It seems to be an obvious statement and indeed may be true in some countries for some periods of time or for some sectors of a community. This is not, however, necessarily true. This view is argued here on the basis of international comparisons as well as the experience in individual countries, including the UK.

International Comparisons

Table 5.6 compares the position in the wealthiest and poorest alcohol-drinking countries (that is, those countries where alcohol consumption is above a minimum level).

Table 5.6: Some of the wealthiest and poorest of alcohol-drinking countries, 1997

	Wealthiest			Poorest	
Country	GDP US$ 000s PPP* (a)	Alcohol Litres per head (b)	Country	GDP US$ 000s PPP* (a)	Alcohol Litres per head (b)
USA	29.4	6.6	Rumania	4.6	9.9
Norway	26.8	4.0	Peru ***	4.4	1.8
Switzerland	25.9	9.4	Croatia	4.3	11.6
Denmark	25.5	10.1	Bulgaria	4.3	8.4
Japan	24.6	6.7	Russia	4.2	5.2
Average**	26.4	7.4	Average	4.4	7.4

Notes: *Purchasing power parity.
**Simple unweighted average.
***Wine and beer only; with spirits the figure may be nearer 4 litres.
Sources: (a) Organization for Economic Co-operation and Development (OECD)/World Bank, as published in the German *National Statistics Yearbook* 1999.
(b) BLRA, table K8 of the 1999 *Statistical Handbook*.

Before preparing Table 5.6, this author had not expected the average consumption of the two groups to be identical, although it had been expected to be close. The conclusion is that alcohol consumption is influenced by factors other than income. The next few paragraphs delve further into this initial thought.

The UK Experience

There are two ways of demonstrating changes in consumer behaviour to show that the income concept is now out of date. It was true that there were similar trends during the 1960s and 1970s in income (measured as personal disposal income – PDI) and volume, but the importance of variables changes as the economic and social environments change. This is shown in Figure 5.8.

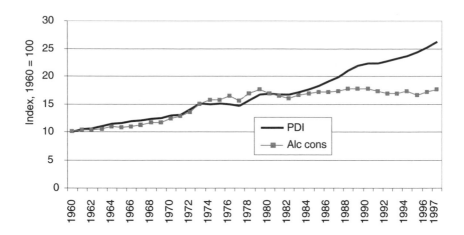

Figure 5.8: Personal disposable income* and alcohol consumption, 1960–97

Note: *Figures are in constant prices, thereby overcoming the problems of inflation.
Sources: Personal disposable income (PDI) is produced by the ONS and published in several of their books, such as the *Annual Abstract of Statistics* and the *National Incomes Blue Book*. It is also published in the BLRA *Statistical Handbook*, table E1. The figure for alcohol consumption is produced by the BLRA and given in its *Statistical Handbook*, with a full explanation of how it is calculated.

Figure 5.9 shows consumer behaviour changing over time. Expenditure on alcohol as a proportion of total consumer expenditure peaked in the late 1970s, but it has since been falling.

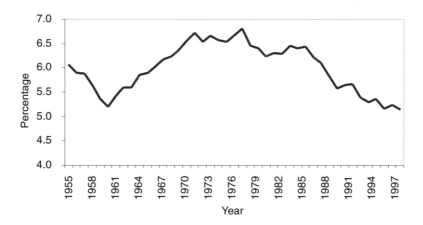

Figure 5.9: Consumer expenditure on alcohol as percentage of PDI, 1955–97

Source: The ONS produces data for both PDI (see Figure 5.8 for publications) and consumer expenditure on alcohol. The latter figure is published in a special quarterly report dealing with consumer expenditure on all items, not just alcoholic drink. All the relevant figures are published in tables E1, E2 and E3 of the BLRA *Statistical Handbook*.

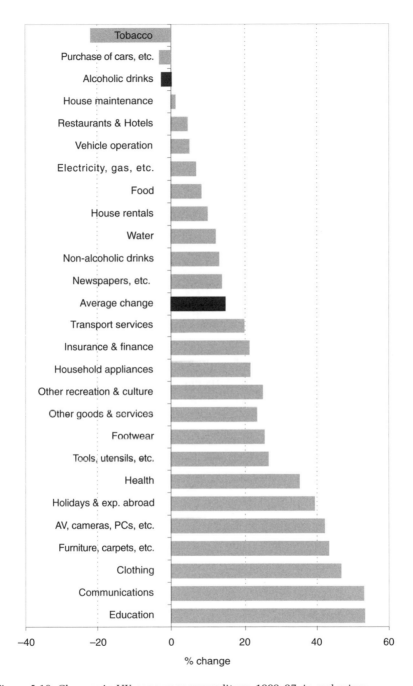

Figure 5.10: Changes in UK consumer expenditure, 1989–97, in real prices

Source: ONS data published in its *Consumer Trends*.

Figure 5.10 shows consumer expenditure between 1989 and 1997 for a wide range of goods and services. While expenditure on most items has risen in real terms, expenditure on alcohol has declined. The enormous growth in telecommunications shows the impact of fashion and new technology, while the growth of expenditure in other areas shows the ever-greater importance given to the home. All of these trends rebound upon more mature markets such as alcohol. Figure 5.10 shows that there has been a remarkable shift in consumer expenditure, from traditional items to the needs of a modern consumer, such as holidays, audio visual equipment, personal computers, furniture, clothing and telecommunications. Quite simply, alcoholic drinks have lost out to the current requirements of today's consumer. Once again there is a clear demonstration that a growth in real income need not be reflected automatically in a growth of alcohol consumption.

All three graphs give the same picture – in recent years the increase in income has not been matched by a corresponding increase in the expenditure on alcohol. Indeed, the exact opposite has happened.

The International Experience

France

In economic terms this is one of the success stories of Europe. From a gross domestic product (GDP) per head below that of the UK in 1960, it has risen to a figure which is now above the UK. And yet with the growth of income, alcohol consumption has fallen by 37% since its peak in 1963. This trend is shown in Figure 5.11.

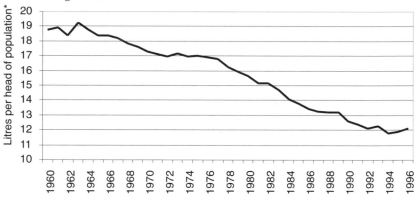

Figure 5.11: Alcohol consumption in France, 1960–96

Note: *The volume for each drink is collected and then integrated into a total alcohol figure using known average strength figures. If these are not known it is assumed that the average strength of beer is 5% and wine 12%.

Source: Canadian Brewers Association, based on industry sources within France. The figures are published by the Canadian Brewers Association in their book *Alcohol Beverage Taxation and Control Policies*, the latest edition being 1997.

Italy

Exactly the same is true in Italy. It has had a rapid rise in its GDP per head until it is now ahead of the UK. And yet its alcohol consumption has declined by 52% since 1970. This dramatic change is shown in Figure 5.12.

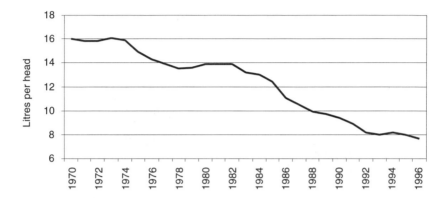

Figure 5.12: Alcohol consumption in Italy, 1970–96

Source: Canadian Brewers Association (as for figure 5.11).

Spuln

The same picture of declining alcohol consumption (–37% since its 1975 peak), set against a growing GDP per head, is evident in Spain. This is shown in Figure 5.13.

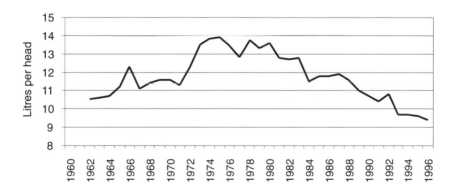

Figure 5.13: Alcohol consumption in Spain, 1960–98

Source: Canadian Brewers Association (as for Figure 5.11).

The US

The countries cited above are similar, being primarily wine consumers and originally having very high per capita volumes. The US does not fall into that category (only 13% of alcohol consumed is wine) and has the biggest economy in the world. The general pattern in the US has been similar to that of France, Italy and Spain. As GDP has grown, alcohol consumption has fallen. This is elaborated on in Figure 5.14.

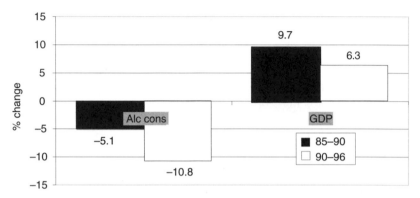

Figure 5.14: Alcohol consumption and GDP in the US, 1985–90, 1990–96

Sources: Canadian Brewers Association (as for Figure 5.11) and OECD/World Bank (as for Table 5.6).

Australia

Australia has traditionally been a beer-drinking country, but now beer accounts for only 55% of alcohol consumed. Nevertheless, the picture is still very similar – as GDP per head has increased, so alcohol consumption has declined, as shown in Figure 5.15.

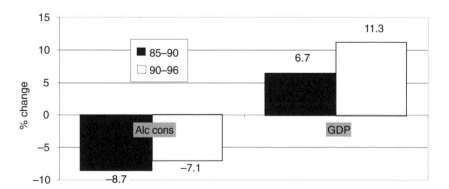

Figure 5.15: Alcohol consumption and GDP in Australia, 1985–90, 1990–96

Sources: Canadian Brewers Association (as for Figure 5.11) and World Bank/OECD (as for Table 5.6).

Some people may suspect that it is contrary to economic theory to have a situation in which an increase in income leads to a fall in demand for a specific good or service. But this is not so, as there is an effect called the 'Giffen paradox'. A simple demonstration of this theory is to consider the position of people who can eat either bread or meat. They will eat mostly bread, but as income improves they will eat more meat and less bread. The falling demand for bread reflects the Giffen paradox.

Available evidence suggests that the relationship between alcohol consumption and income is complicated, and it is a fallacy to assume that an increase in income leads automatically to an increase in consumption. Consumption is clearly influenced by many factors such as taste, fashion, and the alternative attraction of other consumer goods such as mobile phones and personal computers. Moreover, as emphasised in Chapter 4, different sub-groups of people have varied drinking patterns that reflect distinctive factors, such as their life stages.

DEMAND: 'TRADING UP' AND 'TRADING DOWN'

'Trading up' is where a consumer may be said to act irrationally – in other words he or she buys more of a dearer product and less of a cheaper product. This could often be the result of a taste or fashion change.

'Trading down' is where a consumer decides to buy the same product in a cheaper outlet; for example, from pub to club or from pub to drinking at home. This is one way in which a consumer can offset either price increases and/or income decreases and/or decide to reallocate discretionary income among competing leisure activities.

Beer

Quite simply, the overall position is one of trading down. Beer volume has been maintained at a higher rate than expenditure, and the effect of the two major recessions – in the early 1980s and early 1990s – is clearly evident, as shown in Figure 5.16.

A classic case of trading up caused by a taste change reflects the growth of lager compared to the decline of mild. This is shown in Figure 5.17. Lager (the type of beer found in most countries of the world) is the more expensive beer while mild (a traditional dark British beer) is usually the cheapest draught beer in the pubs in which it is served.

Another very relevant factor is the switch to drinking at home, as the take-home price is lower than the pub, bar or club price. This clearly reduces the average price of consumption. There has been a long-term trend to increase in drinking at home – in 1979 the off trade accounted for 12% of total beer sales, but by 1997 the proportion was 28%. The recessions no

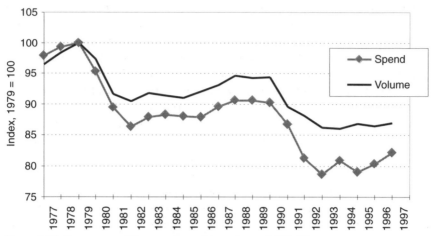

Figure 5.16: Beer: expenditure compared to volume, 1977–97

Sources: ONS for expenditure on beer and HMCE for beer volume. All figures are given in tables
A9 and E3 of the 1999 edition of the BLRA *Statistical Handbook*.

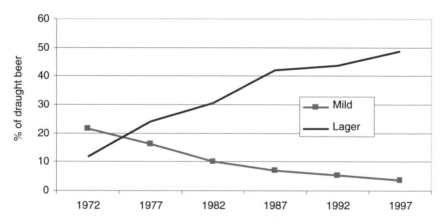

Figure 5.17: Sales of draught lager compared to draught mild, 1972–97

Source: BLRA undertakes a detailed volume survey of members obtaining details of sales by
different types of beer. The data are published in tables 14a and 14b of the 1999 edition of their
Statistical Handbook.

doubt played a part, but the sea change in attitude towards drinking and
driving is also fundamentally important.

Wine

Anyone who has been involved in the wine market over the past 30 years or
so will know intuitively that there has been a trading up in the quality of
wine. In the early days, when wine drinking was still a minority taste, the

market was being developed by the introduction of brand names, such as Blue Nun, White Tower, Hirondelle, Nicolas, Piat d'Or, and so on. However, the British consumer has become much more knowledgeable and now it is often the grape type that determines his or her choice – for example, Chardonnay. The British market is now one of the most cosmopolitan in the world. The problem is how to demonstrate this development numerically. One way is to compare the source by country of still table wines. In 1970, 47% of the volume came from France and 22% from Spain. This is shown in Figure 5.18.

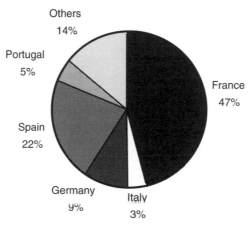

Figure 5.18: UK wine imports, 1970

Source: HMCE (which is the UK's authority dealing with excise and customs duties on imported goods).

But by 1998, the position had completely changed, as indicated in Figure 5.19.

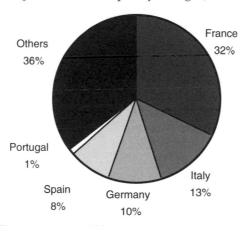

Figure 5.19: UK wine imports, 1998

Source: HMCE.

The French share has declined to 32%, Spain to 8% and 'Other' has climbed to 36%. An indication of the cosmopolitan nature of the UK wine market is that 11% of wine consumed comes from Australia and 6% from the US, while South Africa supplies a further 5%, Chile 4% and Bulgaria 3%. Most (88%) of table and sparkling wines are bottled in the country of origin.

Another example of trading up in the wine sector is the growing volume of (French) champagne. In 1997, this was the most expensive wine among imported sparkling and semi-sparkling wine, and yet the consumer chose to buy more, as shown in Table 5.7.

Table 5.7: Sparkling wine sales, 1997

	Price per litre (£)*	Share of total volume	Volume change between 1992 and 1997
Champagne	9.99	32%	+53%
Other sparkling	5.70	43%	+41%
Semi-sparkling from Italy	1.26	15%	–78%
Other semi-sparkling	1.86	10%	+126%
Overall	4.65	100%	–20%

Source: HMCE.
Note: *Prices include c.i.f. (cost, insurance, freight) only; that is, before duty, VAT and margins added by UK traders.

Spirits

Figure 5.20 shows that expenditure on spirits has moved more or less in parallel to volume. The only period of trading down evident from the graph is in the recession of the early 1980s.

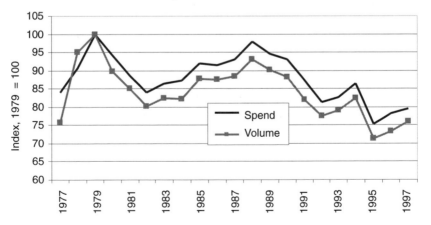

Figure 5.20: Spirits: expenditure compared to volume, 1977–97

Sources: HMCE and ONS produce the series on consumer expenditure; data are published in the 1999 edition of BLRA's *Statistical Handbook*, tables C3 and E3.

In some ways, this is a part of the income section, but it is more complex than that as it also reflects changing tastes and consumer behaviour. It also demonstrates that the consumer will act in a complex manner by sometimes clearly choosing to trade down while on other occasions will act contrarily to 'economic man' by choosing to trade up. The purchase of alcohol in France – cross-border shopping and smuggling – is yet another dimension to this issue, and is considered in depth later in this section of Chapter 5.

DEMAND: OUTLET AVAILABILITY

Outlets Able to Sell/Supply Alcoholic Drinks

It is a requisite of the UK licensing legislation that all premises selling alcoholic drink are either licensed by local magistrates or registered. In 1995, the number of such premises was 201,100. Further details are provided in Table 5.8.

Table 5.8: Number of licensed outlets in the UK, 1995

Outlet	Number
Public houses*	60000
Other full-on licences* **	24800
Restaurant and residential licences***	32300
Licensed and registered clubs****	31400
Off licences	52600
Total	201100

Notes: *Where a customer can consume an alcoholic beverage without any other requirement.
**This covers hotels, wine bars, cocktail bars, etc.
***Where it is a requirement that the customer must either be having food or be a resident. Covers restaurants and private hotels.
****These are mainly members' clubs, which are registered and non-profit making. A few thousand (perhaps) are profit-making clubs, and therefore formally licensed. Examples of profit-making clubs are sports clubs (golf, squash) as well as night clubs.
Sources: Home Office Liquor Licensing Statistics, Scottish Office licensing information and the N. Ireland Office. All these figures are published in the BLRA *Statistical Handbook*, tables G1 to G4 inclusive.

Proportion of Alcohol Consumed at Home

In the past, and in the UK, alcohol consumption was invariably linked in many peoples' minds with drinking in the pub, but this picture is now very outdated. One of the major trends over the past few decades has been the continuous growth of drinking at home. This is not surprising given the growth of take-home beer sales and the large increase in wine consumption, most of which is consumed at home. Indeed, it is possible to calculate that over half the alcohol consumed in the UK is drunk at home. Table 5.9 shows the proportion of specific beverages that was consumed on UK licensed premises in 1997.

Table 5.9: Proportion of alcohol consumed on licensed premises, 1997

	Beer	Cider	Wine	Spirits	Total
% of total alcohol consumed*	54.2	4.5	22.8	18.5	100.0
% of each drink which is consumed 'on' the premises**	73.0	42.0	13.0	21.0	–
Proportion of total alcohol consumed 'on' the premises***	39.6%	1.9%	3.0%	3.9%	48.4%

Notes: *This estimate is produced by BLRA and given in table D3 of its 1999 *Statistical Handbook*. It also describes the methodology for producing this statistic.
**The figure for beer is estimated by the BLRA, while the figures for the other drinks have been produced by Stats(MR) (an independent market research company specialising in the drinks industry and owned by Neilsen) and published in a small book of drink industry statistics produced by NTC publications.
***This is simply line 1 multiplied by line 2; in the case of beer, the calculation is 54.2 x 73.0/100.

Thus over 50% of alcohol is drunk at home, but even this estimate is an understatement as it excludes purchases in France, that is, cross-border shopping, and smuggling. It is interesting to reflect that over half the alcohol consumed is sold through some 25% of the licensed outlets. Furthermore, given the underlying consumption trends, this proportion is bound to grow.

Availability and Alcohol Consumption

Some people argue that the increased number of outlets has led to an increase in the volume consumed. This is a bit like the 'chicken and egg' situation. If the demand were not there, then the supplying outlets would not have opened. The position regarding the availability of alcohol was changed fundamentally by the licensing acts of the early 1960s – new categories of licensed premises were introduced and off licences could be opened in shop hours rather than pub hours. The other major period of change has been in more recent years when pubs became able to open all afternoon, including Sundays. Nevertheless, it is interesting to compare, over a reasonable time period, trends in alcohol consumption and numbers of outlets. This is shown in Figure 5.21.

Basically, the trends in Figure 5.21 split into two. Before the 1979 peak, consumption had risen much faster than the number of outlets; since then the number of outlets has increased by 18%, but alcohol consumption has declined by 5%. Furthermore, the change in hours has been accompanied by a general standstill in alcohol consumption and a continuous decline in beer consumption (this is relevant as it is the main drink in pubs and clubs).

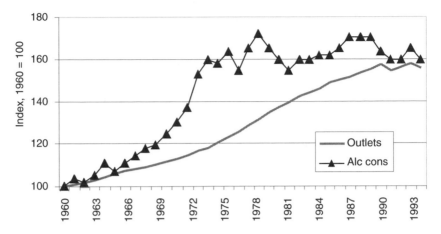

Figure 5.21: Outlets compared to alcohol consumption, 1960–96

Sources: Licensing sources as for Table 5.8; alcohol consumption as for Table 5.9.

The fundamental graph in the preceding discussion is Figure 5.10, which shows how consumer expenditure has changed over the past few years to reflect current aspirations. Despite the relatively large increase in outlets over the past few years, expenditure on alcohol and volume consumed have declined as consumers have chosen to spend their money on alternative competing products.

DEMAND: PRICE AND TAX

The Importance of Price

An econometric study of the UK beer market undertaken for the BLRA by Oxford Economic Forecasting (OEF) showed that price was the most important short-term variable. A brief summary of their research was included in the BLRA duty submission to the Treasury dated July 1996. OEF looked at many different factors that could impact upon the beer market and found price to be the only really significant factor.

There are several ways in which the consumer can try to avoid higher prices.

- Buying a lower-priced product. Interestingly, the evidence shows the opposite – trading up from mild and bitter to lager, or trading up in wine quality.
- Buying in a lower-priced outlet – this is very evident in the beer market with the trend towards take-home sales.

- Buying in a lower-tax environment; for example, buying beer and wine in Calais. This is considered further later in this section of Chapter 5.
- Making illegal purchases; for example, buying on the black market.
- Producing the product at home, either legally or illicitly.

The UK is a high-tax country, and the close relationship between price and tax is shown in Table 5.10.

Table 5.10: Tax as a proportion of UK consumer expenditure, year ending March 1998

Drink	Consumer expenditure (£m)	Total tax (£m)	Tax as % of expenditure
Beer	15911	5125	32.2
Wine and made-wine	6364	2572	40.4
Spirits	5759	2462	42.8
Cider and perry	1199	316	26.4

Sources: ONS produce consumer expenditure data and HMCE publish data on excise duty revenues. BLRA has calculated the VAT take from consumer expenditure. All figures are published in the BLRA *Statistical Handbook*, tables E2, F1 and F7.

This section is concerned with excise duty and VAT, but other taxes also affect the price of drinks, albeit indirectly; for example, the uniform business rate which is especially applicable to pubs and hence beer prices. However, other government action can also have a direct impact on price. Garafas (1995) estimated that the Beer Orders (under which brewers were forced to sell some 11,000 pubs) had increased the price of beer by 4p a pint. Slade (1998) has concluded that 'the recommendation by the MMC to force divestiture resulted in higher retail prices'.

The Taxes

Two taxes directly affect the price of alcoholic drinks sold in the UK:

- Excise duty. This is levied when the alcoholic drinks leave the 'duty ring' and is related to volume and strength (albeit the strength bands are very wide in the case of wine). Excise duty is thus included in the price paid by subsequent purchasers, such as wholesalers and retailers. Exports are duty free.
- Value added tax (VAT). VAT is levied upon the price of the product and is payable at each stage of the distribution chain, although the consumer pays the total amount. While excise duty is related to volume and strength, VAT is a function of price, which means that each time the price is raised the government gets increased revenue from VAT. In addition, while excise duty is levied on a few goods, VAT in the UK is levied across

a much wider range of products and services. Exports are zero-rated for VAT purposes.

In effect there is a tax-on-tax situation, as VAT is levied on the final consumer price, which also includes the duty.

At one time, duty was by far the most important revenue raiser, but nowadays there is little difference in the yield from the two taxes (Table 5.11)

Table 5.11: UK VAT and excise duty revenues, 1997–98

	Excise duty (£m)	VAT (£m)	Total (£m)
Beer	2696	2429	5125
Wine and made-wine	1362	1210	2572
Spirits	1546	916	2462
Cider & perry	137	179	316
Total	5741	4734	10475

Sources: HMCE, ONS and BLRA (as for Table 5.10).

Excise Duty

Excise duties on alcoholic drinks are levied in most countries, although there are some important differences. The UK is one of the 'high duty' countries within the European Union, as will be evident from Tables 5.12, 5.13 and 5.14.

Table 5.12: Excise duty on 5% abv beer, EU, January 1998

Country	Excise duty (pence per pint)
Finland	53.7
Ireland	37.6
UK	31.7*
Sweden	31.4
Denmark	17.4
Netherlands	8.0
Belgium	7.7
Austria	6.5
Italy	6.3
Greece	5.6
Portugal	5.3
France	4.9
Luxembourg	3.6
Germany	3.5
Spain	3.1

Note: *Subsequent to this table duty in the UK rose to 32.7p in January 1999. All these tables are at end 1997 exchange rates – the minimum rates were set in ECUs (now Euros).
Source: The Brewers of Europe (CBMC), which is the European trade body for the brewing industry. It collects this data annually from all its member associations.

The duty rate in Germany rose to 3.5p in 1993 as a result of having to implement the EU Rates Directive; prior to that the amount of duty had been constant since 1952 at a little over a penny a pint. In 1991 and 1992, beer duty in Denmark was reduced by 47% overall to try to curb cross-border shopping and smuggling with Germany. In 1997, Sweden reduced its beer duty by 39% in order to try to reduce cross-border shopping and smuggling occurring between Sweden and a number of countries. Finally, a reduction is anticipated in Finnish duty rates for exactly the same reason.

Table 5.13: Excise duty on a 75 cl bottle of still table wine, EU, January 1998

Country	Excise duty (pence per bottle)
Sweden	153.3
Ireland	136.3
Finland	116.8
UK	108.5*
Denmark	49.6
Netherlands	24.1
Belgium	23.3
France	1.7
Austria	Zero
Germany	Zero
Greece	Zero
Italy	Zero
Luxembourg	Zero
Portugal	Zero
Spain	Zero

Note: *Subsequent to this date, duty in the UK rose to 112p a bottle in January 1999. (Duty on sparkling wine is 160p for a 75 cl bottle.)
Source: CBMC (as for Table 5.12).

The reason why some countries are allowed to charge a zero rate is once more a function of the Rates Directive. While minimum rates of duty for beer and spirits were agreed, the only point of agreement on wine was that the minimum rate should be zero. The rate in France is nominal, and is levied for reasons of quality control rather than as a fiscal measure.

There is another facet resulting from the UK's membership of the EU that has led to a restriction on the ability of the UK government to set duty rates. As a result of a case decided by the European Court of Justice (ECJ) in 1984, the UK has lost its flexibility regarding the relationship between beer and wine rates. The ECJ accepted the argument of the Italian government that the UK's wine duty rate was much higher than beer and that this constituted a barrier to entry to wine, as wine was mainly an imported product, and beer was mainly home produced, and the two products were competitive. The ECJ decision was implemented in the 1984 budget when wine duty was reduced and beer duty was increased.

Table 5.14: Excise duty on 40% abv spirits, EU, January 1998

Country	Excise duty (£ per 70cl bottle)
Sweden	10.55
Finland	9.34
Denmark	6.80
UK	5.48
Ireland	5.17
Portugal	3.76
Belgium	3.06
Netherlands	2.77
France	2.68
Germany	2.40
Luxembourg	1.92
Greece	1.74
Austria	1.34
Spain	1.27
Italy	1.20

Source: CBMC (as for Table 5.12).

High Taxes and Consumption Trends

One argument put forward for high duties is that they restrict consumption, both in terms of absolute level and rates of growth. Are these views supported by available evidence?

The first table in this sequence (Table 5.15) presents information related to growth of consumption in high-duty countries. It should be noted that the figures in the following tables for alcohol consumption are based on total population and exclude unrecorded consumption. The relevance of the latter will be explained later, but the quantities of alcohol shown in the following tables are the amounts that have paid duty. Limiting this comparison to members of the EU means that the underlying economic circumstances over this period are fairly similar.

Table 5.15: Growth of consumption in high-duty EU countries, 1960–96

Country	Alcohol Consumption*					% change	
	1960	1970	1980	1990	1996	1960–80	1980–96
Denmark	4.2	6.8	9.4	9.8	10.1	122	7
Finland	2.4	4.5	6.4	7.8	6.3	171	–2
Ireland	3.0	5.9	7.4	7.2	7.5	142	2
Sweden	3.9	5.8	5.7	5.5	5.3	45	–7
UK	4.3	5.4	7.5	7.7	7.7	73	3
Average	3.6	5.7	7.3	7.6	7.4	103	2

Note: *In litres of alcohol per head.
Sources: Canadian Brewers Association report entitled 'Alcohol Beverage Taxation and Control Policies' 1997, for all countries, except the UK where the source is the BLRA.

By way of contrast, Table 5.16 shows the growth of alcohol consumption in low-duty countries.

Table 5.16: Growth of consumption in low-duty EU countries, 1960–96

Country	Alcohol consumption*					% change	
	1960	1970	1980	1990	1996	1960–80	1980–96
Austria	8.3	10.3	10.8	11.5	11.0	29	2
Belgium	6.4	8.9	10.8	9.9	9.1	70	−16
France	18.8	17.3	15.7	13.2	12.1	−17	−23
Germany	7.3	10.9	12.9	12.6	10.8	78	−16
Italy	12.5	14.1	12.9	8.7	7.7	3	−40
Netherlands	2.6	5.6	8.8	8.5	8.1	239	−8
Portugal	10.8	9.8	10.8	10.5	10.8	−1	0
Spain	8.8	11.4	12.8	10.4	9.4	45	−27
Average	8.7	10.3	11.1	10.0	9.2	27	−17

Note: *In litres of alcohol per head.
Sources: Canadian Brewers Association and BLRA (as for Table 5.15).

Alcohol consumption in the higher-duty countries grew considerably faster in the period 1960–80 than in the low-tax countries. Since 1980 alcohol consumption has remained pretty static in the high-duty countries while falling in the low-duty countries. Thus high taxes have not stemmed the rate of growth.

Of course, one logical reason for the higher growth in the high-duty countries is that alcohol consumption was so low in 1960; the average in the low-duty countries was 2.3 times greater than in the high-duty countries. By 1996 the ratio between the averages of the two groups had fallen to 1:2. Thus high taxes have not restricted the level of consumption but it seems that alcohol consumption was moving to some kind of central level, quite independent of the rates of alcohol duties.

Conclusion

Price is undoubtedly the most important short-term variable. Nevertheless, as shown earlier, consumers do not always act as textbooks might suggest and there are clear examples of trading up in price. In the UK, and in many other countries, a key element in price is tax – whether by way of excise duty or VAT.

TAX EVASION – GENERAL

Nobody likes paying taxes; one of the great attractions of 'duty free' is that it avoids taxes. It is also true that the higher the tax, the greater the incentive to evade paying it. Tax evasion, or trying to reduce the amount of taxes paid, can take many forms. These include:

- Cross-border shopping. Applies to consumers in all the high-tax countries. This is for personal consumption.
- Smuggling. This is deliberate evasion, when the purpose is to resell the goods on the black market.
- Illicit distilling.
- Production of other drinks for personal consumption, although this may not be illegal in all countries.

The amount of 'recorded' consumption in any specific country is defined as the quantity of alcoholic drinks upon which duty has been paid. Some countries try to estimate 'unrecorded' quantities, that is, the amounts which have been subject to cross-border shopping, smuggling, illegal production and distillation. The available figures are given in Table 5.17.

Table 5.17: Comparison between 'recorded' and 'unrecorded' alcohol consumption, Finland, Norway and Sweden, 1997

	Recorded litres of alcohol per head	Unrecorded litres of alcohol per head	Total litres per head	Unrecorded as % of total
Finland	6.9	1.3	8.2	16
Norway	5.3	1.6	6.9	23
Sweden	5.9	3.2	9.1	35

Sources: *Statistical Bulletins* from the Brewers Associations in each country.

Fraud is another problem resulting from high duties and there have been some high-profile cases in the UK courts on this scheme.

In 1997, HM Customs and Excise (HMCE) (which, as described earlier, is the British government body charged with the collection of excise and customs revenues) set up a specialist working party looking at fraud among other issues, and its report was published in 1998. This report chronicles very clearly the criminal aspects of this trade. Just a few of the findings are repeated below:

A clear relationship has been demonstrated between cross-channel smuggling and a deterioration in law and order.

There is concern about the implications of the growing availability of cheap alcohol and tobacco to underage consumers.

The demand for the illicit product is established and the distributional networks set up.

TAX EVASION AND CROSS-BORDER SHOPPING – THE UK EXPERIENCE

Cross-border shopping is the term used to describe the purchases by British residents of beer and wine overseas. These purchases are made in shops and warehouses, and thus the buyer pays the local rate of duty and VAT. Most of this activity takes place in the Calais area, but research by the Brewers and Licensed Retailers Association (BRLA) shows that purchases are made elsewhere in France as well as other countries. The introduction of the Single Market in January 1993 meant that UK citizens returning from another EU member state could import as much drink as they wished provided it was for their *personal use*. However, it soon happened that very large amounts were being imported which were not for personal use but for resale on the black market.

Another phrase used to describe this trade is 'duty-paid imports'. This was used to distinguish these imports from the traditional 'duty-free' purchases made on board ferries and aircraft and at airports. Since the end of June 1999, duty-free purchases are no longer available on journeys between the UK and other member states of the EU.

Why Does it Happen?

Quite simply, beer and wine are available in supermarkets and cash-and-carries at a much lower price in Calais than in the UK. A key reason for this difference is duty. Duty on a pint of beer at 5% alcohol by volume (abv) is 5p in France and currently 32p in the UK. The duty on a bottle of wine in France is some 2p compared to 112p for still table wine and 160p for sparkling wine. It is no wonder that British-owned companies have established outlets in Calais – Tesco and Sainsbury among the supermarkets, while East Enders and the Beer and Wine Company are among the cash-and-carry wholesalers. In other words, this trade is a form of (legal) tax evasion whereby the consumer can stretch his or her discretionary income.

Growth in Passengers

A simple way to demonstrate the fact that UK consumers quickly understood the benefits of buying in Calais is to look at passenger growth. While there has been growth overall, the most significant rise in passenger growth is day-trippers in cars.

BLRA research shows that the biggest buyers are the latter group of people, those on day trips in cars. Between 1993 and 1997 the growth of day-trippers in cars was 178% and the number has continued to grow in 1998. In 1990, day-trippers in cars accounted for 6% of all UK resident adults making a sea crossing to the Continent. By 1993, the proportion had doubled to 13%, and almost doubling again by 1997 when the proportion became 25%. This last figure includes both the ferries and the Channel Tunnel.

The ferry companies, which had spare capacity in the winter months, were quick to utilise this situation. Advertisements were placed on television and cheap fare promotions were sponsored by national newspapers.

Impact on the UK market

In their press release dated 19 November 1998, HMCE gave figures for cross-border shopping and smuggling (Table 5.18).

Table 5.18: Share of UK consumption taken by duty-paid imports, 1998

Product	UK duty paid	Legitimate personal imports	Smuggled goods
Beer	94.5%	1.5%	4%
Wine	89.5%	7.5%	3%
Spirits	95%	3.5%	1.5%

Source: HM Customs and Excise (1998).

The research carried out by BLRA broadly agrees with these findings, particularly in the case of beer. Bearing in mind that 72% of beer sales in 1997 were in the 'on trade' (for consumption on licensed premises), this volume equates to 15% of the take-home trade. In wine, the BLRA research suggests that 14% of UK table (still) wine consumption and 25% of UK sparkling wine consumption were met by these imports. The volume imported of fortified wine and spirits remains relatively small, which in turn means that the market penetration is also low.

The BLRA and HMCE agree that 75% of these imports substitute for UK sales. In the case of smuggled goods, these resales are made outside the controls of the licensing system.

Volume growth

Since 1992, there has been a dramatic growth in the volume of beer, table (still) wine and sparkling wine imported to this country, either as legitimate cross-border shopping or as smuggled goods.

The BLRA has researched this trade since before the introduction of the Single Market in January 1993. Figure 5.22 shows the substantial volume growth in imports of beer, one of the three sectors most affected by cross-border shopping and smuggling.

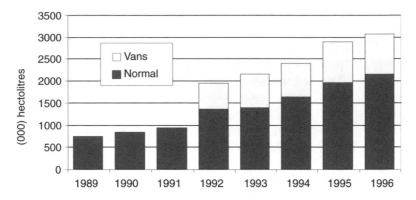

Figure 5.22: Duty-paid imports of beer into the UK, 1989–96

Source: BLRA. The average volumes purchased by normal passengers are established through interviews on Calais dockside, after which they are multiplied by the passenger numbers from the
government's International Passenger Survey. The numbers of vans and their average volume are
calculated by observational research.

There are a number of points:

- the van trade only developed after the introduction of the Single Market.
  This category covers the large-scale imports by people in Ford Transits
  and similar vehicles
- the volume growth in the first year of the Single Market, 1993, was 110%,
  since when it has grown by a further 57% to 1997.

The volume growth is even more striking for wine. Using the same research
technique, the BLRA found that the volume of still table wine increased by
123% in 1993, the first year of the Single Market, and by a further 104%
since then. Increased imports of sparkling wine are even more surprising. In
1993, their growth was 285%; since when they have grown by a further
125%. Very few spirits are purchased in Calais; certainly up to the end of the
duty-free regime.

Conclusion

The introduction of the Single Market in 1993 has had a significant impact
on the UK's wine and beer markets. There are several reasons for this growth:

- the lifting of quantity restrictions on imports for personal use
- the much lower prices available in Calais, a key factor being the much
  lower rates of excise duty in France
- the very low ferry fares brought about by their surplus capacity in off-
  peak times, allied to the competition created by the opening of the
  Channel Tunnel.

SUPPLY: STRUCTURE AND EMPLOYMENT*

Production

Over 90% of the beer sold in the UK is produced in the UK. At present there are just over 80 major breweries located in the UK, and the number rises to more than 500 when the new micro-breweries and pub breweries are included. Breweries are located in every region of the UK and are often the major, or one of the major, employers in their locality.

About 70% of the spirits sold in the UK are produced there. Altogether, there are many distilleries in the UK, most being located in the Highlands and Islands of Scotland and producing whisky. Like breweries, a distiller is often the major employer in its area.

Virtually all cider consumed in the UK is produced here (mainly in the West Country). There are some 380 vineyards in England, but their combined output is a very small proportion of total consumption, as virtually all wine consumed in the UK is imported.

A few years ago, the Henley Centre estimated for the BLRA that there were 39,000 jobs in brewing and distribution (published in the BLRA duty submission to the Treasury, dated June 1995). It is likely that the number has fallen since then, possibly to 33,000.

The Scotch Whisky Association (SWA) has estimated that there are 13,000 people employed in the production of Scotch whisky (SWA Statistical Report, 1996). The number employed is increased by (perhaps) another 5,000 to take account of the production of cider, gin, vodka, and so on.

Wholesaling

There are many wholesalers in the UK, although there is no precise information on the number of operators and employees specifically dealing with alcoholic drinks. Quite often, some of the major brewing companies deal with a wide range of products including alcoholic drinks.

The group of companies in this sector encompass a wide range of activities:

- suppliers of a full range of products such as beer, wines and spirits, as well as non-drink items such as food
- importers; either as a specialist drinks importer or a general importer of a wide range of goods, or a UK subsidiary of a foreign producer (such as Dortmunder Union and Hallgarten)
- specialists in a certain product range; for instance, Beer Sellers and cask-conditioned beers, or Premium Beers Worldwide.

---

*Author's Note: there are many references to the 'Treasury' in the next two sections. This is the title of the UK government's Finance Ministry.

In addition, these companies might give a full delivery service, or be a cash-and-carry outlet.

The Wine and Spirit Association (WSA) has estimated that there are 99,500 people in production, wholesaling and specialist retailers dealing specifically in alcoholic beverages. For the reasons given under 'Off Licences' (below), this figure may be an underestimate. Ignoring off licences, and subtracting the production figures, implies a residual of some 40,000 people.

Pubs and Clubs

While breweries and distilleries are located in specific towns, pubs and clubs are in every town and village throughout the country. They are often the social centre for their locality and can even be the largest employer. As was shown in Table 5.8, there are some 60,000 pubs and 31,000 clubs in the UK.

In September 1998 the Office for National Statistics (ONS) published in *Employment Trends* a figure of 430,000 employees, of which 270,000 were part-time. However, it is necessary to allow for self-employed entrepreneurs, such as tenants, free traders and their spouses. The current BLRA estimate is that there are some 80,000 licensees and their spouses.

Restaurants and Hotels

There are some 57,000 licensed hotels and restaurants in the UK. Clearly, the vast majority of people employed in hotels and restaurants are not dependent upon alcoholic drinks for their livelihood. But this is not true for every employee. The WSA has estimated that there are 26,000 specialist employees in hotels and restaurants dealing specifically with wines and spirits.

Off Licences

There are some 53,000 off-licensed outlets in the UK. Multiple grocers account for a significant proportion of the turnover of the alcoholic drinks sector. At the other end of the scale there are thousands of independent grocers and other small shops with an off licence which account for just a small proportion of the total off-trade turnover. It is hard to argue that there are employees in these outlets whose jobs are directly dependent on alcoholic drinks, although it could be said that employment levels would be lower if they did not sell these beverages. This is especially true of the small general retailer for whom the sale of drinks might make the difference between an outlet being viable or not.

However, there are over 10,000 specialist outlets, which might be independent operators or owned by multiples, which sell only (or mainly) alcoholic drinks. Employment in these outlets is directly related to the industry. A very conservative estimate is to suggest that there are five people per outlet, leading to a total of 50,000. It is true that a proportion of these would be part-time.

Suppliers of Goods and Services

No industry operates in a vacuum. The economic activity generated by the brewing industry is reflected in purchases from farmers, cask and keg manufacturers, and the producers of cans and bottles. Capital investment programmes lead to the purchase of equipment from brewing plant or packaging plant manufacturers, and distribution needs are reflected in the lorry fleets operated by either the brewers themselves or specialist transport companies. Similar requirements and purchases are also made by other drinks producers in the UK (cider, Scotch whisky, gin, vodka, and so on). Wholesalers also have distribution fleets and they will also need to invest in depots and package handling equipment. An independent economics group (Pieda) has calculated for the SWA (report published by SWA) that whisky producers pay £1 billion to their suppliers for goods and services.

While producers tend to purchase from larger companies, retailers (particularly bars and pubs) are very much involved with local entrepreneurs. These people cover services such as cleaning, plumbing, decorating and general maintenance. Of course, operators of pubs and clubs also purchase plant from manufacturers of, for instance, cellar and beer dispensing equipment, but many other purchases – furniture, glasses – may come from specialist suppliers.

Estimating the number of employees whose livelihood is dependent upon the drinks industry is extremely difficult and the relevant concept is 'full-time equivalents'. It may be that there are supplier employees whose full-time work is in the drinks industry, for example, those producing and selling cellar and bar dispensing equipment, but there will be a large proportion whose employment is only partially dependent upon the industry.

Producing such estimates depends to a certain extent upon a detailed analysis of purchases by producers, wholesalers and retailers. Some years ago the Henley Centre estimated for the BLRA that the production and wholesaling of beer created 74,000 jobs, while there were 136,000 jobs among suppliers to pubs and clubs (published in BLRA duty submission to the Treasury, dated June 1994). Pieda has produced an estimate for the SWA that the production of whisky creates 44,000 jobs among suppliers.

The Multiplier Effect

This is economist's jargon, which can best be explained by an example. Suppose a major factory in a town closes. The first effect will be that the ex-employees will curtail their purchases in the local shops, concentrating solely on the essentials, such as food. This cut back will be felt by the suppliers to those shops of non-essentials such as TV manufacturers, carpet

makers, and so on. The downturn in expenditure in that town will rever-
berate to a much wider extent throughout the economy.

The Henley Centre has produced an estimate for the BLRA of 97,000 jobs
full-time equivalents (published in the BLRA July 1994 duty submission to
the Treasury). Pieda has produced an estimate for the SWA of 12,000 jobs
subject to the multiplier effect (published by the SWA in its books on the
economic importance of the Scotch Whisky Industry).

Small and Medium-sized Enterprises (SMEs)

There are some very large companies producing beer and spirits. However,
over half the alcohol consumed in the UK is purchased in the off trade. A
substantial proportion of this is inevitably sold by the multiple grocers and
specialist off-licence chains.

Concentrating on these large companies gives a biased picture. In fact,
the typical operators in this industry are the small and medium-sized enter-
prises (SMEs). A medium-sized company is generally defined to have up to
50 employers, while a small company has 25. The BLRA has recently
reviewed the sector, and concluded that there are over 100,000 such operators. And this excludes suppliers.

Producers

Quite clearly, many brewers do not qualify as an SME, but nevertheless there
are several hundred producers that do qualify. This includes all the new
micro and pub breweries as well as some of the longer-standing, traditional,
local brewers. Little information appears to be available on *wholesalers*, but
there are probably many with less than 50 employees.

Retailers

There are 60,000 *pubs*, and a quarter of these are managed and owned by
brewers or by independent pub companies. A few of the remaining 45,000
will have more than 50 employees, particularly where food or accommoda-
tion is an essential part of their operation, but the vast majority are SMEs.
In addition, there are some 30,000 *clubs*, a substantial proportion of which
are members' non-profit-making clubs. Most of these are SMEs.

Off retailers

The position with *off retailers* is somewhat different. The main sellers are the
multiple grocers, co-ops and specialists, and even the specialists are often
chains. There are, nevertheless, a few SMEs in this sector.

Suppliers

Some of the suppliers will inevitably be large national, or even multinational
companies, but a substantial number are SMEs. Some of these may be

farmers, but many will be the small entrepreneurs that service pubs and clubs, such as cleaners, decorators and plumbers.

Summary

The above discussion has described the structure of the industry meeting the demand for alcoholic drinks. Perhaps one of the most surprising findings is the large number of small and medium-sized operators in this sector. However, from the viewpoint of the economic importance of the industry, it is important to bring together all the employment estimates to try to get a total estimate of the number of people whose livelihood is directly, or indirectly, dependent upon the sales of alcoholic drinks.

It should be noted that the information in Table 5.19 includes a high proportion of part-time employed, particularly in pubs and clubs, hotels and restaurants, and off licences. The reasons for, and benefits of, part-time employment are many, for both the employer as well as the employee. However, a key factor in this sector, particularly pubs and clubs, is the variability of demand, with peaks at lunch-time and evenings.

The WSA has produced an estimate for all drinks of 438,000. The figure in Table 5.19 is 931,000, but subtracting the figure for pubs and clubs gives 421,000, which is remarkably close to the WSA estimate.

Table 5.19: Employment in the UK drinks industry, 1994

Economic sector	Number employed	Comment
Production		
Brewing and distribution	33000	
Scotch whisky	13000	
Other drinks	5000	
Total	51000	
Wholesaling		
Total	40000	Best estimate
Pubs and clubs		
Employees	430000	Under 5 per outlet
Licensees and spouses	80000	
Total	510000	
Hotels and restaurants		
Total	26000	0.5 person per outlet
Specialist off licences		
Total	50000	5 per specialist outlet
Suppliers		
Brewers	74000	1 person per 34000 barrels, or 1 per local brewery

Table 5.19: (cont...)

Economic sector	Number employed	Comment
Suppliers (cont...)		
Pubs and clubs	136000	1.5 people per outlet
Scotch whisky	44000	
Total	254000	
All categories		
Total	931000	

Sources: BLRA, SWA, WSA, GVA, Henley Centre in various publications (often in conjunction with duty submissions) as described within the above text, with additional estimates by the author. The author believes that this is the first time such a detailed picture has been produced.

GENERAL ECONOMIC IMPACT

Consumer Expenditure

The amount spent by consumers on alcoholic drinks was given in Table 5.10 and totalled £29,233 million in 1997. This equalled 5.4% of total consumer expenditure.

Exports

The world-wide success of Scotch whisky exports is well-known; in 1996 the value of these exports was £2,278 million. The SWA points out that this is one of the top five UK exports. Gin and vodka are also exported – the GVA notes that 85% of gin is exported and its value is some £200 million. Beer exports have also been growing and totalled £216 million in 1997. The UK also exports wine, and this could reflect the strength of major brands (such as Harvey's sherries) as well as deliveries to outlets in Calais.

Production in the UK

It is a benefit to the UK economy that such a high proportion of these goods is produced in the UK. One area where the UK industry has responded posi-tively to changing consumer demands has been the brewing industry's response to lager. UK production, and hence employment, has been main-tained as a result of having the major brands produced in the UK, whether under licence or by other arrangements.

Imports

The willingness of the UK consumer to try new products and new tastes is clearly seen, both with the growth of lager and the growth of wine consumption. Indeed, as shown above, one of the features of the wine market over the past few decades has been the increasing diversity of the brands and varieties on sale. This openness of the UK market has been reflected in the emergence of specialist importers as well as benefiting a whole range of importers and wholesalers.

Employment

Employment is the result of people wanting to buy alcoholic drinks, whether in the UK or abroad. Employment figures were summarised in Table 5.19, with the total being 931,000.

Investment

In 1996, according to the ONS, capital expenditure was £123 million by the spirits industry and £31 million by the cider industry. The BLRA regularly collects data on capital expenditure from its members, and in 1996 the figures were £223 million on production, packaging and distribution, and £814 million on retail estate (primarily pubs). In addition, BLRA members invested some £200 million on other items, such as depots, computers and EPOS (electronic point of sale) systems.

Integration within the Economy Overall – Current Expenditure

This was shown above under the heading 'Supply: Structure and Employment', and is also shown in Table 5.20.

Table 5.20: Purchases by the UK brewing industry, pubs and clubs, 1994

Goods or service	Amount spent (£m)
Brewing	
Utilities	132
Raw Materials	424
Packaging	230
Repairs and maintenance	114
Marketing and sponsorship	309
Other goods and services	126
Pubs and clubs	
Utilities	602
Glassware	23
Cleaning, repair and maintenance	555
Pub entertainment	121
Advertising and promotion	110
Insurance and other goods and services	140
Beer dispensing and catering equipment	150
Other fixtures and fittings, and vehicles	201

Sources: Henley Centre, as published by the BLRA in its June 1994 duty submission to the Treasury.

These suppliers and their employees also pay taxes, and the magnitudes are estimated below.

Excise Duty

The amounts were given in Table 5.11; the total amount of excise duty paid on alcoholic products to the UK Treasury was £5,741 million.

VAT

The amounts were given in Table 5.11; the total amount of VAT paid on alcoholic products to the UK Treasury was £4,734 million.

Other Tax Streams

So often, the tax discussions centre on excise duty and VAT, but quite clearly this is only one part of the total tax income to the UK Treasury resulting from the economic activity generated by the production, distribution and sale of alcoholic drinks. The difficulty lies in trying to estimate these other magnitudes.

In 1994, the BLRA published research undertaken by the Henley Centre (published by the BLRA in its June 1994 duty submission to the Treasury) who produced estimates of these other tax streams applicable to brewing and wholesaling and pubs and clubs. Table 5.21 shows the figures calculated by the Henley Centre and, in addition, incorporates estimates for the other sectors covered in Table 5.19. The estimate for other drinks producers and independent wholesalers has been produced using the brewing and whole-saling figure as the base and then grossing this up by the respective numbers employed. Hence the tax per employee is £17,000 in both cases. The figure for income tax and National Insurance contributions for hotels, and so on, was produced using the pubs-and-clubs figure as the base and then reducing it by the respective employment levels. It was further assumed with corpo-ration tax and the uniform business rate that these figures applied mainly to off licences, and so the estimates in Table 5.21 have taken this into account.

This table does not take into account the tax payments made by suppliers to the drinks industries. The Henley Centre calculated that the appropriate figures were £480 million for brewing and wholesaling and £844 million for pubs and clubs. Similar magnitudes must be anticipated for suppliers to the other drinks producers and hotels, and so on.

Table 5.21: Other UK tax streams, 1994

Tax stream	Brewing and wholesaling	Other drinks independent wholesalers	Hotels restaurants, off licences	Pubs and clubs
Excise duties on cigarettes and AWP* Machines (£m)	None	None	None	156
VAT on sales other than alcoholic drinks (£m)	None	None	None	813
Income tax and National Insurance contributions (£m)	175	300	115	783
Oil duties, vehicle licences (£m)	29	50	Neg	10
Corporation tax (£m)	321	560	100	975
Uniform business rate	35	60	60	574
Total (£m)	560	970	275	3311
Tax per employee (£m)	17000	17000	3600	6300

Note: *Amusement with prizes.
Sources: The figures for brewing and pubs and clubs were produced by the Henley Centre and published by the BLRA in its 1994 duty submission to the Treasury. The calculation of the other figures by the author is described in the above text and takes into account the figures in Table 5.19.

Consumer Expenditure Net of Tax

The normal way to show this is to deduct excise duty and VAT from consumer expenditure, but, as Table 5.21 demonstrates, this understates the amount of tax going to the Treasury. The total tax in Table 5.21 is £5.1 billion, but this includes tax revenue derived from non-alcohol sales – mainly in pubs and clubs; for instance, the top two lines are tax revenues due to sales of food, AWP (amusement with prizes) machines, and so on. An estimate of the remaining taxes in pubs and clubs directly due to the sales of alcoholic drinks can be produced by assuming that at least 75% of an average pub's turnover derives from the sale of these products. The result of making these adjustments means that the figure of £5.1 billion is reduced to £3.5 billion.

Thus the calculation of consumer expenditure net of tax becomes £27.2 billion, less duty of £5.7 billion, less VAT of £4.7 billion, less other taxes of £3.5 billion, which is equal to £13.3 billion. And this figure still excludes the taxes paid by suppliers to the industry, which would inevitably be included within the prices they charge. Nevertheless, excluding taxes paid by suppliers, it can be seen that over half the price paid by consumers for their alcoholic drinks goes direct to the Treasury.

This means that under half the amount spent by consumers is used to pay employees, to pay suppliers, to fund the cost of raising capital, to be retained in the business and to pay dividends to shareholders.

Intangible Benefits (Health)

The benefits of moderate consumption of alcoholic drinks are well known and there is respected documented research showing the beneficial effects on health and easing of stress. The above has concentrated on issues that are fairly straightforward to evaluate, and the author has not attempted to put a monetary value on these intangible benefits.

Conclusion

Consuming alcoholic drinks is an integral part of the culture of many countries. Millions of people consume alcoholic drinks with no harm to themselves or to others. Trying to assess the benefit and pleasure these people obtain from, say, having wine with a meal or having a beer when thirsty after going for a walk or playing a sport or working in the garden is not quantifiable in monetary terms. The demand for these drinks exists and the purpose of the above discussion has been to show the employment, economic and tax benefits deriving from that demand.

THE MAIN FINDINGS

If there is a theme to this section of Chapter 5, it is: 'Don't always believe the conventional wisdom.' The author firmly believes that several of the points made above may have come as a surprise to some readers.

The following are some of the key points made.

- The use of per capita consumption to measure long-term alcohol consumption trends is fraught with difficulties, not least the substantial changes in population age structures.
- It is possible for the number of regular drinkers to *increase* when per capita consumption is *falling*.
- There have been major changes in taste and people have been 'trading up' in some areas.
- There is a lack of a positive relationship between rising income and consumption; indeed, in some countries, there is evidence of a negative relationship.
- Alcohol expenditure in the UK is falling in real terms and is falling as a proportion of personal disposable income.

- There is a lack of a positive relationship between the number of outlets and alcohol consumption.
- More alcohol is consumed at home in the UK than in pubs and clubs.
- Price is an important variable and tax is a key element of that.
- The UK is a high-tax country, but high taxes do not appear to have restricted the growth of alcohol consumption either in the UK or in other high-tax countries.
- The impact of high duties in depressing the level of demand has been undermined until consumption levels in EU low-duty countries are now only 20% higher than in EU high-duty countries.
- High taxes lead to substantial tax evasion; as much as 35% of alcohol consumption in Sweden involves drink on which Swedish duty has not been paid.
- The UK has seen substantial tax evasion by people buying their drinks in Calais; it accounts for some 5% of beer and spirits and over 10% of wine consumption.
- HM Customs and Excise estimate that over 70% of this beer is smuggled. A similar high proportion is applicable to wines and spirits.
- High duties encourage fraud, which is another problem, both in the UK and other EU countries.
- One way of showing the growth of tax evasion is that between 1990 and 1997 there was a sevenfold increase in people taking their cars to France for a day trip.
- The producers, wholesalers and retailers of alcoholic drinks employ over 900,000 people, either directly or indirectly.
- The typical operator in the sector is an SME, which is due to the large number of pubs operated by individual licensees as well as the large number of small businesses acting as suppliers to the industry, particularly local tradesmen.
- The producers, wholesalers and retailers of alcoholic drinks purchase goods and services from a wide range of organisations, including local tradesmen.
- Over half the amount spent by UK consumers on alcoholic drinks goes straight to the UK Treasury.

LIST OF ABBREVIATIONS

abv	alcohol by volume
AWP	Amusement with prizes machines
BLRA	Brewers and Licensed Retailers Association. This is the UK trade association for the brewing and pub industries. At one time it was known as the Brewers' Society

CBMC	The Brewers of Europe (Confederation des Brasseurs du Marche Commun). This is the trade body representing all the brewing industries within the European Union and additionally Norway and Switzerland
c.i.f.	cost, insurance, freight
ECJ	European Court of Justice
ECU	European Currency Unit – now succeeded by the Euro
EPOS	Electronic point of sale
EU	European Union
GDP	Gross domestic product. This is the concept used by economists to measure the total economic activity in a country, and UK figures are produced by the ONS
GHS	General Household Survey
GVA	Gin and Vodka Association. This is the UK trade association for these products
HMCE	Her Majesty's Customs and Excise. This is the government department responsible for the collection of excise and customs duties, and it deals with issues such as smuggling and tax avoidance through fraud
Lpa	Litres of pure (100%) alcohol. This concept is used to amalgamate the volumes of the different drinks to give an overall figure of total consumption
OECD	Organization for Economic Co-operation and Development
OEF	Oxford Economic Forecasting. An independent economics research body that has undertaken studies for the BLRA
ONS	Office for National Statistics. The government body which deals with all UK official statistics
PAS	Public Attitude Surveys. An independent market research company that has specialised in researching the UK drinks market for some three decades
PDI	Personal disposable income, a statistic produced by the ONS
PPP	Purchasing power parity
SME	Small and medium-sized enterprises
SWA	Scotch Whisky Association. This is the UK trade body for the producers of Scotch whisky
VAT	Value added tax
WSA	Wine and Spirit Association of Great Britain and Northern Ireland. This is the UK trade body representing the importers of wines into the UK, and the producers/importers of spirits and liqueurs other than gin, vodka and Scotch whisky

B: The Positive and Negative Impacts of Alcohol Use

Eric Single

> *Of course there are benefits to drinking – otherwise, people wouldn't do it so much …*
>
> (Poikolainen 1995)

INTRODUCTION

There is a growing recognition that the consumption of small amounts of alcohol has a protective effect against heart disease and stroke (for example, Poikolainen 1995). Poikolainen's simple but eloquent statement reminds us, however, that alcohol has conveyed a wide variety of subjective benefits to the drinker since long before there was any evidence that low-level drinking conveys objective physiological benefits. There are also clearly psychological effects such as an improved sense of well-being and quality of life, as well as evidence of potential cognitive effects in enhancing creativity and therapeutic impacts in times of stress (Baum-Baicker 1985, Mäkelä and Mustonen 1988, Midanik 1995). Peele (1997) maintains that it is critical in terms of recognising the reality of traditional social alcohol use to go beyond the therapeutics of alcohol for heart disease and recognise that alcohol accompanies, encourages, and in some sense leads to good times, sociability, shared experiences, and personal enjoyment and well-being. Ironically, these benefits are so widely accepted as to be somewhat invisible.

Thus, research is a long way from quantifying the subjective benefits of alcohol in a manner that can be compared to the costs of alcohol misuse.[1] Nonetheless, it is possible to derive estimates of the number of deaths and hospitalisations prevented by low-level alcohol use and compare these numbers to the number of deaths and hospitalisations caused by alcohol misuse. This information helps to complete the picture of how alcohol use impacts upon a society and it helps to prioritise alcohol prevention policies towards those prevention strategies which not only reduce adverse consequences but also maximise (or at least do not reduce) the benefits of alcohol use.

However, the reader is warned that comparing the costs and benefits of alcohol use to population health is *not* a zero-sum game where the object is to achieve parity between the two sets of figures. There is little purpose in 'balancing' the number of deaths caused by alcohol with the number of deaths prevented by alcohol. Regardless of the number of lives and hospitalisations averted by moderate use of alcohol, the goal of public policy should be to minimise the harm caused by alcohol misuse. The objective of alcohol prevention is to reduce deaths, hospitalisations and other adverse consequences of alcohol misuse, regardless of the number of lives and hospitalisations prevented by moderate use.

The purpose of this section of Chapter 5 is to present estimates of the numbers of deaths and hospitalisations caused and prevented by alcohol use. I begin with a description of the negative impacts of alcohol use in Canada, in terms of mortality, morbidity and economic costs. Estimates of the number of lives and hospitalisations saved by moderate alcohol use is then presented and compared with similar estimates from Finland. I conclude with a discussion of the implications of these findings for prevention policy and for future epidemiological research.

THE NEGATIVE IMPACT OF ALCOHOL MISUSE: MORBIDITY, MORTALITY AND ECONOMIC COSTS IN THE CANADIAN CONTEXT

A useful way to summarise the negative impact of alcohol use to a society is to estimate the economic costs of alcohol. Regardless of the approach taken, economic cost estimation first requires estimation of the number of deaths and hospitalisations caused by alcohol use. Utilising international guidelines for estimating the costs of substance abuse (Single et al. 1996a), a major study was undertaken to estimate morbidity, mortality and economic costs attributable to substance abuse in Canada in 1992 (Single et al. 1996b). Only the results regarding alcohol are summarised below.

As with all cost-estimation studies, the first step in estimating the costs of alcohol was to estimate the number of deaths and hospitalisations attributable to alcohol misuse. The methodology is described elsewhere (Single et al. 1996b, Single et al. 1999). Briefly put, information on relative risks for different causes of disease and death (using *ICD*-9 categories) were estimated from meta-analyses (particularly Fox et al. 1995 and English et al. 1995). Controlling for age and gender, pooled estimates of relative risk were combined with prevalence data to generate 'aetiologic fractions' or attributable proportions of the total deaths and hospitalisations for those causes. These were then applied to reported numbers of deaths and hospitalisations due to each cause (controlling again for age and gender). An important limitation to this method is that the risk posed by alcohol consumption is estimated solely from individuals' mean total consumption in the epidemiological studies that provide estimates of relative risk, without taking the individual's drinking pattern into account.

It was estimated that 6,701 Canadians lost their lives as a result of alcohol consumption in 1992. The largest number of alcohol-related deaths stemmed from impaired-driving accidents. It was estimated that 1,021 Canadian men and 456 women died in motor vehicle accidents in 1992 as the result of drinking. Alcoholic liver cirrhosis accounted for 960 deaths and there were 918 alcohol-related suicides.

Furthermore, the findings regarding years of life lost indicate that many of these deaths involved relatively young persons. Due to the high incidence of alcohol-related accidental deaths and suicides, the number of potential years of life lost was relatively high at 186,257 (134,495 years for men and 51,762 for women). This represented 27.8 years lost per alcohol-related death. Motor vehicle deaths represented 22% of all alcohol-related deaths and 33% of productive life years lost, indicating the relatively young age of alcohol-related traffic fatalities.

It was further estimated that there were 86,076 hospital separations (56,474 for men and 29,602 for women) due to alcohol in 1992. Not taking co-morbidity into account, the number of alcohol-related hospital days was estimated at 1,149,106 (755,205 for men and 393,902 for women[2]). The greatest number of alcohol-related hospital separations was for accidental falls (16,901), alcohol dependence syndrome (14,316) and motor vehicle accidents (11,154). The greatest number of hospital days was for accidental falls (308,224 days), indicating the debilitating nature of many such injuries. Thus, accidental falls accounted for 6% of deaths, 20% of hospital separations and 27% of hospital days attributed to alcohol. In contrast, motor vehicle accidents accounted for 22% of deaths but only 13% of hospital separations and 12% of hospital days due to alcohol.

The estimated 6,701 deaths due to alcohol represented 3% of total mortality in Canada for 1992. The 186,257 years of potential life lost due to alcohol represented 6% of the total years of potential life lost due to any cause, the 86,076 hospitalisations due to alcohol constituted 2% of all hospitalisations, and the 1.15 million days of hospitalisation due to alcohol represented 3% of the total days spent in hospital for any cause.

Based on these estimates of mortality and morbidity, it was estimated that alcohol accounts for more than C$7.5 billion in economic costs, or C$265 per capita, in Canada in 1992. The largest economic costs of alcohol were C$4.14 billion for lost productivity due to morbidity and premature mortality, C$1.36 billion for law enforcement and C$1.30 billion in direct health care costs. These figures should not be taken as precise estimates of the economic impacts of alcohol misuse. The size of the figures will vary according to several dimensions, including the choice of discount rate for valuing lost income in the future in current dollars, the choice of consumption measure in the prevalence estimates and whether or not costs take specific diagnosis into account (Single et al. 1998). The Canadian study included sensitivity analyses on these three aspects of the study methodology, and reported the findings under alternative assumptions. The sensitivity analyses found considerable variation in the results, depending on the operational assumptions used. Nonetheless, it is reasonable to conclude that alcohol misuse represents a major cause of mortality and morbidity in Canada, with enormous consequent costs to the Canadian economy.

THE POSITIVE IMPACT OF ALCOHOL USE: LIVES SAVED AND HOSPITALISATIONS AVERTED FROM LOW-LEVEL ALCOHOL USE

Before presenting some recent findings regarding the positive impacts of alcohol use, it is important to note some caveats concerning the estimates of deaths and hospitalisations saved by moderate alcohol use. First, as stated at the outset, there is no standard by which to judge what is an appropriate or desired number. The fact that moderate alcohol use may cause a significant reduction in deaths and hospitalisations does not mean that there should be any diminution of effort to reduce the deaths and hospitalisations caused by alcohol misuse.

Second, our consideration of the benefits of alcohol is limited to estimates of morbidity and mortality averted by low-level use. There is nothing comparable to the estimated economic costs of alcohol misuse, as there has never been a published study on the economic benefits of alcohol consumption. This is in large part due to the lack of a scientifically accepted model for estimating benefits. Whereas the costs of alcohol misuse are able to draw upon the reasonably well-established 'cost-of-illness' methodology as well as other approaches (Rice 1986, Single et al. 1996a), there is no comparable methodology in common usage to estimate the benefits of consuming psychoactive substances.

Finally, as with estimation of mortality and morbidity caused by alcohol, estimates of the deaths and hospitalisations saved by moderate alcohol use are based solely on consideration of an individual's mean level of consumption – the individual's drinking pattern is not taken into account.

Scientific awareness of the cardiovascular benefits of alcohol consumption is still relatively new, and estimates of the number of lives saved by moderate use have only been reported in Canada (Single et al. 1999) and in Finland (Mäkelä et al. 1997). In the Canadian study, it was estimated that alcohol prevented 7,401 deaths in 1992 (5,162 males and 2,239 females). This includes deaths due to ischaemic heart disease (4,205 deaths prevented), stroke (2,965 deaths prevented), heart failure and ill-defined heart conditions (183 deaths prevented), and from various other causes (47 deaths prevented). The number of deaths averted by the use of alcohol is therefore greater than the number of deaths caused by alcohol use.

However, the Canadian study also found that alcohol-related mortality frequently involves young adults, while the benefits of low-level consumption to preventing heart disease generally involves preventing the loss of life among older adults. Thus, the years of potential life lost due to alcohol (186,257) is more than twice as large as the number of years of potential life saved by the beneficial effects of alcohol (88,656). With regard to morbidity, while alcohol accounts for approximately 86,000 hospitalisations in 1992, it is estimated that 45,414 hospitalisations (31,270 for males and 14,114 for females) were prevented by low-level alcohol use in the same year. These were mainly due to the benefits of drinking to ischaemic heart disease (18,705), stroke (16,138), cholelithiasis (7,722), and heart failure and ill-defined heart conditions (2,312). Therefore, the number of hospitalisations caused by alcohol far outnumbers the number prevented by alcohol use.

The Finnish study (Mäkelä et al. 1997) focused solely on cardiovascular disease caused and prevented by alcohol misuse. It was found that the number of lives saved by low-level alcohol use in Finland was nearly equal to the number of deaths caused by alcohol in older age groups, but the overall number saved was much smaller than the number of deaths caused by alcohol use. This finding contrasts with that of the Canadian study. As noted above, in Canada it was found that the number of lives saved was higher than the number of deaths caused by alcohol use, although years of life lost and hospitalisations caused by alcohol were much greater than the years of life and hospitalisations saved.

Although the overall rate of consumption in Finland was slightly below that in Canada, it is likely that the well-documented Finnish pattern of drinking (for example, Mäkelä et al. 1983) may also account for at least part of these divergent results. A Finn who consumes seven drinks a week often does so at one sitting, while a Canadian who averages seven drinks a week tends to have one or two drinks on several days of the week. Given the manner in which Finns drink, even an average of one drink per day is often not 'moderate' at all. Thus the more sporadic, binge-drinking patterns among Finns may be an important reason why they appear to obtain fewer cardiovascular benefits from drinking compared with Canadians.

CONCLUSIONS

The first and foremost conclusion is that alcohol has both significant costs and benefits. Alcohol misuse is a major cause of preventable death in many societies and it accounts for substantial hospitalisations and economic costs. By the same token, however, as noted in Chapter 2, low-level use of alcohol entails considerable benefits. In the Canadian context, alcohol actually saves more lives than the number of deaths it causes. Even in Finland, where the number of deaths caused by alcohol far outnumbers the number of lives saved, low-level alcohol use accounts for substantial reductions in deaths. Furthermore, these benefits do not include the intangible positive effects of alcohol use.

Second, although the object of alcohol policy is not to equalise the magnitude of benefits and costs related to alcohol use, the existence of significant positive impacts on population health has important policy implications. The existence of significant benefits of alcohol use to public health influences strategies that favour reducing adverse consequences without necessarily restricting access to alcohol. These measures, sometimes referred to as 'harm-reduction' measures, include server-intervention programmes, impaired-driving countermeasures, the promotion of low-strength beverages, the enforcement of licensing regulations and modifications of the drinking environment. Where moderate alcohol use leads to significant reductions in mortality and morbidity, it would seem logical that these harm-reduction measures be given priority over policies which focus on restricted access to alcohol and which may thus reduce the benefits of alcohol consumption to population health.[3] In a situation where alcohol is demonstrably beneficial to the health of a significant proportion of a population, it is more difficult to argue that public policy should make it less available (Stockwell et al. 1997). On the other hand, harm-reduction measures generally reduce the likelihood or severity of alcohol problems without restricting access to alcohol or reducing the positive benefits of consumption.

The third conclusion is that despite the very limited nature of the evidence at this point, there are strong indications that drinking pattern has a significant impact not only on the nature and magnitude of adverse consequences, but also on the benefits of alcohol consumption. Prospective and case-control studies on the risk of cardiovascular disease and other consequences of alcohol consumption generally examine an individual's average drinking level without taking drinking patterns into account. Thus, the estimates of mortality and morbidity caused or prevented by alcohol use must necessarily rely on a summary measure of an individual's overall level of drinking to assess risk. But the finding of a much lower cardiovascular benefit in Finland compared to Canada strongly suggests that it may be important to consider more than the average ethanol intake in future studies. The binge-drinking pattern common in Finland (and in other countries, including the UK) may not only result in greater alcohol problems, particularly acute problems arising from intoxication, but it may also greatly limit the benefits of low-level drinking. Thus, drinking patterns are not only important in predicting adverse consequences, they may also be just as important in determining the magnitude of the benefits from drinking.

Virtually all of our information on the consequences of drinking focuses on negative effects. We know what to avoid, but we know little about positive features of drinking or what constitutes a beneficial pattern of drinking. There is an old story about an inebriated man who looks for his lost keys under a street lamp, not because he lost them there but because that is where the light is best. The search for evidence regarding a beneficial pattern of drinking is analogous to this proverbial drunkard unsuccessfully looking for his keys under the street lamp. Research has understandably focused its light on problem drinking and there is an extensive literature on patterns of alcohol consumption which involve serious risk of harm. We have solid evidence on risk avoidance but we know little about normal, unproblematic drinking and the patterns that maximise subjective and physiological benefits. Until researchers point their torches on normal, unproblematic drinking, our understanding of beneficial patterns of consumption will necessarily focus on the avoidance of risk rather than the positive benefits of drinking.

NOTES

1. Alcohol misuse encompasses any consumption which involves a social cost additional to the resource costs of the provision of that drug (Single et al. 1996a). Thus, the costs of alcohol 'misuse' or 'abuse' include costs associated with moderate levels of use if such use incurs social costs to the community. The operational definitions of 'low-level' or 'moderate' use are taken from English et al. (1995).
2. Total estimates may equal one case more or less than the sum of males and females due to rounding.
3. Of course, other considerations such as effectiveness also play a key role in prioritising policy alternatives.

6
Consequences: Patterns and Trends

Martin Plant, Moira Plant, Christine Thornton and Henk Garretsen

Throughout recorded history, humanity has had an ambivalent relationship with alcohol. It has already been emphasised in Chapter 4 that drinking patterns vary considerably internationally and within specific population sub-groups. Moreover, it has been stressed that the types of consequences that ensue from alcohol consumption are influenced by social setting, drinker characteristics and pattern of drinking (Grant and Litvak 1998).

THE INTERNATIONAL PICTURE

It is not easy to compare rates of 'alcohol problems' or adverse consequences of drinking internationally. Even so, one useful indicator of the adverse effects of prolonged heavy alcohol consumption is provided by rates of liver cirrhosis mortality (Table 6.1). It is, however, emphasised that the contribution of heavy drinking to such statistics varies from country to country.

Table 6.1: Deaths from chronic liver disease and cirrhosis rates per 100,000, 1993/94/95

Country	Year	Females	Males	Totals
Argentina	1993	3.2	12.9	7.6
Australia	1994	2.7	6.8	4.7
Austria	1995	9.1	27.8	17.7
Bahamas	1995	10.8	23.2	16.7
Barbados	1995	4.2	22.4	12.1
Belgium	1992	5.4	10.5	7.8
Belize	1995	5.4	3.6	4.6
Brazil, South, South-East & South-West	1992	4.7	20.6	12.2
Canada	1995	3.3	8.2	5.6
Chile	1994	12.6	36.8	23.8
Colombia	1994	3.5	8.6	5.9
Costa Rica	1994	10.0	19.6	14.7

Country	Year	Females	Males	Totals
Cuba	1995	4.9	9.3	7.1
Estonia	1995	8.1	13.4	10.5
Finland	1995	3.4	11.7	7.4
France	1994	6.5	16.1	11.0
Germany	1995	8.9	22.2	15.1
Greece	1995	1.9	5.6	3.6
Hungary	1995	31.0	96.4	61.0
Ireland	1993	2.1	3.7	2.9
Israel	1995	2.9	7.4	5.0
Italy	1993	9.2	20.3	14.3
Kazakhstan	1995	14.2	26.5	19.5
Lithuania	1995	6.4	15.8	10.5
Luxembourg	1995	5.3	17.4	11.0
The Former Yugoslav Republic of Macedonia	1995	3.0	10.2	6.4
Mauritius	1995	3.5	35.7	18.9
Mexico	1995	16.1	55.7	34.9
Republic of Moldova	1995	75.3	87.7	80.8
Netherlands	1995	2.6	4.5	3.5
Norway	1994	2.7	4.2	3.4
Poland	1995	5.1	15.7	10.0
Portugal	1995	7.3	24.9	15.3
Romania	1995	24.5	51.3	37.1
Singapore	1995	3.1	7.9	5.4
Slovenia	1995	16.0	36.4	25.1
Spain	1994	5.7	18.1	11.5
Sweden	1995	2.9	5.5	4.1
Trinidad & Tobago	1994	3.5	11.6	7.7
UK	1995	3.9	6.6	5.2
UK – England & Wales	1995	3.6	6.2	4.9
UK – N. Ireland	1995	2.9	4.4	3.6
UK – Scotland	1995	6.4	10.9	8.5
USA	1994	4.6	10.8	7.5
Venezuela	1994	5.4	20.5	12.7

Source: World Health Organization (1998).

As noted earlier, levels of per capita alcohol consumption vary considerably between different countries (Table 4.1). It has previously been claimed that the relationship between alcohol consumption levels and liver cirrhosis is fairly straightforward. In fact, the picture is now rather confused. Some remarkably high levels of cirrhosis have recently become evident in Eastern Europe (Moldova, Hungary and Romania). Moreover, there are differences in cirrhosis rates in countries that have recently reported similar per capita alcohol consumption levels (such as the UK and Italy). Presumably such peculiarities reflect variations in patterns of drinking, the quality of alcoholic beverages and a number of other factors, such as diet and general health.

Some useful information about the consequences of drinking amongst teenagers in Europe has been provided by the ESPAD survey already cited in Chapter 4 (Hibell et al. 1997). This study showed that amongst 15–16-year-olds in 26 countries, the highest rates of adverse 'individual' or 'relationship' consequences associated with their own drinking were reported by those in Denmark, Finland, Lithuania, Sweden, the UK and the Ukraine. Countries in which rates of such problems were reportedly low included Portugal and Turkey (Istanbul). Countries in which the highest proportions of teenagers reported adverse sexual experiences associated with their own drinking included the Czech Republic, Iceland, the UK and the Ukraine. Countries with the highest rates of teenage delinquency problems ascribed to their own drinking included Estonia, Finland, Iceland, Poland, the UK and the Ukraine. Most of these 'high-risk' countries were also those in which teenagers had reported relatively high levels of periodic heavy drinking and drinking to intoxication. The latter have long been associated with acute problems of the type noted above. As noted in Chapter 4, alcohol consumption amongst UK teenagers has been rising for some time. A Dutch study by Garretsen et al. (2000) found that the proportion of those aged 16–24 in Rotterdam who were defined as being 'problem drinkers' rose from 8.6% in 1980/81 to 14.8% in 1994.

Another study that has provided an international perspective on alcohol problems among people in different countries involved examining gender differences in 'acute' problems (such as intoxication) amongst adults in eight European countries. This showed that, contrary to what has sometimes been suggested in the past, women had *fewer* such problems than men at any given level of alcohol consumption (Bloomfield et al. 1999, Plant et al. 2000). Similar findings have also been produced by a Dutch study (Bongers et al. 1998).

SEEKING HELP FOR ALCOHOL-RELATED PROBLEMS

The true extent of 'psychiatric symptoms' of alcohol dependence in the general population is unknown. One British survey into this topic was conducted in 1993. This indicated that nearly one-fifth of men aged 20–24 reported having experienced three or more symptoms of alcohol dependence in the past year (OPCS 1995). It should be emphasised, first, that this evidence does not form a robust basis for stating that these people were 'alcohol dependent' in any clinical sense. Second, it should also be emphasised that the overwhelming majority of those who seek help for serious or chronic alcohol problems are older than 24 years of age. Oddly, 'alcohol dependence', as measured by this survey, declined steadily beyond the age of 24. Not only does this pattern not fit the profile of people who seek agency help for alcohol problems; it does reflect the fact that young people are those particularly likely to report periodic heavy drinking and acute adverse consequences. As noted in Chapter 4, some elderly people do drink heavily; some also experience problems due to their drinking. Even so, the elderly in general are less likely than younger people either to drink at all, or to experience alcohol problems. In The Netherlands there has recently been a sharp rise in heavy and problem drinking amongst those in the age range 45–54 years (San José et al. 2000).

It has frequently been noted that women constitute a minority of those who seek help for alcohol-related problems from the various 'alcohol agencies' in the UK (Royal College of Psychiatrists 1986). Information is available which charts the gender ratio amongst those who are admitted to hospitals with primary or secondary diagnoses of alcohol psychosis, alcohol dependence syndrome or the non-dependent abuse of alcohol. Such admissions have been rising fairly steadily in England and Wales. This trend is shown in Figure 6.1. Throughout the period shown, from 1970 to 1994, females constituted a slowly increasing minority of these admissions. In 1970, women accounted for 25% of admissions, while in 1994 they accounted for 30% (DoH 1999).

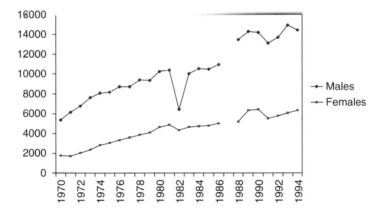

Figure 6.1: Admissions to mental hospitals and psychiatric units in England and Wales for alcoholic psychosis, alcohol dependence syndrome and non-dependent abuse of alcohol, 1970–94

In Scotland, a different general pattern has been evident, with admissions rising until 1977, then declining since then. In fact, as shown in Figure 6.2, the number of male admissions has fluctuated more markedly over the period 1970–94 than that for women. Even so, as in England and Wales, there has been an increase in the proportion of such admissions involving women. The latter accounted for 19% of admissions in 1970 and 30% in 1994.

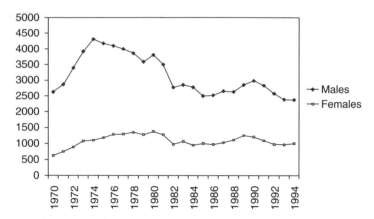

Figure 6.2: Admissions to mental hospitals and psychiatric units in Scotland for alcoholic psychosis and alcohol dependence syndrome, 1970–94

As Figure 6.2 shows, the proportion of females amongst hospital admissions for the diagnoses noted above has fluctuated from 29–31% in any year over the past decade. It was 30% in 1988, and 31% in 1995 (BLRA 1998, Scottish Executive 1999). The pattern noted in Figure 6.2 is rather different from that reported in relation to some Scottish alcohol treatment agencies in the 1970s. At that time women constituted approximately 25% of clients (Plant and Plant 1979).

ALCOHOL-RELATED DEATHS

The precise number of 'alcohol-related' deaths is unknown since the degree to which alcohol consumption may be a factor in many premature fatalities is uncertain (Giesbrecht et al. 1989, M.L. Plant 1997, Raistrick et al. 1999). Even so, a useful indication of the trends in some forms of alcohol-related deaths is provided by statistics related to diagnoses such as alcoholic psychosis, alcohol dependence syndrome, cardiomyopathy, alcoholic fatty liver, acute alcoholic hepatitis, alcoholic cirrhosis of the liver, and acci-dental, suicidal or undetermined poisoning by alcohol. Since 1970 such rates have been rising, both in England and Wales and in Scotland. These trends are shown in Figures 6.3 and 6.4:

Throughout Britain, the number of alcohol-related deaths amongst men has been higher than that amongst women. In 1970, women constituted 40% of such deaths in England and Wales. By 1993, this proportion had *fallen* to 36% (Scottish Council on Alcohol 1997). A quite different pattern was evident in Scotland: women accounted for 27% of deaths in 1970 and this proportion had *risen* to 33% by 1995. Even so, as noted in Chapter 2, information recently produced by the Medical Council on Alcoholism (2000) has indicated that the rate of increase in liver cirrhosis mortality in England and Wales amongst men has been rather more marked than that amongst women.

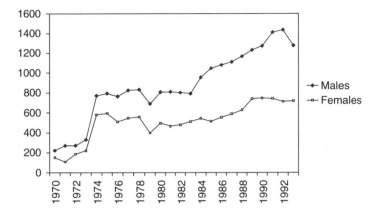

Figure 6.3: Number of alcohol-related deaths in England and Wales, 1970–93

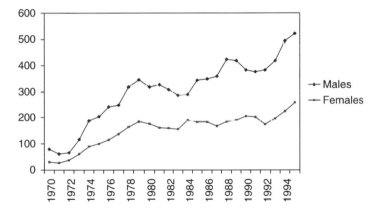

Figure 6.4: Number of alcohol-related deaths in Scotland, 1970–95

Additional useful information about alcohol-related mortality has been periodically produced in relation to occupation. Table 6.2 shows occupational groups in England and Wales that had high ratios of liver cirrhosis mortality (the average occupation has a ratio of 100).

The occupational groups noted in Table 6.2 include several that have long been noted as having high rates of alcohol problems. Moreover, these occupations also featured as having high mortality ratios related to other alcohol-related causes. The latter include cancers of the oral cavity, pharynx, oesophagus, liver and larynx, and also falls down the stairs (Drever 1995).

The relationship of alcohol problems to occupation has been commented upon many times. It has been suggested that some jobs are characterised by stress, insecurity, lack of supervision, pressure to drink heavily and other factors (such as the availability of alcohol at work) that may foster heavy or problematic alcohol consumption (Plant 1979, Hore and Plant 1981).

Table 6.2: Occupations with high rates of liver cirrhosis mortality, 1979–80 and 1982–90

Occupation	Mortality Ratio
Men	
Lawyers	233
Doctors	341
Literary & artistic	198
Sea farers	265
Publicans & bar staff	383
Caterers	171
Armed forces	182
Cooks & kitchen porters	140
Dockers & goods porters	144
Women	
Literary & artistic	215
Publicans & bar staff	378
Hairdressers	211

Source: Drever (1995).

ALCOHOL-RELATED CRIME

Drunkenness

As in relation to mortality, the link between alcohol and crime is often far from clear. However, some offences are, by definition, alcohol-related. Chief among these are 'drunkenness', and driving while under the influence of alcohol (Collins 1982, Stewart and Sweedler 1997). In recent years, the overall number of people convicted of 'drunkenness' offences has declined. This is shown in Figures 6.5 and 6.6. Both Figures relate to the period 1972–96.

Throughout Britain, women are a minority of drunkenness offenders. In England and Wales, females constituted 6.8% of such offenders in 1972. By 1996 this proportion had risen to 9.2%. The number of women convicted of this offence has risen slowly but steadily, while there was more fluctuation in the generally rising trend amongst men. In Scotland, women constituted 8.9% of offenders in 1972; by 1996, this proportion had *declined* slightly to 8.2% (BLRA 1998).

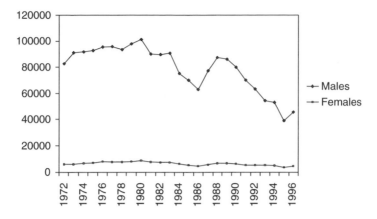

Figure 6.5: Drunkenness offenders in England and Wales, 1972–96

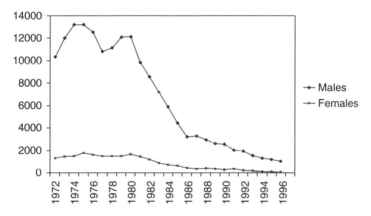

Figure 6.6: Drunkenness offenders in Scotland, 1972–96

Drinking and Driving

Convictions of drivers for being over the permitted blood alcohol level have exhibited a different pattern in England and Wales from that evident in Scotland. The numbers of persons so convicted has been *rising* in England and Wales and *falling* 'North of the Border'. These differing trends are illustrated in Figures 6.7 and 6.8.

Referring to Figure 6.7, only 1.5% of offenders were women in 1972. By 1996, this proportion had grown to 8.5%. In Scotland, women also constituted 1.5% of those convicted of drinking and driving in 1972. This proportion had grown to 7.9% by 1996 (BLRA 1998).

In conclusion, the international pattern of alcohol problems is complex and varied. It is simply not possible to compare many problem indicators because of poor data and incompatible recording methods or service provision.

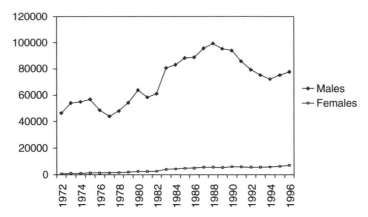

Figure 6.7: Persons convicted of drinking and driving in England and Wales, 1972–96

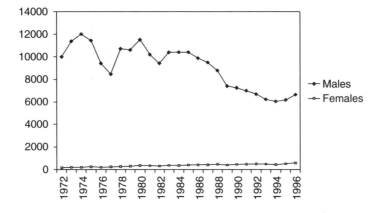

Figure 6.8: Persons convicted of drinking and driving in Scotland, 1972–96

In Scotland, there had been a degree of 'gender convergence' in relation to admissions to mental hospitals and psychiatric units for alcoholic dependence and alcohol dependence syndrome. The numbers of male and female drunkenness offenders in both England and Wales and in Scotland have also converged, though this was mainly due to a fall in the massive preponderance of such people who were males. The same applied to drink driving convictions in Scotland.

In relation to some of the variables considered, the gender gap appears to have widened. This was evident in respect of alcohol-related deaths and hospital admissions in England and Wales and Scotland and drinking and driving convictions in England and Wales. These findings therefore do provide qualified support for the conclusion that there has been a degree, albeit fairly modest, of convergence in the levels of alcohol-related problems of British women and men. This evidence needs to be interpreted with caution. First, the survey data considered above may be subject to differential reporting bias for females and males. Females may be more likely than males to under-report their true levels of alcohol-related problems or adverse consequences, due to the double standards and stigmatisation which persist in relation to female drinking. Second, the official figures related to morbidity, mortality and criminal offences may reflect a host of procedural and administrative factors. The latter may seriously obscure the real picture of alcohol-related problems amongst males and females. It has also been stressed that the positive and negative effects of alcohol consumption vary markedly in relation to pattern of consumption, setting, and a host of contextual factors (Grant and Litvak 1997, M.L. Plant 1997, Plant et al. 1997, Hibell et al. 1997).

7
Harm Minimisation

Kathryn Graham and Martin Plant

As noted earlier in this book, concern about drinking has very ancient origins and throughout human history there have been numerous attempts to control or curb various aspects of drinking which have been regarded as undesirable or unacceptable (see Berridge 1989, Musto 1997). Temperance movements have periodically risen and fallen in response to high levels of heavy or problematic drinking. A famous drastic twentieth-century example of such an attempt at control is provided by the American experience of Prohibition between 1920 and 1933. However, temperance has not been the only approach taken to addressing alcohol consumption and problems. Attempts at reducing the level of alcohol-related problems may be broadly dichotomised into strategies designed to reduce or even eradicate alcohol consumption (the most extreme example being prohibition) and those intended to reduce the harmful effects associated with drinking, while not necessarily reducing drinking *per se.*

REDUCING THE LEVEL OF ALCOHOL CONSUMPTION IN SOCIETY AS A WHOLE

Following on from the 'public health' traditions of the nineteenth century, a number of influential commentators have put forward detailed policy recommendations involving as a key policy aim the reduction of national per capita alcohol consumption (Bruun et al. 1975, Edwards et al. 1994, World Health Organization 1994a). There are at least two principles justifying a focus on *overall* alcohol consumption: the way that alcohol consumption is distributed in the general population, and the benefits of broadly focused prevention.

Ledermann (1956) identified the connection between general levels of alcohol consumption in the population and the levels of alcohol-related harm, such as liver cirrhosis. In particular, he demonstrated that as the level of consumption increases within a society, the proportion of persons drinking heavily and at higher risk of problems increases as well. Thus, some policies have been implemented to reduce alcohol consumption overall with the assumption that the number of persons engaging in problematic drinking would also be reduced.

Another reason for focusing on the general population rather than solely on problem drinkers is that although the heaviest drinkers have the most problems related to alcohol, the greatest burden to society comes from less heavy drinkers who have a moderate number of alcohol-related problems but are vastly larger in number. Therefore, the greatest impact on society as a whole will be felt by focusing on the large group of moderately heavy drinkers rather than the smaller group of very heavy drinkers even though they have the most extreme problems. This has been referred to as the 'preventive paradox' (Kreitman 1986). One example might be the tremendous reduction in harm in many countries achieved by reducing drink driving among all drinking drivers.

HARM MINIMISATION

Other authors have suggested a rather different approach (Plant et al. 1997) which also sets out to reduce or minimise the level of alcohol-related problems, but without having the reduction of per capita alcohol consumption as the *primary* objective. During recent years the latter perspective has been called 'harm reduction' or 'harm minimisation'. This approach has evolved in parallel to a similar approach to the reduction of harm associated with illicit drugs or to HIV and AIDS. In relation to the spread of HIV/AIDS and intravenous drug use, harm reduction has involved measures such as the distribution of condoms and information on 'safer sex', needle exchange programmes which supply clean needles to drug users in order to limit the spread of disease through sharing of infected needles, and the provision of bleach to facilitate the sterilisation of injecting equipment (Strang and Stimson 1990, O'Hare et al. 1992, Erickson et al. 1997). Tigerstedt has described these recent approaches to alcohol control policies as 'the new public health':

> The new public health movement dates back to the 1960s and 1970s when most of the infectious diseases had been fought back in Western countries ... Such an understanding of the new public health movement indicates that public health is part of a more general strategic shift in society. Notably, this shift makes it possible to 'go beyond an understanding of human biology', as it 'recognises the importance of those social aspects of health problems which are caused by life styles. In

turning the attention towards the social and physical environment' (the
new public health) seeks to avoid blaming the victim. (1999: 2)

He further notes the following with regards to approaches to problems that
focus on reducing overall consumption:

Quite recently, ambitions to formulate new research-based strategies have
appeared. There are several reasons for this. The health protective effect
is one of them, negative attitudes towards governmental regulations is
another (the latter was mentioned by Bruun et al. in 1975). Further,
important specifications have been made concerning per capita alcohol
consumption and particular alcohol-related problems, indicating a more
complex relationship between volume and harm than was previously
assumed. (1999: 12)

With regards to the focus on per capita consumption, Tigerstedt cites a
conference paper by Rehm (1999) ironically entitled 'Draining the ocean to
prevent shark attacks?' This paper criticised the overly simple view (a) that
per capita alcohol consumption and alcohol-related problems have a close
and inevitable relationship, and (b) that the key to reducing problems is to
cut per capita consumption. As indicated by some of the evidence cited in
Chapter 6 of this book, this relationship is, in fact, quite complex. Specific
types of alcohol problem appear to reflect the alcohol consumption patterns
of specific subgroups of drinkers in different contexts. Moreover, trends in
specific alcohol problems over time can be quite different from each other.
This has also been shown in relation to some of the UK evidence cited in
Chapter 6 (see Plant et al. 1997, Grant and Litvak 1998).

There is no single, simple solution to alcohol problems. As outlined by
Linda Wright in Chapter 9, alcohol education and health promotion alone
are not panaceas. This chapter describes some alternative approaches that
involve strategies designed to prevent or minimise specific types of alcohol
problems. Many of these approaches have been described in more detail
elsewhere (Single and Storm 1985, Tether and Robinson 1986, Plant et al.
1997). The defining feature of harm minimisation has been described by
Plant et al. as follows:

The characteristic feature of harm minimisation which distinguishes it
from other public health approaches to alcohol is that it attempts to
reduce the harmful consequences of drinking in situations where the
drinking can be expected to take place. The decision to drink is accepted
as a fact. This does not imply approval (or disapproval) of alcohol
consumption. It is simply presumed that people will be drinking in a

particular situation and effort should be made to reduce the potential harmful consequences that may occur. (1997: 6)

Examples of harm minimisation strategies which will be described briefly in this chapter relate to two general categories: (1) those aimed at increasing safety in and around bars, pubs or dance clubs, and (2) multifaceted community interventions aimed at reducing harm generally in the community.

SAFER BARS AND SAFER STREETS

Many of the approaches to prevent or reduce alcohol-related problems have been designed to either construct or reinforce some form of controls in and around the places in which people gather to drink and enjoy themselves. For example, during 1993, a UK-based charity, the Addictions Forum, in association with several other agencies, staged a conference in London under the title 'Safer Bars and Safer Streets'. This meeting served to bring together some of the research and prevention efforts directed toward drinking in licensed premises and the behaviour that takes place in and around licensed premises. Some of the major efforts in this direction are described below.

Community Approaches to Safety In and Around Bars

Community approaches to reducing problems related to drinking in licensed premises have included town or city planning committees to address transportation, location of fast food outlets and density of licensed premises (MCM Research 1993, Stockwell et al. 1993b); policing task forces to monitor disorder and violence and to develop strategies such as neighbourhood watch, transportation alternatives and training for door staff (Homel et al. 1997); enforcement campaigns (Stockwell et al. 1993b); development of a local committee to develop a code of practice and monitoring strategies for licensed premises (Homel et al. 1997); use of Safety Audit Committees to identify and propose suggestions such as increased lighting or policing for high risk areas (Homel et al. 1997, Lang and Rumbold 1997); training and registration of door staff (MCM Research 1993); use of incidence registers (Arnold and Laidler 1994) and the development of house policies for bars (Homel et al. 1997); and pub-ban and pub-watch schemes for identifying and banning troublemakers from all bars in a specific area (MCM Research 1993). The following describes some specific community-based interventions directed towards the broader context of bars.

The Torquay experiment

The police in the English coastal town of Torquay conducted a one-year experiment. This was prompted by concerns about violence and intoxication in and around harbour area bars, especially in the summer when this area was busy with tourists. In response to these concerns, the police carried out a scheme that involved the rigorous enforcement of the existing liquor licensing laws. Uniformed police maintained a frequent and visible presence in the target area. Bar owners were advised that laws relating to opening hours, serving alcohol to those below the minimum legal age of alcohol purchase and serving alcohol to people who were intoxicated, would all be monitored closely. During the year of the operation of this experiment, crimes including those associated with public drunkenness declined by one-fifth. In a nearby 'control' town no such improvement was noted. Once the experiment was abandoned, local crime rates rose again (Jeffs and Saunders 1983). Oddly, this clearly productive experiment was not sustained. Only one British police force, in Sussex, is known to the authors to have made a concerted and explicit attempt at adopting the Torquay approach as part of their long-term policy. This apparent lack of enthusiasm for what appears to be a good idea serves to emphasise two practical points: first, that research findings frequently fail to become widely known; second, alcohol policy has to compete with many other issues as either a local, national or international priority.

The 'Surfers Paradise' project and other community-based initiatives in Australia

The 'Surfers Paradise Safety Action Project' was initiated in 1993 in response to concern about the level of violence associated with the high density of bars in the core area and the effects of this violence not only on the local community but also on tourism. The project involved the police, business owners (including licensees), representatives of the Council, community groups, taxi operators, researchers and others. As described in Graham and Homel:

> A key element of the project was that it provided a structure for focussing the community militancy about safety and security by channelling energy into a Steering Committee, three major task groups, and a Monitoring Committee responsible for overseeing adherence to a Code of Practice developed by night club managers. (1997: 184)

A Project Officer was appointed to oversee all aspects of the project, including setting up three Task Groups (Public Spaces, Security and Policing, and Venue Management), helping to develop ways of increasing levels of awareness and compliance, and implementing the use of a Risk Assessment Policy Checklist for assessing policy compliance by venues. As part of the project, the licensees themselves developed a Code of Practice.

The project was evaluated using a number of different types of data, including police statistics and direct observations by researchers in bars

(Homel and Clark, 1994) and indicated a substantial immediate impact of the programme in terms of both drunkenness and violence. However, as reported by Homel et al.:

> observational data collected over the summer of 1996 indicate that violence has returned to pre-project levels, and that compliance with the Code of Practice has almost ceased. 'It is hypothesized that only a system of regulation that integrates self-regulation, community monitoring, and formal enforcement can ensure that achievements of community interventions are maintained on an indefinite basis.' (1997: 36)

Similar community-based initiatives were developed concurrently with the Surfers Paradise project (Lang and Rumbold 1997) and the approach used in Surfers Paradise has since been replicated in other communities (Hauritz et al. forthcoming). Through these projects, a number of critical features of successful projects have been identified. Homel et al. described the following characteristics of successful community interventions:

> strong directive leadership during the establishment period; the mobilisation of community groups concerned about violence and disorder; the implementation of a multi-agency approach involving licensees, local government, police, health and other groups; the use of safety audits to engage the local community and identify risks; a focus on the way that licensed venues are managed [particularly those that cater to large numbers of young people]; the 're-education' of patrons concerning their role as consumers of 'quality hospitality'; and attention to situational factors, including serving practices that promote intoxication and violent confrontations. (1997: 43)

Lang and Rumbold (1997) noted that several community interventions in Australia showed positive short-term results but these results were not sustained, including the changes that occurred as part of the Surfers Paradise project. Their review identified critical features involved in sustainability of such interventions. First, they recommend that programmes need to change cultural attitudes toward the acceptability of alcohol-related violence. Although regulation and enforcement are a necessary part of community approaches, they are not enough to sustain changes. In addition, ownership of the project by the local community is also a necessary feature for sustainability. They also recommend that licensees must also 'buy into' or 'own' the project and that there needs to be good cooperation between licensees and police. These are similar to factors in sustainability identified generally for community action projects (Holder and Moore forthcoming), including cultural relevance, key leader support, development of local resources, and policy and structural change.

Inside the Bars

Drinking in licensed premises has been associated with problem behaviours including both aggression and drink driving (O'Donnell 1985, Homel et al. 1992). However, there is considerable variability in terms of the 'riskiness' of bars. For example, Stockwell et al. (1991b) found that a sub-sample of bars could be identified whose customers were more likely than customers of other bars to be involved in both assault and drink driving. Observational studies of bar-room aggression have identified some of the characteristics of licensed premises associated with higher levels of aggression and other problem behaviours (Graham et al. 1980, Marsh and Fox-Kibby 1992, Homel and Clark 1994). These include aspects of the physical environment such as care and maintenance of the bar, layout, crowding and noise levels, as well as aspects of the social environment such as low social control and an 'anything goes' atmosphere, poorly trained staff or too few staff, and a high level of intoxication of patrons generally. Accordingly, a recent review (Graham and Homel 1997) recommended the following ways of structuring bars to minimise aggression and other problems: have clean, well-maintained environments that create the expectation that patrons will behave properly (see also Leather and Lawrence 1995 regarding expectations for bar environments); avoid physical environment features that irritate or frustrate people such as extremely loud low-quality music, uncomfortable seating, poor ventilation or line-ups; minimise provocation related to games and entertainment by ensuring that there are clear and well-enforced rules around signing up for turns and expected games behaviour; minimise the potential use of glassware, bottles and furnishings as weapons (for example, using plastic or tempered glass, keeping empty bottles and glasses cleared away); encourage eating with drinking to help keep patrons from becoming intoxicated; foster a positive and pleasant social atmosphere but with clear limits; discourage drinking to intoxication; hire bar staff who are skilled at communicating with people and can be firm in managing problem behaviour while avoiding aggressive encounters (and avoid security staff who like to fight); and ban patrons who are known to be aggressive. The research identifying risky bars provided the basis for the development of an intervention directed at individual bars rather than the community. This intervention, called 'Safer Bars', is described below.

Server Intervention or Responsible Beverage Service Programmes

The 'Safer Bars' programme for reducing aggression and injury in bars was developed in Canada using research summarised by Graham and Homel (1997) which identified the characteristics associated with violence as well as more recent observational studies of bar-room aggression (Wells et al. 1998, Graham et al. forthcoming, Wells and Graham forthcoming). The programme, still in the evaluation phase, includes the following components:

1. *'Assessing and Reducing Risks of Violence'*. This workbook is structured as a self-administered questionnaire and contains the following sections: (a) entering the bar; (b) a safe and friendly atmosphere; (c) layout; (d) physical comfort and safety of customers; (e) setting rules and keeping order; (f) servers and bartenders; (g) security staff; (h) minimising problems; (i) closing time; and a miscellaneous section. The bar owner and/or manager rates his or her bar by answering the questions on the left side of the booklet and then calculates a score for each section with the help of explanations on the right side of the booklet. Each item in the workbook identifies an area of the bar that presents possible risk factors and is potentially changeable, although some aspects may be more difficult or costly to change than others. The intended use of the workbook is to make bar owners *more aware of risk factors and the range of options for them to consider in reducing aggression*. From these options, the bar owner can identify areas where change is most feasible.

2. *'Safer Bars training for bar owners, managers and staff'*. Developed from existing research on bar-room aggression, social psychology, police training and aggression prevention training, the training uses an *experiential peer learning model* which is generally found to be more effective in changing attitudes and building skills than approaches focused simply on learning factual material. The format of the training is mainly interactive, using group discussion, role-play and small group exercises to develop and reinforce changes in knowledge, attitudes and skills. Content of the training includes understanding bar-room aggression, assessing the situation, knowing yourself and keeping your cool, non-verbal communication, responding to problem situations, and legal issues. The training includes a video ('Just Another Night') describing in story format the first few nights' work of a new doorman and a Participant's Workbook, including exercises.

3. *'Do You Know the Law?'* A booklet that provides a summary of legal issues and case studies regarding the laws applying to violence and injury associated with drinking in licensed premises.

The Safer Bars programme is in the final stages of development and evaluation. Interviews with bar owners indicate that they find the workbook for assessing risks to be very thorough and useful. Evaluation of the preliminary training programme received very positive feedback from bar staff who participated in the training and showed a measurable change in knowledge

(Chandler Coutts et al. forthcoming). Research is being planned to evaluate the effectiveness of the programme on actually reducing violence in bars.

Other initiatives directed specifically toward bars have been included in community initiatives described earlier in this chapter. A few stand-alone initiatives include training and certification of door staff in legal issues, fire, and health safety and communication skills (implemented in a number of communities in the UK), and guidelines for model policies addressing such issues as door monitoring, promoting food, staff training and other aspects of bar management prepared by the Responsible Beverage Service Council in Scotts Valley, California.

BROADER COMMUNITY INITIATIVES

Harm minimisation of alcohol-related problems often involves community interventions with multiple components including but not restricted to a focus on bars. The most common issues addressed by these projects are high-risk drinking practices (for example, increased risk of injury associated with drinking to intoxication), underage drinking, drink driving and violence. These projects typically take a number of years to implement (five or more) and, for even highly successful projects, it is often difficult to demonstrate a measurable impact on outcomes (Graham and Chandler Coutts forth-coming), possibly because the impact of the project is weak compared to countervailing forces or because there is a time lag before the full impact of the project is realised (Midford et al. 1998). The following describes several major community-based initiatives designed to reduce harm from alcohol consumption.

Preventing Alcohol Trauma: A Community Trial

From 1991 to 1996, Holder and his colleagues conducted a large-scale evaluation of a community approach to reducing alcohol-related trauma (Holder et al. 1997, *Addiction*, special issue). The project was designed to assess whether a comprehensive community approach could produce measurable effects on key outcomes. The approach involved five components: (1) community mobilisation to increase awareness of alcohol-involved trauma, increase support for interventions that involve structural change in the community environment (such as policy changes), and support for the other components included as part of the programme; (2) responsible beverage service training to reduce intoxication of patrons of licensed establishments and lower the rate of driving or engaging in other risky behaviours while impaired; (3) drink driving interventions aimed at increasing support for enforcement, increasing enforcement and increasing perceptions of the risk of getting caught for impaired driving; (4) interventions to prevent underage drinking, including increased enforcement, training of off-sales clerks and media advocacy to increase attention to the problem; and (5) restricting alcohol access by controlling outlet density. As described in the special issue of *Addiction*, the project included substantial process and outcome evaluation. Measurable impacts were found on alcohol-involved traffic crashes (Voas et al. 1997) and on community support for responsible beverage service training, development of prevention policies (Saltz and Stanghetta 1997) and sales to minors (Grube 1997).

The Lahti Project

This was a collaborative project involving the Finnish Foundation for Alcohol Studies and the World Health Organization's European Office in Copenhagen designed to raise awareness of alcohol issues and to reduce heavy and problematic drinking in a Finnish city during 1993 and 1994. The project differed somewhat from the American trial led by Holder in that the components were not defined in advance. Rather, as described by Holmila (forthcoming), the project involved 'reflexive problem prevention' in that the project incorporated an action research paradigm in which research results were constantly fed back to the community and formed part of the thinking for subsequent definitions of problems. The project involved a range of community-based actions including examining views on alcohol policies by key local people, a brief intervention in primary health care, educational events, youth and family work, sales surveillance, and the promotion of the responsible service of alcohol and server training for bar staff (Holmila 1997). The main impact of the project was on increased awareness of defining and addressing alcohol problems at the community level rather than an exclusive focus on alcohol control policies. As described by Holmila:

> Attitudes to alcohol problems changed. The proportion of those citizens who considered drinking to be a serious problem grew during the project. There were system-level changes amongst the municipality's employees and the voluntary groups in the community in the ways of seeing the prevention of alcohol problems as part of ordinary daily work and changes in the community's response to alcohol problems were achieved. Mini-intervention for heavy drinkers spread from a few experimental centres to include all the primary health care centres in the city. (1997: 204)

Overall consumption did not decrease as a result of the intervention; however, there was a significant decrease in alcohol consumption by the heaviest-drinking group compared to a similar group in a comparison community.

Community Mobilisation for the Prevention of Alcohol-Related Injury (COMPARI)

The COMPARI project was begun as a university-initiated, three-year demonstration project in 1991 in Western Australia and provides a good example of a project that involved successful transfer from university-based research to community ownership (Boots and Midford 1998), a key factor in sustainability of interventions. The initial project was undertaken to demonstrate that alcohol-related injury could be reduced using a community mobilisation approach involving community development, environmental change, mass media campaigns and health education. The project developed over 22 different activities related to these goals during the three-year implementation phase. In subsequent years, many activities were continued and the COMPARI programme developed into an ongoing community-based programme. Boots and Midford (1998) attributed the success of the programme to a focus on action, financial support from various agencies at crucial junctures, competent and dedicated staff, a powerful and diverse steering committee, and exploitation of opportunities by those involved in the project.

Although the COMPARI project was hugely successful in its adoption by the local community, it was more difficult to demonstrate effects on the overall rate of alcohol-related injury. Midford et al. (1998) conducted time series analyses on the rate of night-time assaults and traffic crashes, hospital morbidity related to alcohol use, and hospital emergency use for the period 1991–6. They found no significant effects for the time period under study, but some data for subsequent years indicated a possible emerging impact of the intervention following 1996. They concluded that monitoring change over a longer period than the typical duration of a project may be needed to demonstrate the effects of community mobilisation projects.

Alcohol-Impaired Driving

In many countries, the reduction in drink driving has been one of the most successful alcohol-related harm reduction efforts to date (Homel et al. 1988, Beirness et al. 1993, Mathijssen and Wesemann 1993, Berger and Marelich 1997). It is likely that many factors have contributed to this reduction (see Williams 1992), including grassroots movements such as Mothers Against Drunk Driving (MADD) and a related growing intolerance on the part of the public, increased risks or perceptions of risk of getting caught through random breath-testing and other increased enforcement by police (Homel et al. 1988), increased penalties for drink driving, and increased legal liability (and increased awareness of liability) of alcohol servers for injuries resulting from irresponsible serving.

The North Karelia Project

A fine example from outside the alcohol field of what may be achieved by wide-ranging and sustained community action has been provided by the Finnish North Karelia Project. This famous health promotion initiative succeeded in reducing levels of mortality from heart disease by 70% over a period of more than 20 years. The project involved mobilising key people and agencies in whole communities in order to change lifestyles, diet, and the type of food being produced, distributed and consumed. It also involved persuading people to abandon traditional unhealthy diets including too much salt and dairy fats and to transform both eating and smoking habits (Puska et al. 1995).

The examples included in the present study also provide promise of new methods to decrease alcohol-related harm. The community studies directed toward reducing problems in and around bars have demonstrated that these approaches can be highly successful; however, more work needs to be done to ensure the sustainability of such projects. Means of institutionalising successful interventions might include building continuing community support, implementing and enforcing policies that extend beyond the project, and making effective training programmes for bar staff part of standard licensing criteria, as has been done for Responsible Beverage Service programmes in some American states. The examples of community initiatives from the US, Australia and Finland also provide promise of successful approaches to reducing harm. While reductions in harm demonstrated within a particular project tend to be modest, the evidence from these efforts suggests that the projects may help to change the overall attitudes and structure of communities in ways that facilitate future prevention. It should be noted that dramatic decreases in tobacco smoking and drink driving that have occurred over the past 20 or so years did not develop from a single project; rather there appeared to be a cumulative effect of attitude change and environmental policies that ultimately showed a major impact.

In conclusion, it should be noted that there have been a vast number of local attempts to 'do something about alcohol problems'. Many – probably the vast majority – of these have not been documented, and relatively few have ever appeared in scientific journals. Even so, there is a growing body of documented examples that provide useful models for harm minimisation. Three considerations are crucial to the value of measures intended to reduce or minimise the level of specific alcohol problems. First, such strategies have to be socially or politically acceptable in the context in which they are implemented. Countries and localities within countries often have very varied traditions and beliefs about both drinking and how to keep alcohol-related problems in check. Strategies are needed which are socially and culturally appropriate. Second, there should be at least some evidence that a strategy is likely to be effective. Third, to retain its value, any successful strategy must be sustained. Key factors in the success of community action projects are described in more detail by Graham and Chandler Coutts (forth-coming) and Holder and Moore (forthcoming) as part of a future special issue of the journal *Substance Use and Misuse*.

8
Clinical Responses

This chapter explores the issue of the management of people who present with drinking problems. It is important to recognise that the views of many professionals have changed greatly in the past 20 years or so. There is more evidence, but also fewer certainties, than previously. For this reason, this chapter is in three distinct sections.

Section A, by Nick Heather, is, as one would expect from him, an elegant and erudite exploration of the current literature on psychosocial interventions. It is notable that whereas we used to believe that some treatments were better than others, people in the treatment field are having to acknowledge that there may be precious little to choose between them. In terms of one- or two-year outcomes, one intervention seems to produce much the same results as another, as do so-called 'spontaneous remission' rates. So it might be that what we need to look at more rigorously is what people do with treatment, what treatments people perceive to be beneficial, and why. In other words, we need to look at what people do with treatment, rather than what treatment does to people.

Section B, by Colin Bennie, Iain McKinney and David Campbell, describes a home detoxification service. In the UK, such agencies are burgeoning, often as an alternative to in-patient care. They have shown a high degree of customer satisfaction, are popular with health care professionals and, as one would now expect, their outcomes appear to be as good as those obtained by in-patient drying-out facilities. Home detoxification is also possibly cheaper than some alternative modes of management.

Section C of this chapter takes us somewhere quite different. 'Complementary' or 'alternative' therapies are becoming increasingly popular in many fields, including that of alcohol problems. Such approaches have been gaining ground for a variety of medical and psychological problems, and many 'conventional' practitioners now acknowledge that such approaches may be of value, either as stand-alone interventions or as adjuncts to existing interventions. Good alternative practitioners operate from a coherent, often ancient, set of beliefs about the nature of humankind. Although these beliefs are a long way from conventional Western medicine, they have a history long antedating our current beliefs and methods. It is appropriate that in this age of uncertainty the views of alternative practitioners are not discounted out of hand. Hence the inclusion of a wide-ranging introduction to this field by Diwakar Sukul, a practitioner who is a specialist in this area.

Perhaps there is something very basic that we need to attend to in our treatment efforts. That it is up to us to instil hope. Whether the interventions are psychosocial, medical or 'alternative', it is our job as practitioners to enable people to see that, with or without our various diverse forms of help, change is possible.

A: Psychosocial Treatment Approaches and the Findings of Project MATCH*

Nick Heather

Project MATCH in the US was the largest and most expensive evaluation of treatment for alcohol problems, or indeed of psychosocial treatment for any kind of disorder, ever carried out, involving 1,726 problem drinkers at a cost of over US$27 million. If for no other reason, the sheer size of this project demands that its findings should be taken very seriously when considering the effectiveness of different approaches to the treatment of alcohol problems.

However, before discussing the implications of MATCH findings for treatment practice, this section of Chapter 8 will trace the history, development and current status of two of the treatment approaches included in Project MATCH. The project was designed to compare three types of psychosocial (that is, non-drug) treatments:

1. cognitive-behavioural therapy (CBT)
2. motivational enhancement therapy (MET) and
3. twelve-step facilitation therapy (TSF) which was based on the philosophy and methods of Alcoholics Anonymous and its famous 'Twelve-step' recovery programme.

Although other broad approaches to the treatment of alcohol problems could be identified, these three were considered to be either the most popular forms of treatment in the US or those with the greatest support from the research literature, thus representing in the minds of the MATCH investigators those treatment approaches most relevant to progress in the field. We will now consider the provenance, the underlying treatment philosophy and the research evidence relevant to CBT and MET.

COGNITIVE-BEHAVIOURAL THERAPY

Origins

The beginnings of CBT in the alcohol field coincided with the introduction following the Second World War of behaviour therapy methods, based on theories of learning developed by psychologists, for a range of psychiatric disorders. This culminated in a wave of enthusiasm for behavioural treatments during the 1960s. At this time, however, these methods were sometimes crude and were derived from a mechanistic learning theory founded mainly on the results of experiments with infra-human species (notably the white Norwegian rat). In the alcohol field, chemical aversion therapy, based on the principles of Pavlovian conditioning theory and using emetine to induce nausea after drinking alcohol, was being given to problem drinkers as early as the 1940s. This type of aversion therapy was reported to yield very encouraging success rates but none of the research studies in question used control groups and they were all concerned with well-off, fee-paying clients who would probably have done well with any kind of treatment. While advocates for aversion therapy may still be found (for example, Rimmele et al. 1995), this general treatment method has been largely abandoned in the UK, chiefly because it is thought that there are more effective and less unpleasant ways of achieving the same goal of a reduction in alcohol problems.

Following the first wave of behavioural treatments, there occurred a revolutionary change in psychology and behavioural science, with profound implications for the treatment of many disorders. On the theoretical level, this took the form of a rejection of the mechanistic, animal-based learning theory on which the earlier forms of behaviour therapy had been based. In its place, Albert Bandura (1969) in particular, but many other scientists too, advocated a conception of the learning process in which its specifically human aspects were represented. Thus, this new theory recognised that much human learning was acquired by observation and modelling (that is, imitation) of other human beings. So too, the role of cognitions – expectancies, causal attributions and beliefs related to the self or to others and both conscious and unconscious – was incorporated into learning theory. This does not mean that more basic forms of learning – chiefly classical (Pavlovian) and operant (Skinnerian) conditioning – were now seen as irrelevant; rather, these more primitive conditioning processes were seen as finding expression in behaviour via the human capacity for thought and language. This new account of human learning was called *social learning theory* (Bandura 1977).

On a more practical level, 'the cognitive revolution' in learning theory led to the introduction of much more sophisticated forms of behaviour therapy. The central place of cognitions in behaviour change was emphasised and methods were developed aimed at modifying distorted and otherwise unhelpful expectations and beliefs, together with their maladaptive effects on behaviour. However, a distinction must immediately be made between what has become known as *cognitive therapy* and the *cognitive-behavioural therapy* with which we are concerned here. The former was developed mainly by Aaron Beck and his followers and was initially focused on the treatment of depression (see, for example, Beck et al. 1979) where it has achieved considerable success. The aim of cognitive therapy is to modify maladaptive beliefs and other cognitions that are thought to underlie the disorder without attempting directly to change behaviour itself; the assumption is that if the maladaptive cognitions can be reversed, the emotional and behavioural problems will resolve themselves. Cognitive therapy has been applied to substance-use disorders (Beck et al. 1993), but a recent review of the available evidence (Miller et al. 1998) shows that this approach had only limited success in treating alcohol problems.

CBT, on the other hand, places more emphasis on the direct modification of behaviour in the treatment process. One way of putting this is that cognitive-behaviour therapy owes much to the older behaviour therapy tradition of encouraging altered *performance*, whereas cognitive therapy lies within the psychotherapeutic tradition of 'talk therapy'. Thus CBT relies heavily on performance-based methods such as relaxation, behaviour rehearsal, role-play and homework assignments in which new ways of behaving are tried out. Rather than Beck's work, the main theoretical influences on CBT were Thoresen and Mahoney's (1974) self-control theory, Meichenbaum's (1977) work on 'self-talk', D'Zurilla and Goldfried's (1971) problem-solving principles and Bandura's (1978) self-efficacy theory, as well as, more directly, Marlatt and Gordon's (1985) relapse-prevention approach to addictive disorders. The distinction between the two types of therapy should not be overstretched; cognitive therapists often set their clients homework assignments, and cognitive-behavioural therapists may use 'cognitive restructuring' to modify expectations that may interfere with recovery, such as the belief that a full relapse is inevitable after any amount to drink (see

Marlatt and Gordon 1985). Nevertheless, the distinction in principle is clear and these two approaches to the treatment of alcohol problems should not be confused.

Treatment Philosophy and Components

The basic philosophy underlying CBT has already been touched on in the preceding paragraphs. The cognitive-behavioural perspective is based on the assumption that problem drinking, like any kind of drinking, is predominantly learned behaviour. (The role of genetic predisposition to develop alcohol dependence or problems would be conceded by most cognitive-behavioural therapists, but they would still insist that the individual form that the drinking takes, and whether or not the inherited predisposition actually results in problem drinking, must be learned in a particular environmental and social context.) The broad aim of CBT, therefore, is to achieve an 'unlearning' of destructive or maladaptive patterns of behaviour and replace them with healthier and more adaptive patterns associated with the improved quality of life the client desires. This improved quality of life can be sought, depending on client characteristics and circumstances, either by aiming the client at total abstinence from alcohol or at moderate drinking. But these are not, as is often implied in discussions of treatment for alcohol problems, the goals of treatment, they are merely the means by which the ultimate goal of the client's improved satisfaction with life is brought about.

As also noted above, another crucial assumption of CBT is that performance-based methods are superior to talk-based methods in producing the desired changes in behaviour, at least as far as the treatment of alcohol problems and other forms of addictive behaviour is concerned. There is indeed evidence to support this assumption, both from comparative studies of treatment for behavioural disorders in general (see Bandura 1977) and specifically in the treatment of alcohol problems (for example, Chaney et al. 1978, Oei and Jackson 1980).

Another crucial feature of the CBT approach to alcohol problems is that it covers a wide diversity of specific modalities and methods, although all of these subscribe to the underlying treatment philosophy just sketched. CBT modalities include behavioural marital therapy, the community reinforcement approach, skills training (including social skills, assertiveness and communications skills training), anxiety management, anger management, behavioural self-control training, covert sensitisation (a form of aversion therapy conducted entirely in imagination), cue exposure and several others. Among the many therapeutic methods and procedures commonly employed in CBT are relaxation training, behaviour contracting, problem-solving skills training, behaviour rehearsal, role-play, role-reversal, self-monitoring, self-reinforcement training, functional analysis of high-risk situations, drink refusal skills, and so on (for a fuller description of these various modalities and methods, see Heather 1995; for a detailed discussion of some of the more prominent modalities, see Hester and Miller 1995; for a more 'how-to-do-it' coverage, see Jarvis et al. 1995).

Sometimes the distinction between modalities and methods is hard to sustain because many of the methods have at some time been elevated to the status of self-contained treatment modalities. The important point here, though, is that the CBT approach offers the therapist a wide range of thera-peutic procedures and specific targets that can be adjusted to the needs, circumstances or preferences of the individual client. This stands in contrast to many treatment philosophies that preceded CBT in which one standard approach was offered to all clients, irrespective of their needs or wishes. During the 1970s, the CBT feature of multimodal treatment was dignified by the term *broad spectrum approach*. While this term is now seldom used, the principle still very much applies: CBT offers a rich variety of aims and methods that can be tailored to the requirements of the individual client.

A final, general feature of CBT should be noted before moving on. This is that it is intimately linked with a much wider body of behavioural theory and research. This includes basic research on the determinants of human behaviour and the conditions under which changes in behaviour occur, as well as more clinical research on interventions for a wide range of psychi-atric disorders and other types of problem. Thus, for the first time in the history of treatment for alcohol problems, CBT can claim to be a genuinely *scientific* approach to treatment, one that is responsive to research evidence and to theoretical advances. Advocates of CBT do not claim that it is the last word on effective treatment for problem drinking but would assert that, because of its scientific foundations and commitment to objective evalua-tion, it has a built-in potential for improvement.

Coping Skills Therapy

One type of CBT modality will be described in more detail because it formed the basis of the CBT intervention that was examined in Project MATCH. This is the coping skills programme developed by Peter Monti and his colleagues (1989). This approach sees problem drinking and alcohol depen-dence essentially as a habitual, maladaptive way of coping with stress. Stress may occur for a variety of reasons – as a result of particular life events, more general lifestyle factors, acute situational factors, behavioural deficits deriving from the individual's social learning history, or a biological vulner-ability to stress. 'Coping' is the individual's attempt to meet the demands placed upon him or her by the stressor. However, if the individual's coping skills are inadequate to meet these demands, and depending again on the person's learning history, alcohol may be used in an attempt to reduce stress. The task in treatment therefore is to train the individual in ways of coping with identified stressors without resort to drinking.

Monti et al.'s programme is intended to be delivered on a group basis and is divided into two main components: interpersonal skills and intrapersonal skills. In the interpersonal component, following an introductory session aimed at building group cohesion and assessing individual problems, further sessions are targeted at various aspects of communications skills, assertiveness training, drink refusal skills and enhancing social networks. Such interpersonal skills are seen as important both because they improve the client's ability to cope with high-risk situations and because they provide a means of attracting the social support that is critical to recovery. The intrapersonal component includes many of the standard ingredients of CBT packages: managing thoughts about alcohol, problem solving, increasing pleasant activities, relaxation training, anger management, managing negative thinking and coping with persistent problems. Good evidence for the clinical effectiveness of this coping skills approach was obtained by Monti et al. (1990).

Relapse Prevention

The coping skills approach was also heavily influenced by Marlatt and Gordon's (1985) work on relapse prevention and this has been of major importance for the development of CBT generally. The relapse prevention (RP) perspective begins with the observation that alcohol dependence, like all addictive behaviours, is a highly relapsing condition; the main challenge in treatment is not so much to bring about an initial change in drinking behaviour, which is relatively easy, but to ensure that this change persists after treatment has ended. A key concept here is the 'high-risk situation', that is, situations with a high probability of relapse in the individual case. Research (for example, Cummings et al. 1980) has established that the most common high-risk situations for problem drinkers are negative emotional states (frustration, anger, anxiety, depression, boredom, and so on), interpersonal conflicts and social pressure (either direct or indirect in the sense of simply observing others drinking). If the client is able to perform an effective coping response to the high-risk situation, he or she will experience a sense of mastery and control over that situation, and an increase in 'self-efficacy' for dealing with future high-risk situations of the same kind; the probability of relapse will be reduced. When the person does not possess an adequate coping response, he or she is likely to experience a decrease in self-efficacy and a feeling of helplessness in dealing with the situation. Moreover, if the person holds 'positive outcome expectancies' regarding the effects of alcohol (that is, has learned to expect that drinking will provide an immediate and temporary way of coping with stress), the likelihood of a return to drinking will be much increased.

Whether or not this initial 'lapse' leads to further drinking depends on how it is perceived by the client. The *abstinence violation effect* (AVE), which is more or less equivalent to the belief that 'one may as well be hanged for a sheep as a lamb', will move the client towards a full relapse.

RP methods can be divided into *specific intervention strategies* and *global self-control strategies*. The goal of the specific strategies is to help the client to recognise and anticipate high-risk situations, to teach alternative ways of coping with these situations and to modify cognitive and emotional responses to them. In RP training, clients are taught to be their own thera-pists because the situations for which coping is necessary will continue to crop up after the formal treatment programme has ended. It is assumed that, having successfully practised them in particular high-risk situations, the client will be able to generalise coping skills to other tempting situations.

A second set of techniques belonging to the specific strategies is concerned with the client's reactions after a lapse or temporary return to drinking has taken place, as it probably will. Cognitive restructuring tech-niques, together with more practical plans for dealing with emergency situations, are aimed at helping the client to counteract the cognitive and emotional aspects of the AVE and preventing the lapse from turning into a full-blown relapse to heavy drinking.

The global self-control part of the RP programme is aimed at encouraging a comprehensive change in lifestyle so that relapse is made less likely. The client is encouraged to find avenues for rewarding experiences that do not involve drinking. This may involve taking up old hobbies and interests, or 'positive addictions' like meditation or physical exercise. Finally, the client may be given help to control the occasional urges and cravings for alcohol that will inevitably arise despite carefully planned avoidance and coping strategies.

The main principle underlying all these techniques is that it is in the client's best interests to anticipate and fully discuss the possibilities for relapse with the therapist during the active treatment phase as a preparation for the temptation that will undoubtedly arise in the real world. In tradi-tional treatment programmes, discussion of relapse was eschewed because it was believed that such discussion would somehow give the client 'permis-sion' to relapse. The RP treatment philosophy is based on the very different assumption that anticipating and preparing for high-risk relapse situations, in the same way perhaps that a fire-drill anticipates and prepares for a fire, is the best way to avoid their destructive consequences.

Effectiveness of Cognitive-Behavioural Therapy

Over the past 20 years, W.R. Miller and his colleagues from the University of New Mexico have compiled, up-dated and periodically published reviews of research on the outcome of treatment for alcohol problems. The latest and most ambitious of these reviews (Miller et al. 1998) resulted in a large table (or, in Spanish, *Mesa Grande*) in which the results of 302 controlled trials of treatment outcome were summarised. Studies entering the *Mesa Grande* were confined to controlled trials, usually *randomised* controlled trials, in which characteristics of clients receiving the treatments to be compared were equated before treatment began. Because of the ethical impossibility of withholding treatment from those who need or request it, the great majority of studies compared different types or intensities of treatment or the same type of treatment with and without the addition of a special therapeutic component. All controlled trials published up to 1996 comparing at least two treatment or control conditions and reporting post-treatment outcome on at least one measure of alcohol consumption or alcohol-related problems were included in the review. Unpublished studies were also included if a full report describing the results was available. The *Mesa Grande* is reproduced in Table 8.1.

Table 8.1: The *Mesa Grande*

Modality	% Clinical	MQS	N+	N–	CES
Brief Intervention	46%	12.68	19	9	+221
Motivational Enhancement	54%	13.31	10	3	+145
Social Skills Training	88%	10.94	11	6	+120
Community Reinforcement Approach	75%	13.25	4	0	+80
GABA Agonist Medication	100%	12.00	3	0	+72
Opioid Antagonist Medication	100%	11.00	3	0	+66
Behaviour Contracting	100%	10.40	4	1	+64
Client-Centered Therapy	80%	10.40	4	1	+47
Aversion Therapy (Nausea)	100%	10.05	3	3	+36
Marital Therapy (Cognitive-Behavioural)	100%	12.86	4	3	+34
Behavioural Self-Control Training	68%	12.94	17	17	+25
Cognitive Therapy	86%	10.26	3	4	+22
Aversion Therapy (Apnea)	100%	9.66	2	1	+18
Covert Sensitisation	100%	10.88	3	5	+18
Acupuncture	100%	9.67	2	1	+14
Antidipsotropic-Disulfiram	100%	10.76	10	11	+09
Self-Help Manual	60%	12.00	2	3	+01
Aversion Therapy (Electrical)	100%	11.13	7	9	–03
Marital Therapy (Other)	100%	12.25	4	4	–11
Placebo Medication	100%	13.00	1	2	–27
Stress Management	80%	11.00	1	4	–29
Lithium Medication	100%	11.43	3	4	–32
Functional Analysis	67%	12.00	0	3	–36
Relapse Prevention	75%	11.75	5	11	–37

Table 8.1: (*cont...*)

Modality	% Clinical	MQS	N+	N–	CES
Self-Monitoring	100%	13.00	1	2	–37
Antidepressant (SSRI)	36%	8.45	5	6	–38
Hypnosis	100%	10.25	0	4	–41
Psychedelic Medication	100%	9.88	2	6	–45
Antidipsotropic-Calcium Carbamide	100%	10.00	0	3	–52
Antidepressant Medication (non-SSRI)	100%	8.75	0	4	–59
'Standard' Treatment	80%	10.20	1	4	–67
Milieu Therapy	93%	11.00	3	11	–78
Anxiolytic Medication	100%	8.25	3	9	–79
Videotape Self-Confrontation	100%	10.29	0	7	–84
Alcoholics Anonymous (mandated)	80%	11.40	1	4	–90
Antidipsotropic Metronidazole	100%	9.64	1	10	–102
Relaxation Training	69%	10.81	3	13	–135
Confrontational Counselling	67%	11.67	0	9	–155
Psychotherapy	86%	11.21	2	12	–163
General Alcoholism Counselling	84%	11.20	2	17	–226
Educational Lectures/Films	35%	9.68	4	27	–364
Treatment Methods With Only One or Two Outcome Studies					
Sensory Deprivation	0	10.00	2	0	+40
Biofeedback	100%	13.00	2	0	+38
Cue Exposure	100%	10.00	2	0	+32
Developmental Counselling	0	14.00	1	0	+28
Meditation	100%	12.00	1	0	+24
Assessment Only	0	11.00	1	0	+22
Dopamine Antagonist	100%	11.00	1	0	+22
Sedative-Hypnotic Medication	100%	11.00	1	0	+22
Feedback	0	10.00	1	0	+20
Unilateral Family Therapy	0	10.00	1	0	+20
Case Management	100%	11.00	1	0	+11
Exercise	50%	10.50	1	1	+09
Twelve-Step Facilitation	100%	17.00	1	1	00
Tobacco Cessation	100%	6.00	0	1	–06
Minnesota Model	100%	11.50	1	1	–10
Surveillance	100%	11.00	0	1	–11
Neurotherapy	100%	12.00	0	1	–12
Problem Solving	100%	12.00	0	1	–12
Legal Interventions	0	11.00	0	1	–22
BAC Discrimination Training	100%	12.00	0	2	–24
Choice of Treatments	50%	8.00	1	1	–24
Beta Blocker Medication	100%	13.00	0	1	–26
Serotonin Agonist Medication	50%	11.50	0	2	–34
Antipsychotic Medication	100%	9.00	0	2	–36
Dopamine Agonist Medication	100%	9.00	0	2	–36
Placebo Medication	100%	11.00	0	2	–44

Source: Reproduced with permission from W.R. Miller, N.R. Andrews, P. Wilbourne and M.E. Bennett (1998), 'A wealth of alternatives: effective treatments for alcohol problems', in W.R. Miller and N. Heather (eds), *Treating Addictive Behaviors*, 2nd edition. New York: Plenum, pp. 203–16.

Two independent raters judged the methodological quality of all studies included in the *Mesa Grande* on 12 dimensions, resulting in a methodological quality score (MQS) for each study. Outcome logic scores (OLS) were arrived at by a similar rating process and resulted in a classification of each study as providing strong positive evidence (+2), positive evidence (+1), negative evidence (–1) or strong negative evidence (–2) for a particular treatment modality. The MQS and OLS were then multiplied for each study to arrive at a weighting of the study's contribution to the evidence on treatment outcome by its methodological quality. These products were then summed across all studies bearing on the effectiveness of a specific treatment modality, resulting in the cumulative evidence score (CES) for each modality shown in Table 8.1.

The CES can be interpreted as summarising the balance of evidence for and against the effectiveness of a particular treatment approach, with high positive scores reflecting treatments with a large amount of evidence in their favour, high negative scores reflecting treatments associated with a large amount of mainly unfavourable evidence, and intermediate scores reflecting either a small number of studies in total or a larger number of studies with conflicting evidence.

To avoid the temptation of drawing inferences from a very small number of studies, the *Mesa Grande* has a separate section for modalities tested in only one or two studies at the time the review was concluded. If any modality is not mentioned at all in Table 8.1, it is because there had been no controlled evaluations of its effectiveness at the time. Also shown in Table 8.1 are: (i) the number of positive (N+) and negative (N–) studies reviewed for each modality, (ii) the mean MQS (range 0–17) reflecting the overall quality of research on each modality; and (iii) a rating of the severity of problems in the client population for each modality, expressed as a percentage of studies dealing with a clinical population of individuals seeking treatment for significant alcohol problems or dependence (as opposed to a non-clinical population of problem drinkers or 'normal controls').

One of the most striking aspects of the *Mesa Grande* is that most of the modalities obtaining the highest CESs are CBT approaches. These include some of the modalities that have already been mentioned: social skills training (3rd), the community reinforcement approach (4th), behaviour contracting (7th), cognitive-behavioural marital therapy (10th) and behavioural self-control training (11th). All these treatments are based on the principles of social learning theory and all are performance-based. There is some evidence to support purely cognitive treatment methods, grouped under the modality 'cognitive therapy' (12th in Table 8.1), but this is less consistent and impressive than the evidence in favour of cognitive-behavioural methods. One of the new pharmacotherapies that have recently been developed to treat alcohol problems (opioid antagonist medication (that is, Naltrexone), 5th in Table 8.1) has been shown to work best if used in combination with cognitive-behavioural methods (O'Malley et al 1992).

The modality that obtains the highest CES in the *Mesa Grande* is 'brief intervention'. This covers a wide range of methods directed at problem drinkers with relatively mild alcohol problems and levels of dependence. They are often delivered by non-specialists, mainly general medical practitioners, following screening for excessive drinking among people who are not seeking help for drinking problems. The point for present purposes is that many of these brief interventions take the form of condensed versions of CBT (see, for example, Sanchez-Craig et al. 1987), although, as we shall see, motivational components feature very prominently in brief interventions too.

It will also be seen that the category 'relapse prevention' obtains a negative CES in the *Mesa Grande*. This occurs because when RP has been evaluated as a treatment modality in its own right, it has obtained mixed support (for example, Annis and Chan 1983). However, as indicated above, the chief influence of RP has been as a therapeutic principle that is used to inform demonstrably effective coping skills programmes (Chaney et al. 1978, Monti et al. 1990).

The evidence of the *Mesa Grande* supports the conclusion that CBT modalities in general represent the most effective forms of treatment for alcohol problems. This has indeed been the conclusion of other (for example, Heather and Tebbutt 1989, Mattick and Jarvis 1993), although not all (Riley et al. 1987), reviews of the alcohol treatment literature. But a caveat must be introduced here. In addition to their being well-supported by the evidence, CBT modalities are also the most intensively researched forms of treatment in the field. This is because they were initiated as treatments after the widespread introduction of clinical trial methodology and also because they were developed by behavioural scientists whose training emphasised the need for rigorous evaluation. It may be that the reason some other treatment modalities fare poorly in the *Mesa Grande* is because they are under-researched and there is little evidence either for or against their effectiveness. This may apply to 'Twelve-step facilitation' which has a very low positive CES in Table 8.1 but has only two studies making up this CES, therefore placing it in the section of the *Mesa Grande* for modalities 'with only one or two outcome studies'. In any event, as we shall see below, the results of Project MATCH have considerably changed the verdict on the effectiveness of Twelve-step facilitation.

MOTIVATIONAL INTERVIEWING/ MOTIVATIONAL ENHANCEMENT THERAPY

Origins

Anyone involved in treating alcohol problems will know that people who present to agencies do not all come with a definite commitment to change. Even when a problem drinker seems to be convinced that some change is necessary, there is nearly always a lingering attachment to heavy drinking and intoxication, and a profound ambivalence towards alcohol; according to one of the most influential accounts of addictive behaviour presented in recent years (Orford 1985), conflict and ambivalence are at the heart of the addictive experience.

These observations formed the background for the development of a relatively new approach to alcohol problems treatment, called *motivational interviewing* (MI), which was first described in a classic paper by William R. Miller in 1983. Miller was initially influenced by the client-centred therapy of Carl Rogers (1951), but MI differs from the classical, non-directive counselling style and is a unique treatment approach in its own right. The rationale, applications and effectiveness of motivational interviewing have been explored over the last decade by Miller and his co-workers and it has become increasingly widely used during that time. It is one of the most important, if not *the* most important, innovation in the field in recent times. MET, which is one of the foci of this section, is the version of MI that was evaluated in Project MATCH.

Part of the appeal of MI may be ascribed to the popularity of another innovation in the addictions field occurring during the 1980s – the *stages of change model* developed by James Prochaska and Carlo DiClemente (1986, 1992). The model is based on observations that, when changing behaviour in significant ways, people pass through similar stages and use similar processes of change. The key concept is 'readiness for change', which is seen as an internal state influenced by outside factors. The traditional concept of treatment motivation can be seen as the person's readiness to change the specific behaviour in question. Thus the theoretical basis of MI fits very neatly with Prochaska and DiClemente's model, especially given the importance in the model of the *contemplation* stage of change; MI is the principal way in which therapists attempt to move people from the contemplation stage to the preparation and action stages of change.

Treatment Philosophy

Before stating what MI is, it will be useful to say what it is not. A traditional view in the alcohol treatment field is that the problem drinker (or 'alcoholic') is someone who shows denial of his or her disease of alcoholism, a resistance to being helped to recover from it and a number of other defence mechanisms all aimed at insulating the person from reality and the need for change. These defence mechanisms are said to be deeply ingrained in the alcoholic's character and, indeed, define the nature of the condition. As a result, the alcoholic client is regarded as a habitual liar who cannot be trusted to cooperate with treatment, and his or her lack of contact with reality can be used as a justification for 'treatment' against his or her will, something that is commonplace in the US (see Weisner 1990). The only possible way of overcoming the alcoholic's rigid defences is to batter the alcoholic into submission and an acceptance of the label of alcoholism by a process of aggressive confrontation with the reality of his or her situation.

Given the popularity of this kind of confrontational approach to helping problem drinkers, particularly in the US, it is perhaps surprising that there is no evidence whatever to support it. It appears that problem drinkers at all levels of severity do not show more 'denial' and 'resistance' than people without drinking problems; and that those who accept the label of 'alcoholism' do no better, and may actually do worse, than those who reject it (see Miller and Rollnick 1991). When compared to alternative approaches to counselling, confrontation has been found to be less effective and to be harmful for clients with low self-esteem (Annis and Chan 1983). Although often associated with the Twelve-step philosophy, the confrontational approach runs entirely counter to the spirit of the writings of Bill Wilson, the co-founder of Alcoholics Anonymous (Alcoholics Anonymous 1980).

In view of the lack of evidence to justify it, the popularity of the confrontational approach is mysterious but there are ways of trying to explain it. One possibility is that confrontation actually creates the very behaviour it seeks to overcome in the manner of a self-fulfilling prophecy. If the therapist adopts a hostile and authoritarian posture towards the client, insisting that the client is fundamentally misguided and that only the therapist knows best, the client is likely to respond in an opposite direction by denying that the problem is as serious as the therapist asserts. This is because of a basic psychological mechanism called *reactance* in which people react to a perception that their autonomy is being threatened by a spirited assertion of their personal freedom and individuality. This is especially likely given the profoundly ambivalent feelings the client will usually have about drinking alcohol.

Hence the so-called denial and resistance shown by the client, and taken by the therapist as confirmation of a pre-existing personality disorder, is not some inherent ingredient of the client's character structure but rather a product of a particular kind of interaction between therapist and client. More generally, motivation is not an immutable personality trait residing *inside* the individual which different clients possess to a greater or lesser degree; it is, at least in significant part, a variable property of the interaction between the individual and those attempting to alter his or her behaviour.

Principles and Strategies of Motivational Interviewing

It will not be possible here to give anything like an adequate account of the thinking behind motivational interviewing or the guiding principles, strategies and methods that form part of this general approach to counselling in the addictions. Only the main general features of motivational interviewing and its differences from other perspectives on counselling will be briefly mentioned. For a detailed introduction to motivational interviewing, the interested reader is referred to Miller and Rollnick (1991).

In relation to problem drinking, MI is a highly practical approach to counselling which aims to help clients build commitment and reach a firm decision to change harmful drinking patterns. It is a general method for helping people to recognise the nature of their actual or potential problems with alcohol and take action to solve these problems. One of the keys to understanding the approach is the rule that responsibility for change is left with the client, because that is the only way in which genuine change can occur. The therapist's or counsellor's overriding task is to create an atmosphere in which the client can freely explore his or her concerns and take the first steps towards making lifestyle changes.

The counsellor has a clear agenda in MI which is to actively direct the client, albeit subtly and persuasively, towards change. Although empathic reflection of the client's concerns is a cornerstone of both client-centred counselling and MI, in the latter, reflection is used selectively and is combined with a number of other techniques and skills aimed at tipping the motivational balance in the direction of change. At appropriate points, the counsellor can provide feedback on the consequences of the client's drinking and, when asked, advice. Rather than passively following the client's own directions, the counsellor actively attempts to create a discrepancy between what the client is and what he or she would like to be, and strengthens the client's confidence in being able to do something about his or her drinking.

Thus MI differs sharply from the confrontational style of counselling in ways that have already been described. It also differs from the cognitive-behavioural (or coping skills training) approach in that it avoids teaching and prescribing specific coping strategies. MI can be used as a forerunner to skills training for those clients who reach the action or maintenance stages of change. Often, however, and especially for those whose problems are less severe, a relatively short course of MI will be all that is needed to propel the client along the path towards change. As hopefully has been made clear, MI is ideally suited to those clients who express ambivalence about the need to change drinking behaviour, that is, those in the contemplation stage of change.

Applications of Motivational Interviewing

MI is important as a general approach to counselling and an overall style of interaction which can and should permeate all interviews with problem drinkers. However, its main principles have also been translated into special intervention programmes for specific purposes.

The leading example here is the *Drinker's Check-up* (DCU) described by Miller et al. (1988). The complete DCU consists of two sessions: a two-hour comprehensive assessment, and a return visit a week later when clients receive feedback of assessment results as part of a motivational interview. The assessment measures include a comprehensive profile of drinking behaviour, blood tests for the measurement of liver enzymes indicating excessive drinking, neuropsychological tests sensitive to alcohol's effects on the brain, and a survey of reasons for drinking and measures of alcohol-related problems. Thus, this intervention emphasises the feedback aspects of MI. Miller and colleagues promoted the DCU through advertisements in the local news media as a health check-up focused on drinking and stressed that it was intended for drinkers in general, not for alcoholics. The intervention was made as non-threatening as possible to attract those in early stages of problems. The results of an evaluation of the DCU were encouraging (Miller et al. 1988).

Despite the fact that it was originally developed as a preventive measure for application among drinkers with early and mild problems, some of the ingredients of the DCU were expanded to form MET, as studied in Project MATCH. MET consists of four individualised treatment sessions spread over twelve weeks and, whenever possible, includes the client's spouse or another significant person in the client's life. The first session (week 1) provides structured feedback from an initial assessment of problems related to drinking, level of consumption and other relevant issues, and begins the attempt to build clients' motivation. The second session in week 2 continues the motivational enhancement process and works towards a definite commitment to change. The remaining two sessions (weeks 6 and 12) are follow-up sessions in which the therapist continues to monitor and encourage change.

Evidence for the Effectiveness of Motivational Interviewing

The main reason that MI has captured the imagination of many people working in the alcohol problems field is that it makes excellent clinical sense and fits with their experience of dealing with problem drinkers. However, research evidence in support of its effectiveness has been accumulating for some time. For example, Miller and colleagues (1993) provided strong support for the interactional view of client motivation. They randomly assigned problem drinkers to receive confrontational counselling or a client-centred motivational counselling style. Clients in the confrontation group showed a much higher level of resistance during counselling sessions than those in the other group. In addition, the more the counsellor had used a confrontational style during counselling, the more the client was drinking at follow-up over a year later. This and other evidence (see Miller and Rollnick 1991) strongly suggests that confrontation is counterproductive in the attempt to motivate the client for treatment and that a non-confrontational approach should be preferred.

In terms of a stand-alone treatment modality, it will have been noted that MI comes at the very top of the *Mesa Grande* (see Table 8.1), with ten studies in its favour as opposed to three against. As an example of the favourable studies, Brown and Miller (1993) randomly assigned 28 consecutive admissions to a private psychiatric hospital to receive or not receive a two-session motivational assessment and interview shortly after intake, in addition to standard evaluation and treatment. Those receiving the motivational intervention participated more fully in treatment and showed a significantly lower level of alcohol consumption at a three-month follow-up. Similar findings using the same design were reported by Bien et al. (1993a) for out-patient problem drinkers.

As noted above, MI principles have been a strong influence on the development of brief interventions in the alcohol field. In a review of this topic, Bien et al. (1993b) isolated six key ingredients which they claim were common to effective brief interventions. These were summarised by the acronym FRAMES:

- Feedback of personal risk or impairment
- Emphasis on personal Responsibility for change
- Clear Advice to change
- A Menu of alternative change options
- Therapeutic Empathy as a counselling style
- Enhancement of Self-efficacy or optimism.

These ingredients are clearly consistent with the philosophy, style and methods of MI. To the extent that this hypothesis about effective brief intervention is correct, the placement of 'brief interventions' in first place in the *Mesa Grande* league table adds to evidence for the effectiveness of MI.

PROJECT MATCH

Background

The rationale, methods and main findings of Project MATCH have been published and should be consulted by the interested reader (Project MATCH Research Group 1993, 1997a, 1997b, 1998a, 1998b, Donovan and Mattson 1994). In addition, a summary of the project and its findings, together with commentaries from 14 leading authorities in the field, was published in the January 1999 edition of the journal *Addiction*. Here we shall be able to present only an abbreviated version of this immense project.

Before summarising the findings of Project MATCH, it will be helpful to describe the background to the project and the thinking behind its development. There would be wide agreement among treatment providers that no single approach is likely to be effective for *all* problem drinkers. The obvious conclusion is to look for treatment methods or approaches that are especially suited to the needs and characteristics of individual clients, that is, to 'match' different clients to different treatments. This is hardly a new or revolutionary principle; the idea has a long history in the literature on treatment of alcohol problems (Institute of Medicine 1990) and is, of course, commonplace in many areas of medical treatment.

During the late 1970s and 1980s, the potential benefits of treatment matching attracted a good deal of attention in the alcohol problems field and a fairly extensive literature was devoted to this topic (see, for example, Lindstrom 1992). This was mainly prompted by a perception that the results of treatment, especially for more severe alcohol problems, were relatively poor. It was thought that failure to match clients appropriately to treatments had contributed to the negative or inconsistent results of many outcome studies and also that skilful matching in future could produce a significant improvement in success rates. Moreover, a collection of studies seemed to confirm the promise of this matching approach (see Mattson and Allen 1991). During the 1980s, in short, the 'matching hypothesis' seemed to many in the field to offer the best hope for a marked improvement in treatment effectiveness, and Project MATCH was funded to establish whether or not this optimism was justified.

Design and Methods

Project MATCH (Matching Alcoholism Treatment to Client Heterogeneity) involved ten treatment sites in the US and a total of 1,726 clients, divided into two parallel but independent clinical trials – an out-patient arm (n = 952) and an aftercare arm (n = 774). The two arms of the study were included because of the different client populations sampled and to enable a check on possible findings from the study by seeing whether they generalised across these two client populations.

The study was designed to assess the benefits of matching clients showing alcohol dependence or abuse to three different treatments with respect to a variety of client attributes. Clients within each arm of the study were randomly assigned to three twelve-week, manual-guided interventions: Twelve-step facilitation therapy (TSF) – an approach following the principles of Alcoholics Anonymous and founded on the idea that alcoholism is a spiritual and medical disease; cognitive-behavioural coping skills therapy (CBT) – an approach based on social learning theory; and motivational enhancement therapy (MET) – a less intensive form of therapy based on the principles of motivational psychology. Each of these modalities was delivered by trained therapists on a one-to-one basis. CBT and TSF consisted of twelve weekly sessions while MET consisted of four sessions spread over twelve weeks. Treatment was preceded by eight hours of assessment over three sessions. There were five follow-up assessments, at post-treatment and at three-monthly intervals thereafter. The main outcome measures were *percent days abstinent* and *drinks per drinking day* during the one-year post-treatment period.

Findings

Matching clients to treatments

As we have seen, the overall objective of Project MATCH was to determine whether the careful matching of particular characteristics of clients to different forms of treatment would result in a significant improvement in the effectiveness of treatment for alcohol problems in general. To this end, the investigators identified over 20 client attributes that the literature suggested could potentially lead to matching effects. This resulted in 16 primary and 11 secondary specific matching hypotheses (that is, hypotheses that clients with certain characteristics would do better with one form of treatment than another) which were stated before data collection began. As is now well-known, few of these matching hypotheses were confirmed. But despite the general failure to find an overall improvement in treatment effectiveness through matching, the project did come up with a few matching effects that can be applied in treatment programmes.

(a) *Psychiatric severity.* In the out-patient arm, it was found that clients who were low in psychiatric severity at the beginning of the trial (that is, those with low psychiatric co-morbidity) reported more days abstinence after TSF than after CBT. There was also a tendency for those with high psychiatric severity to do better with CBT than TSF but this was not statistically significant, possibly because of the relatively low numbers of clients in the out-patient arm with high psychiatric severity. The advantage for TSF among those with low psychiatric severity had disappeared by the time of the three-year follow-up and this matching effect was not present at all in the aftercare arm. (None of the matching effects discovered in the project appeared in both arms of the study.) Nevertheless, this finding indicates that a Twelve-step approach may be especially suited to out-patients with few or no psychiatric problems.

(b) *Network support for drinking.* Again in the out-patient arm only, those individuals with a social network supportive of drinking (that is, those with a lot of heavy-drinking friends) did better with TSF than MET. Interestingly, this effect did not emerge until the three-year follow-up, implying that it took time for the behavioural changes in question to become evident, but when it did emerge it was the largest matching effect identified in the trial. The clear implication here is that out-patients with social networks supportive of drinking will benefit especially from a Twelve-step programme because that is the most effective means of ridding the social network of heavy-drinking friends and acquaintances.

(c) *Client anger.* Also specific to the out-patient arm, the finding here was that clients initially high in anger reported more days of abstinence and fewer drinks per drinking day if they had received MET than if they had received CBT. This effect persisted from the one-year to the three-year follow-up point. This makes perfect sense in view of the deliberately non-confrontational nature of MET, and high client anger at initial assessment is clearly a positive indicator for the offer of MET.

(d) *Alcohol dependence.* The only statistically significant matching effect to emerge in the aftercare arm of the study was that clients low in dependence at intake reported more days abstinence with CBT than with TSF, whereas those high in dependence reported more abstinent days with TSF than with CBT. Since clients in the aftercare arm were not followed up at three years post-treatment, it is not possible to say whether this effect was a lasting one. The finding can presumably be explained by the fact that TSF places more emphasis on total abstinence than CBT and that abstinence becomes more necessary to recovery as dependence rises. Whatever the explanation, it suggests that, following in-patient detoxification or day care, individuals with high levels of dependence should be offered a Twelve-step programme and those with lower dependence should be offered cognitive-behavioural therapy. It is relevant here to point out that MATCH findings have no bearing on the outcome of clients in moderation-oriented programmes since, although abstinence may have been urged with different degrees of emphasis in the three treatments, moderation was never an explicit goal for any of the treatments studied.

Main effects of treatment

Although main effects of treatment (that is, comparisons involving the overall effectiveness of the three treatments) were not the focus of Project MATCH, these main effects are of considerable interest – possibly of greater interest as it transpired – than the matching effects. Put simply, the study showed that there were no clinically meaningful differences in success rates among the three treatments studied. This basic finding, which was undoubtedly surprising to many in the field, has two important implications for treatment practice.

First, the MATCH results clearly support the effectiveness of Twelve-step programmes in general. It is important to stress here that TSF cannot be regarded as equivalent to Alcoholics Anonymous. Although it was usually delivered by 'recovering alcoholics', TSF was run on an individual basis and did not include many of the important features of AA group meetings and sponsorship. As its name suggests, TSF was intended merely to facilitate attendance at AA. However, this aim appears to have been successful since clients who had received TSF attended significantly more AA meetings in the post-treatment period than those who had received the other two treatments.

The important point here, though, is that Project MATCH represented the first time that a treatment programme based on Twelve-step principles had been compared in a randomised trial with commonly used and scientifically based non-Twelve-step treatments among the average run of people attending for specialist treatment for alcohol problems. As was noted above, many authorities in the alcohol field would have predicted that CBT, in particular, would be superior in outcome to TSF, but this was clearly not the case. This equivalence of effectiveness on the part of Twelve-step treatment has recently been supported by another large study using a very different methodology. In a naturalistic study of results from 15 substance-abuse treatment programmes in the US, Ouimette et al. (1997) found that cognitive-behavioural and Twelve-step treatments were of equal effectiveness.

The other important implication of the MATCH main effects finding concerns the fact that a briefer treatment, MET, was no less effective than two more intensive treatments, CBT and TSF. This applied to the entire range of clients in the sample and not only to those of lower dependence or problem severity. This is an important point because the consensus on the effectiveness of briefer treatments before Project MATCH was that they should be confined to clients with lower levels of dependence and problems. Although MET was somewhat more than one-third as expensive to deliver than the other treatments (Cisler et al. 1998), it was clearly more cost-effective.

Implications for Treatment Practice

Quite apart from its substantive findings, Project MATCH is likely to influence treatment provision simply because of the high standards of training and quality assurance it set itself. Since there was no non-treatment control group in the MATCH design, it cannot, strictly speaking, be concluded that the treatment delivered in the project was highly successful. However, this is a pedantic point because anyone familiar with conventional rates of success from alcohol treatment programmes cannot fail to be impressed by the general level of improvement shown by MATCH clients. These impressive results were almost certainly due to the careful selection and thorough training of therapists and the fact that all three treatments were comprehensively laid out in treatment manuals. This was accompanied by rigorous quality-assurance methods which ensured that treatment was delivered in the ways intended and was of generally high quality.

A direct spin-off from Project MATCH is the availability of manuals describing in detailed specification each of the three treatments (Kadden et al. 1992, Miller et al. 1992, Nowinski et al. 1992). These can be obtained at no cost from the body responsible for funding the study, the National Institute on Alcohol Abuse and Alcoholism. The potential usefulness of these manuals is shown by the fact that over 35,000 requests for them had already been received by 1998 (Gordis and Fuller 1999).

The main direct implications of the MATCH findings for clinical practice are that:

(i)   levels of psychiatric severity, network support for drinking and client anger should be considered when assigning clients to out-patient treatment
(ii) level of alcohol dependence should be considered when assigning clients to aftercare treatment
(iii) apart from these variables, treatment providers need not take into account the client characteristics examined in the project when deciding a client's best treatment from among those studied in Project MATCH.

Despite evidence for some client–treatment matches, however, it is fair to say that Project MATCH did not in general confirm the high expectations about the value of treatment matching that were current before the project began. As the MATCH investigators themselves write: 'Despite the promise of earlier matching studies … the intuitively appealing notion that matching can appreciably enhance treatment effectiveness has been severely challenged' (Project MATCH Research Group 1997b). However, it is important to understand that this general failure of treatment matching applies only to *systematic* matching, in the sense of a formal treatment system with rules to channel clients into specific forms of treatment – for example, a system in which all clients entering treatment are assessed for level of alcohol problems and those showing severe problems (that is, above a certain cut-off point) are assigned to one form of treatment, while those showing less severe problems (that is, below the cut-off point) are assigned to another. The findings are not relevant to other matters that might be included under the general heading of 'treatment matching' and it is important to be clear what these are.

(i)   They have no bearing on the traditional clinical skill of tailoring treatment to the unique needs and goals of a particular client in the individual case. Whether or not this kind of clinical skill adds to the effectiveness of treatment is unknown but confidently assumed. In any event, its place in treatment is untouched by the results of Project MATCH.

(ii) Neither do the results affect the kind of client–treatment matching that informally occurs when therapeutic services dealing with medical, economic, psychiatric, family or legal problems are *added on* to a basic treatment programme – for example, when it is evident that a client has a special need for vocational counselling or when the marital relationship is obviously contributing to the client's problem and marital therapy would be acceptable to the client and partner. The validity of the kind of matching approach seems obvious and there is good evidence at least that it is effective among people with polydrug problems (see McKay and McLellan 1998).

(iii) Possibilities for treatment matching were clearly not exhausted by the Project MATCH design. For example, the findings have no bearing on the possible effectiveness of matching to in-patient versus out-patient treatment settings, to face-to-face versus group therapies, or to pharmacotherapy versus psychosocial treatment. There are also other *forms* of matching that were not studied in Project MATCH – for example, client–therapist interactions (that is, the possibility that certain types of client do better with certain types of therapist) or client self-matching (giving clients the opportunity to select what they think is the best treatment for them). Although the Project MATCH sample was representative of typical treatment attenders in the US, certain types of problem drinker were excluded (that is, those with concomitant dependence on other drugs, homeless problem drinkers and those with co-morbid psychoses), and some kinds of matching procedure may yet prove effective for these other groups. Finally, although the project included a representative type of cognitive-behavioural therapy, it clearly did not exhaust the possibilities under this broad category of treatment approaches; other types of cognitive-behavioural therapy may have produced different results.

CONCLUSIONS REGARDING TREATMENT EFFECTIVENESS

So, how do the findings of Project MATCH affect a comparative evaluation of general approaches to the treatment of alcohol problems? First, it is clear that the results have added substantially to the evidence in favour of the Twelve-step approach. To repeat, there was no evidence that TSF was inferior in general to CBT or MET for a broad range of clients presenting for treatment. In addition, some client characteristics were identified that suggested TSF as the treatment of choice for those clients (low psychiatric severity and high network support for drinking among out-patients, and high alcohol dependence among in-patients). But one important caveat should be borne in mind here. The MATCH results were obtained in the US where there is a high degree of familiarity among the general public with the tenets of the Twelve-step philosophy and probably much greater acceptance of AA teaching than in other countries. Further, the abstinence treatment goal, for people with all levels of alcohol dependence and problems, is more dominant in the public understanding of problem drinking and more subscribed to in treatment circles than, for example, in the UK (Rosenberg et al. 1992, Rosenberg and Davis 1994). Thus it is possible that TSF might not have worked so well in other, perhaps more secular, cultures and considerable caution should be exercised, in the absence of directly relevant research, before applying the apparent consequences of MATCH findings to treatment delivery in the UK.

Another caveat is that the support for TSF found in the MATCH results in no way strengthens the validity of the underlying theoretical assumptions on which the Twelve-step approach is based, particularly the notion that alcoholism is 'a spiritual disease'. These disease theory assumptions are subject to many cogent criticisms (see Heather and Robertson 1997) which are unaffected by these findings. An analysis of the MATCH data by Longabaugh and colleagues (1998) strongly suggests that the crucial element in the success of TSF was its ability to change the client's social network away from heavy-drinking companions, a change that is obviously not unique in principle to the Twelve-step approach.

The second conclusion is that the MATCH findings have considerably increased the basis for using MET and other treatment methods based on motivational interviewing principles. This does not apply merely to clients with relatively mild dependence and problems, as was previously thought to be the case, but to problem drinkers at all levels of severity of problems. The basis for this statement is that the MATCH findings showed MET to be as effective overall as two more intensive and expensive treatments and therefore more *cost-effective*. In times of burgeoning health budgets, increasing restrictions on health service spending and fierce competition for resources from numerous health care sectors, this is a conclusion of considerable practical importance. Indeed, it is likely that if and when the MATCH findings become widely known among health commissioners in the UK, there will be a strong temptation to make a form of MET the standard treatment for alcohol problems. There is some anecdotal evidence that this is already happening. Once more, however, the lack of relevant research in the UK health care setting makes this conclusion hazardous. (It should also be noted that AA is also a highly cost-effective resource from both the individual problem drinker's perspective and from the perspective of health care services – see Humphreys and Moos 1996.)

THE UK ALCOHOL TREATMENT TRIAL

Partly as a response to the need for a large British trial following on from the findings of Project MATCH, in 1998 the Medical Research Council funded a multicentre trial of treatment for alcohol problems in the UK, and this has become known as the *UK Alcohol Treatment Trial* (UKATT). It will not be possible here to describe the design and methods of the UKATT, and only its basic rationale will be briefly sketched.

The main aim of the UKATT is to test the hypothesis that a briefer treatment in the form of MET is all that is needed to bring about the recovery of the majority of problem drinkers seeking help in UK specialist treatment services. To this end, a British adaptation of MET has been developed and this is one of two treatments to which clients will be randomly assigned.

The other randomised treatment is known as *Social Behaviour and Network Therapy* (SBNT). Another glance at the *Mesa Grande* in Table 8.1 will show that some of the most successful treatment modalities are those that include a social, or at least interpersonal, component (social skills training, community reinforcement approach, behaviour contracting, cognitive-behavioural marital therapy). Added to this, there is the important evidence cited above from the Longabaugh et al. (1998) study that the strongest predictor of recovery in the MATCH findings was a beneficial change in the client's social network. SBNT is an amalgam of social network and standard cognitive-behavioural methods and is claimed by the investigators to be the intensive treatment modality that is best supported by the literature on treatment outcome. Thus SBNT represents the most stringent test available at the present time of the hypothesis that MET should become the standard treatment for alcohol problems. Needless to say, the attempt is also being made to discover the characteristics of clients who are best suited to either of the two treatment approaches, MET or SBNT, under study.

In a nutshell, the UKATT is designed to ask whether the most promising form of intensive treatment for alcohol problems is more effective and cost-effective that MET. Unfortunately, a valid answer to this question requires a multicentre trial that will take several years to complete. The findings from the UKATT will become available early in the new millennium.

NOTE

*Parts of this section of Chapter 8 have been adapted from N. Heather (1995), *Treatment Approaches to Alcohol Problems* (WHO Regional Publications, European Series, No. 65). Copenhagen: World Health Organization.

B: Home Detoxification for Problem Drinkers

Colin Bennie, Iain McKinney and David Campbell

The following section describes the operation of a home detoxification service (HDS) in one area of the UK. Many problem drinkers stop drinking spontaneously. It is also true, as noted earlier in this book, that binge drinkers drift in and out of heavy drinking periods and are able to have alcohol-free spells. They may during this time experience mild to moderate alcohol withdrawal symptoms, but are able to tolerate and control these without medical intervention or specialist help.

Many dependent drinkers are able to control withdrawal symptoms with reduced amounts of alcohol until they are alcohol-free. This comes with practise and the knowledge that they require periods of abstinence to allow physical recovery from the effects of excessive alcohol consumption.

However, many problem drinkers cannot cease drinking without experiencing moderate to severe alcohol withdrawal effects (see Chapter 2). These can present as shakes, profuse sweating, nausea, vomiting, disturbance of blood pressure, irritation, anxiety, sleep disturbance, loss of appetite and, in severe cases, auditory and visual hallucinations and delirium tremens.

Until around 20 years ago it was generally standard practice in the UK and in some other countries that the management of withdrawal symptoms required medical intervention, either in specialist alcohol treatment units, medical wards of district general hospitals, or most commonly in acute admission wards in psychiatric hospitals.

The detoxification consisted of assessment, control of withdrawal symptoms with the prescribing of Chlormethiazole or benzodiazepines and attention to the drinker's physical and psychological health. On discharge, follow-up was either through the general practitioner (GP) (family doctor) or attendance at alcohol out-patient clinics.

During the past two decades, however, there has been a shift in emphasis in the treatment of problem drinkers away from intensive in-patient care towards the development and delivery of non-residential and community-based services.

Over this period influential studies into the effectiveness of treatment of problem drinking have demonstrated that in certain circumstances there is no difference in outcome between intensive in-patient programmes and less intense out-patient approaches (Stein et al. 1975, Edwards et al. 1977, Orford and Edwards 1977, Chapman and Huygens 1988).

This precipitated much consideration of the way in which services for problem drinkers were to be developed in the forthcoming years. With the evidence from these earlier studies, the emergence of 'brief interventions' consisting of assessment, advice about drinking and follow-up, proved to be effective in encouraging positive changes in drinking behaviour for many problem drinkers (Chick et al. 1985, Babor et al. 1986, Heather 1986, Robertson et al. 1986). Brief interventions provided a practical and effective response that encouraged earlier detection and early intervention with problem drinkers.

With the development of community-based services there was increasing interest in the role of primary care in response to alcohol problems. Again in the 1970s, studies conducted in general practice (Pollak 1975, Wilkins and Hore 1977, Boothman 1979) highlighted that problem drinkers consult with their GP three times more often than the population in general. Moreover, in the majority of cases it is the GP who is the first point of contact for many problem drinkers seeking help.

The role of the GP has been widely studied in relation to responding to alcohol problems (Clement 1986, King 1986a, 1986b, Wallace et al. 1988, Anderson and Scott 1992) and, importantly, how the GP's response can be most effective in the primary care setting. Much of the work conducted into brief interventions was done so within general practice (Babor et al. 1986, Murray 1991, Anderson and Scott 1992) and suggests that the GP is ideally placed not only to enhance the early identification of drinking problems in primary care but also to respond to them.

However, as these studies highlight, whilst this response is effective with many problem drinkers there are also many who will require more intensive intervention of specialist alcohol services. Here the GP has an important part to play in the early referral to these agencies. Community-based services operating in tandem with primary care should provide a rapid, easy access response.

In relation to detoxification there is a small proportion of problem drinkers who, due to severe physical and psychological problems, will require hospitalisation for a short period in order that the alcohol withdrawal is as safe as possible. The majority, however, who require detoxification can be treated effectively on an out-patient basis. Several authors (Stinnet 1982, Webb and Unwin 1988, Hayashida et al. 1989, Collins et al. 1990, Stockwell et al. 1990) have demonstrated the safety and effectiveness of out-patient alcohol detoxification.

More recently, the development of domiciliary-based alcohol detoxification (Stockwell 1987, Stockwell et al. 1990, Bennie 1992, 1997, Cooper 1994) has proved effective and efficient in providing accessible and convenient treatment options which reduce the stigma of hospitalisation and remove many of the barriers in the help-seeking process.

As noted above, this section of the current chapter describes the experience of providing an HDS in Forth Valley in central Scotland for the past ten years; the rationale for the service, treatment delivery, the detoxification process and, importantly, the lessons learned in that time. It is emphasised that local conditions and community needs influence the ways in which alcohol services operate in specific settings. It is, however, hoped that the following account will provide an example of how one particular type of service has operated.

As mentioned above, a high proportion of alcohol-dependent drinkers do not require controlled alcohol withdrawal, but for those who do, home detoxification has many benefits:

- It is convenient for patients and their families
- It reduces the stigma associated with hospital admission
- It provides a rapid response to patients
- It involves relatives at an early stage
- It provides direct and easy access to local general practitioners
- It involves a short, sharp initial intervention with longer-term follow-up
- It is cost-effective.

THE SCENE IN FORTH VALLEY

This part of Scotland has a population of 274,000 in an extensive catchment area consisting of urban and rural communities. The three main towns are Stirling, Falkirk and Alloa. The Scottish capital, Edinburgh, is 30 miles (45 km) to the east and Glasgow is a similar distance to the west.

There is no residential alcohol facility in Forth Valley, the alcohol problems unit closed in 1978. There is a large Alcoholics Anonymous network and a well-developed Council on Alcohol. The latter type of agency, very important in the UK, provides a counselling service for problem drinkers.

People requiring in-patient care for alcohol problems are admitted to the acute psychiatric wards attached to the general hospitals in each of the three main towns. There are no dedicated beds within these wards for alcohol problems.

REVIEW OF SERVICE PROVISION

Whilst attendance of patients with drinking problems was high at the day centre, there was concern at the considerable default rate (50%) of new referrals and return appointments at the out-patient clinics. A follow-up survey of new referrals to the clinics in 1985 revealed that patients found the clinics inaccessible and expensive to travel to. Other factors associated with non-attendance were that some patients had stopped drinking prior to their appointment and did not feel they needed to attend, and conversely that they were still drinking whilst in treatment and were embarrassed to attend.

A further survey of annual alcohol-related admissions to the acute psychiatric wards in 1987, 1988 and 1989 showed that 20% of all patients admitted in these years had a primary diagnosis of alcohol dependence and a further 5% had this as a secondary diagnosis. Further investigation revealed that a high proportion of these admissions occurred 'out of hours' and were precipitated by social or domestic crisis. The average length of stay for detoxification was 14 days and there was a high readmission rate with this patient group.

The treatment programme was rudimentary, consisting of assisted alcohol withdrawal with benzodiazepines, physical and psychological checks and then, when appetite and sleep had returned, discharge. Follow-up was via the out-patient clinics, but with lengthy waiting times for appointments.

Examination of case records highlighted that a high percentage of patients would not actually have required hospitalisation, but this provided respite from excessive drinking and respite for relatives. Heavy drinking was generally reinstated within two to four weeks of discharge and a high readmission rate after three months. The in-patient stay did not address alcohol-related issues, promote positive changes in drinking behaviour or prepare for discharge back to the home and drinking environment. They could, however, have been treated at home, possibly with a better outcome.

A study was conducted with the 200 GPs in Forth Valley (Bennie 1987). This examined their role security, therapeutic commitment and intervention with problem drinkers. The findings from this exercise mirrored the results of earlier studies of GPs (Cartwright 1977, Shaw et al. 1978, Clement 1984, 1986). It emerged that whilst GPs demonstrated positive role security, their therapeutic commitment towards dealing with problem drinkers was low. This was attributed essentially to lack of training and lack of time to deal with these patients. What they clearly highlighted was the fact that they considered that their most effective intervention was to refer problem drinkers on to the local specialist services, and indeed, in a high number of cases, for in-patient treatment. The responses further revealed that they would welcome the development of a community-based service which would support them in their efforts with problem drinkers in primary care.

WHY A HOME DETOXIFICATION SERVICE?

Taking account of the local and national information and guidance to service providers, there was clearly a demonstrable need within Forth Valley for a community-orientated service for problem drinkers and their families. This clearly had to respond effectively to their needs.

Encouraged by the positive outcome described in Stockwell's research into home detoxification treatment, it was anticipated that the development of a domiciliary detoxification service would provide a more appropriate response, demonstrate positive outcomes and reduce the admission rate to the psychiatric wards.

PLANNING AND PROVIDING THE HOME DETOXIFICATION SERVICE

Many factors were considered when planning the HDS service in Forth Valley:

- It would be a nurse-led service
- Local GPs were consulted and involved from the outset
- The large geographic catchment area and potential referral rates determined that there would be a Clinical Nurse Specialist and five RMN qualified psychiatric nurses
- The emphasis of the service would be on 'shared care' with GPs who would maintain medical responsibility
- It would be a service operating seven days a week
- It would be evaluated
- There would be clear referral criteria, and service protocols.

In the first instance it was agreed that the initial twelve months would be a pilot project and experienced nurses were recruited on a secondment basis. A training programme for the nurses was devised and provided by the Clinical Nurse Specialist. The content of this was varied but concentrated on the clinical and practical issues relating to domiciliary detoxification.

Proforma concerning referral, service standards, assessment schedules, clinical procedures, medication regimes and data collection were devised.

Prior to introducing the service in January 1991, every GP in Forth Valley was provided with information about the service and was visited by the team for a personal discussion about the service, their involvement, and to respond to any queries raised by them. The local Area Medical Committee, General Practitioner Sub-Group had already been informed of and approved the introduction of the new service.

REFERRAL CRITERIA

The referral criteria are essentially self-explanatory and are required to ensure that alcohol withdrawal is as safe as possible for the patient. Detailed information is collected at the point of assessment and it is the nurse's decision as to whether a patient is suitable for treatment.

- The GP considers the patient to be alcohol dependent and requires assessment for detoxification
- The GP conducts brief physical and psychological examinations to exclude serious problems
- The GP arranges biochemistry tests for LFTs (liver function test), GGT (gamma glutamyl transferase) and FBC (full blood count)
- A brief drinking history is provided
- There is no history of alcohol withdrawal seizures or epilepsy
- The patient has someone to act as supporter during the detoxification period.

ASSESSMENT

Initially every referral is responded to within 72 hours with an assessment appointment at the home which involves relatives as well. Referring GPs are asked to telephone patient details in the first instance in order that the response times are maintained and that the service is able to 'strike while the iron is hot'. This is backed up by the referral form.

The assessment interview lasts approximately one hour, and includes:

- full drinking history
- a record of the previous week's alcohol consumption

- medical history
- experience of previous withdrawal symptoms
- existence and measurement of degree of alcohol dependence using the Severity of Alcohol Dependence Questionnaire (SADQ) (Stockwell et al. 1983)
- Severity of Alcohol Withdrawal Symptom Checklist (SAWSC)
- home environment assessment
- previous help sought with the drinking problem.

When the assessment is complete the nurse decides on the patient's suitability for home detoxification treatment.

THE DETOXIFICATION PROCEDURE

The initial and probably the most important aspect of the detoxification is to explain it fully to the patient and his or her supporter. It is essential that the patient is comfortable with the treatment and what is involved. A patient information leaflet is extremely useful and can be referred to at any time. If the patient is aware of what to expect, he or she is less likely to be anxious should some withdrawal effects be experienced. If patients know how to deal with them, they are more likely to tolerate some discomfort than resort to medication.

If it has been considered necessary for the patient to have medication during the detoxification, this is arranged with the GP. The initial dose of medication and the reducing regime are decided by the nurse according to the likelihood of withdrawal symptoms indicated by the SADQ and SAWSC scores obtained.

The HDS uses Chlordiazepoxide generally in a five- to seven-day reducing regime (see Tables 8.2 and 8.3). The prescription is made out by the GP and kept with the patient or supporter. It is also explained to patients that this is a single prescription and will not be extended.

Table 8.2: Chlordiazepoxide five-day reducing course

Day	Medication	Time	Time	Time	Time	Total
1	Chlordiazepoxide 15 mg	10.00 a.m.	–	3.00 p.m.	10.00 p.m.	45 mg
2	Chlordiazepoxide 10 mg	10.00 a.m.	–	3.00 p.m.	10.00 p.m.	30 mg
3	Chlordiazepoxide 5 mg	10.00 a.m.	–	3.00 p.m.	10.00 p.m.	15 mg
4	Chlordiazepoxide 5 mg	10.00 a.m.	–	–	10.00 p.m.	10 mg
5	Chlordiazepoxide 5 mg	–	–	–	10.00 p.m.	5 mg

Table 8.3: Chlordiazepoxide seven-day reducing course

Day	Medication	Time	Time	Time	Time	Total
1	Chlordiazepoxide 20 mg	10.00 a.m.	2.00 p.m.	6.00 p.m.	10.00 p.m.	80 mg
2	Chlordiazepoxide 20 mg	10.00 a.m.	–	3.00 p.m.	10.00 p.m.	60 mg
3	Chlordiazepoxide 15 mg	10.00 a.m.	–	3.00 p.m.	10.00 p.m.	45 mg
4	Chlordiazepoxide 10 mg	10.00 a.m.	–	3.00 p.m.	10.00 p.m.	30 mg
5	Chlordiazepoxide 5 mg	10.00 a.m.	–	3.00 p.m.	10.00 p.m.	15 mg
6	Chlordiazepoxide 5 mg	10.00 a.m.	–	–	10.00 p.m.	10 mg
7	Chlordiazepoxide 5 mg	10.00 a.m.	–	–	10.00 p.m.	5 mg

When this is arranged, the daily visits to the patient are organised. For the first 72 hours there are twice-daily visits, reducing to once daily thereafter until the fifth or seventh day. On each visit the nurse makes several checks:

• blood pressure
• Severity of Alcohol Withdrawal Score
• breath sample
• reduction in medication
• check for irregularities.

Prior to the detoxification, the GP is informed by letter of the outcome of assessment. Similar information is also supplied to the GP on the patient's completion of the detoxification.

During the once-daily visits the nurse continues to assess the post-detoxification needs and formulates the care plan. On completion of the detoxification the follow-up arrangements are made. This can either be in the patient's home or through the network of nurse out-patient clinics in health centres in Forth Valley. Cognitive-behavioural approaches are utilised in the post-detoxification phase and address issues such as abstinence maintenance, relapse prevention, cue identification and lifestyle and drinking behaviour changes.

SOME BASIC INFORMATION

The HDS receives *800* referrals per year from GPs; 35% are *women* (Madden et al. 2000). Referrals to the service have *trebled* since 1991. The average duration of contact with the service is *six months*. Only *38%* of patients referred actually require full detoxification. Every detoxification treatment is completed in between *five and seven days*, except in exceptional or difficult circumstances such as a coexisting dependence on other drugs such as benzodiazepines, opiates, and so on.

EVALUATION OF THE SERVICE

Alongside the initial pilot project, a randomised control trial was conducted comparing home detoxification treatment with minimal intervention strategies designed to help people stop drinking. Patients were randomly assigned to either group. The home detoxification group were treated with the programme described here, the only difference being that one home visit per week was made for four weeks after detoxification to monitor progress and assist the patients to develop a plan for immediate behaviour change. Within the minimal intervention group the patients were assessed using the same schedule and on a separate occasion given advice about stopping drinking. They were also given the booklet from the DRAMS package, *Breaking the Habit: Coming Off*, produced for the Health Education Board for Scotland (HEBS) by Murray (1991) and instructed in its use. The booklet gives sound practical advice on stopping drinking and helps people to plan longer-term behavioural strategies for dealing with abstinence. No medication was given to the patients in this group. They were paid one other home visit one month later to check on their progress. All patients were followed up six months later when information was obtained relating to achievement and duration of abstinence, description of drinking spells, their perceived improvement in physical, psychological and social health, and the use of other supporting agencies. If the patient reported drinking at that time a further SADQ and note of the previous seven days' consumption was taken.

Seventy-six patients were successfully followed up at six months. There were 40 subjects in the home detoxification group and 36 in the minimal intervention group. Pre- and post-treatment information was examined.

The results in relation to treatment outcome highlighted negligible differences in abstinence rates between the groups for the duration of the six-month period before follow-up. However, of those who had returned to drinking during the post-treatment period, the patients in the home detox-ification group had achieved and maintained abstinence for significantly longer. The mean number of weeks' abstinence in the home detoxification group was 16.3 in comparison to 9.6 weeks in the minimal intervention group.

There was also a similar pattern of levels of alcohol consumption in the week prior to the follow-up interview with corresponding similar SADQ scores. Among those returning to drinking in the post-treatment period there was a significant reduction in their average weekly consumption in both groups.

In relation to perceived improvement after treatment, a small percentage of the patients reported no real change, although it was discovered that they had returned to drinking almost immediately after treatment. When information was analysed concerning post-treatment improvement and the responses of improved, unchanged or worse, there were significant rates of perceived improvement in the physical, psychological and social health categories.

Inevitably, the results produced many more questions than answers. It was impossible to say whether one treatment strategy demonstrated a superior outcome to the other. However, this does highlight the necessity for longer-term study of domiciliary detoxification. The operation of the HDS is illustrated by the following two case histories.

Case 1: Mrs W

This 65-year-old, recently retired school teacher was referred by her GP for assessment of her suitability for home detoxification. 'Mrs W' had requested referral, having heard of the service from a friend.

Contact was made initially by telephone and a mutually agreed date and time for assessment was arranged. Mrs W was advised to reduce her alcohol intake in the interim but not to abstain until seen. At assessment she had indeed managed a reduction in her daily consumption from 30 'units' of alcohol to around 15 units (one bottle of vodka to half a bottle of vodka). On that morning she had not had any alcohol and was exhibiting moderate withdrawal symptoms, that is, tremor, sweating, loss of appetite and restlessness. She had a SAWSC score of 12, blood pressure and pulse were within normal limits, and breathalyser reading was 0.00 mg/litre which confirmed her abstinence that day. Administration of the SADQ showed a moderate-to-high physical dependency and she scored high on the home environment assessment, her husband being very supportive and well-informed.

Despite a 15-year history of heavy drinking (average 30 units per day), Mrs W had successfully maintained a career in teaching and had managed to conceal her drinking to all but her closest friends and family. She pinpointed the breakdown of a relationship as the reason she started consuming alcohol in such quantities. Continued heavy drinking was attributed to habit and anxieties surrounding coping without alcohol as a 'crutch'. She also reported no significant periods of abstinence in 15 years.

The detoxification procedure was fully explained and Mrs W's anxieties were addressed by team members. The referring GP was contacted and a five-day reducing course of Chlordiazepoxide was arranged. Detoxification was commenced that afternoon and passed without incident. Following detoxification we discussed the options available to her. Mrs W was confident that, having broken the cycle of daily drinking, she could maintain abstinence and rejected a return to controlled drinking as being too risky.

Throughout our contact (three months) she remained abstinent and, by agreement, at the end of that time her HDS nurse withdrew support.

Case 2: Mr A

This 50-year-old man was referred to the HDS by his GP following his attending a hospital accident and emergency unit with chest pains. LFTs taken showed AST (aspartate transferase) 151, ALT (alanine aminotransferase) 163 and GGT 236.

Mr A was employed as a training facilitator with a large multinational company, having been promoted to this job some three years before. He found his job satisfying but stressful, and it involved a considerable amount of 'socialising', especially on residential courses. In 1998 his marriage broke down and he separated from his wife. He also incurred debts of approximately £30,000 at about the same time as the failure of his marriage. He subsequently met and moved in with his current partner who has been supportive towards him and who drinks, but only in moderation.

Assessment revealed a two-year history of problem drinking. This had been especially severe in the most recent six months. He was drinking approximately 32 units of alcohol per day – usually vodka – from his morning 'eye-opener' until going to bed. He continued to work but latterly found himself drinking during working hours. He cited effect, relaxation (lessening stress) and habit as his reasons for continued heavy drinking. His SADQ score was 32, which showed a high degree of physical dependence on alcohol, and he suffered related withdrawal symptoms. His physical health had started to deteriorate and he experienced daily low mood with suicidal ideation. He had not abstained from drinking for any period in the past two years. His SAWSC score was 12, and his home environment assessment score was 20.

Initially he was offered a seven-day reducing course of Chlordiazepoxide as a detoxification regime. A full explanation of the treatment plan was provided to Mr A and his partner, who agreed to support him. He was also signed off work by his GP. His detoxification proved to be uneventful, with his SAWSC scores quickly coming down over several days and a marked improvement noted in his physical and psychological health.

After detoxification he was offered a series of treatment sessions to tackle problems detected at assessment. This treatment included relaxation techniques to lessen stress, debt counselling to address his financial situation, relapse prevention techniques to promote abstinence, together with encouragement to make positive lifestyle changes – again to promote abstinence.

Mr A responded well to this regime, initially returning to work then, of his own volition, procuring early retirement from his job. This major change to his lifestyle has allowed him to resolve his financial situation as well as to reduce stress. He has started his own consultancy firm. He has been enjoying this work. He no longer has to undertake residential courses and, approximately five months' post-detoxification, is still abstinent.

C: Complementary Therapies for the Treatment of Alcohol Dependence

Diwakar Sukul

INTRODUCTION

This section of Chapter 8 provides an introduction to a body of therapeutic approaches that have been gaining far greater acceptance alongside more 'traditional' Western therapies (BMA 1993, Woodham 1994). It is emphasised, for those who may doubt the value of such approaches, that they should be subjected to the same criteria of effectiveness as those applied to other approaches, such as have been outlined in sections A and B of this chapter. 'Complementary medicine (or 'alternative medicine') is a term used to describe treatments that are generally used alongside orthodox medical treatment. In all discussion of orthodox and complementary medicine it should be remembered that the terms are necessarily relative. What is classed as 'orthodox' with reference to medical matters varies from one country to another: what is considered orthodox in India or Russia, for instance, may well be regarded as alternative or complementary elsewhere. According to Ernst (2000), the prevalence of the use of complementary/alternative medicine ranged from 9% to 65%. Even for a given form of treatment such as chiropractic, as used in the US, considerable discrepancies emerged. Evidence suggests that complementary/alternative therapies are used frequently and increasingly.

Eisenberg et al. (1998), in a survey of 1,539 adults in 1991 and 2,055 in 1997, found that the probability of users visiting an alternative medicine practitioner increased from 36.3% to 46.3%. These authors also found that the use of at least one of 16 alternative therapies during the previous year increased from 33.8% in 1990 to 42% in 1997. The therapies increasing the most included herbal medicine, massage, megavitamins, self-help groups, folk remedies, energy healing and homeopathy. It is now open to any UK family doctor to employ a complementary therapist to offer treatment on the National Health Service so long as the doctor remains accountable.

Ironically, the global rise of the traditional therapies has itself highlighted the importance of linking these treatments with conventional medical practice to create a complementary approach to health care. In the UK this supposition has attracted many multidisciplinary approaches from a cross-section of medical and social-work practitioners, and even the Prince of Wales has suggested that 'orthodox medicine may not have all the answers'.

According to Jobst:

> [As] alternative or complementary medicine becomes more mainstream or orthodox, the practices central to some CAM (complementary and alternative) therapies such as electronic diagnosis, herbal preparations, zone pressure effects and even visualization, will increasingly be packaged for mass marketing. (1998: 123)

The competence of complementary practitioners has steadily gained recognition in the field of medicine since the 1970s. Whatever the reasons for this, it has resulted in alternative medicine having an increasing presence on the political stage, largely due to its non-invasive, therapeutic intimacy and the autonomous decision of the patient to personally invest in his or her recovery process. For example, Rankin-Box has noted that 'a total of 92 districts in England are funding complementary therapies for patients via contracts or extra contractual referrals' (1995: 25).

Complementary medicine creates an awareness of holism by bringing spirituality and medicine together into a whole or holistic attitude to health care. It is helping to create an entirely new attitude to the human experience of health; namely, that the physical, mental, emotional and spiritual dimensions each represent a different view of the same person. Changes in one aspect catalyse changes in the other parts of the organism. Dependence or 'addiction' to alcohol and other drugs is never simply only a physical or a psychological condition. Such dependence involves and affects the whole person, and if treatment is to be truly successful it must necessarily take this fact into account.

Let us then briefly review the elements of 'dependence' as seen from the holistic point of view. The word 'addiction' itself is a direct descendant from the Latin *addicts*, 'to favour'. The latter implies choice. Somewhere, most often at first quite consciously, a choice was made to do something, to take a step. This point of involvement had both psychological and spiritual elements. Something is forbidden, or at least known to be ill-advised, and yet the temptation to 'give it a try' overwhelms the wisdom that would say 'No!' People meet these tests of character daily all the way through life. Sometimes they listen more to the 'still, quiet voice' of wisdom, while at other times to the insistence of temptation. This is both natural and normal and is to be expected. Some people, however, seem to be predisposed to taking the fateful and harmful steps that lead down the path to dependence or addiction, the prolonged harmful use of alcohol or other mind-altering drugs.

At this point it is all too easy to blame and to assign guilt. Often the most harmful expression of blame comes from the problem user him- or herself. Practitioners all too commonly come across the person who has lost every last trace of self-esteem and who drinks, smokes, 'pops' or 'snorts' to hide from him- or herself the unbearable and assumed 'truth' of worthlessness.

Of course, no one is completely worthless, but judgements of the value of self or other influence character more fundamentally than perhaps anything else. Ancient religions provide a legacy of wise voices from a long-ago past offering guidance on this matter that contemporary wisdom would do well to recall.

So, where does complementary medicine begin? What are some of the many ways in which complementary medicine can throw new (and ancient) light on the problem of problematic substance use?

First must come the question: 'What, for this person, is the first cause?' What is the basis, in a lifetime flavoured with a cocktail of pain and joy, of this person's tendency to problem drinking or other forms of drug use? Was it already a question of low self-esteem deriving from a lifetime of condemnation, or did it jump out of a moment of sheer bravado? What are the elements for *this person* of his or her predisposition to drinking or drug use with harmful consequences? Is the predisposition purely an individual matter, or is it influenced socially in terms of family or peer group dynamics? Is it more a question of what might be considered the current norms of society at large? Without first addressing this question no regime of treatment can be initiated that has any real hope of success.

Ultimately, therapists must ask: 'What is the need that this pattern of alcohol consumption or other drug use would meet?' That need lies at the bottom of every case of addiction, even if the drinking/drug use is iatrogenic, the result of having taken certain necessary medications over too long a period of time. The need might not have been present initially but has come about due to continual and necessary practice. In a case such as this, there may still be blame: this time either for a doctor or 'the system', although both might in fact be entirely blameless. Depending upon the character of this 'addict', the blame could either enhance or weaken the resolve to break free and so would still need to be taken into consideration.

THE ELEMENTS OF COMPLEMENTARY MEDICINE

These elements, summarised here, are regarded as the essentials of complementary practice.

- Physical detoxification
- Psychological or spiritual empowerment to the degree necessary for the 'addict' to reach a point of determination to break free and initiate the healing process
- Assistance from counselling or other psychotherapeutic modalities to fill the perceived or felt 'black hole of need' which led to the problem use/addiction in the first place

- Physical, psychological and spiritual integration of the whole and healed person – ideally to the point where he or she can feel grateful for the experience, lessons learnt and wisdom gained, of having once, in the past, been a problem drinker or problem drug-user.

THERAPEUTIC APPROACHES

As emphasised in Chapters 1, 2 and 3, the problematic consumption of alcohol develops and is sustained against a background of multiple causative factors. The person's life may be disturbed on all levels, for example, social, psychological, physical and energetic, and any treatment approach should therefore address as many different aspects as possible in order to success-fully fight and overcome the harmful use of alcohol or other drugs.

Orthodox or 'Western' medicine is extremely effective in treating acute and life-threatening conditions and, as such, is an ideal 'safety net' in the detoxification process. Conventional psychology, for example, is an excel-lent tool for revealing underlying conscious and subconscious problems and cognitively dealing with them. However, more deeply rooted disturbances such as low self-esteem or a lifestyle that is completely adapted to substance abuse, are not fully addressed by this method. This may explain why conventional therapies alone may fail to succeed in sustaining freedom from the harmful use of alcohol, tobacco and other drugs.

Complementary medicine, by design, treats the person in the context of his or her environment as a multidimensional organism. Practitioners draw on a variety of health-promoting and curative techniques. These systems are meant to acknowledge the patient's emotional, mental, social and spiritual as well as physical needs. Complementary and alternative medicine, when used holistically with conventional medicine, can treat the addiction as whole to part, not part to whole.

In the following pages, the principles behind a number of so-called 'alter-native' approaches will be discussed, together with an illustration of how they work and an explanation of how they can be used and integrated into an holistic treatment approach.

Acupuncture and Auriculotherapy

Acupuncture is an ancient technique, which has been used in traditional Chinese medicine for centuries. The basic idea behind the treatment is that an individual's physical, emotional and spiritual well-being is a reflection of an harmonic flow of life energy through the organs and energy channels (meridians). Any health problems or unhealthy habits are both caused by, and result in, changes in this energy flow. Stimulation of defined acupunc-ture points on the body with needles restores the proper flow of energy; the points are carefully selected to correspond to the energy disturbance in the person.

Auriculotherapy is of similar ancient origin but had practically been ignored until its 'rediscovery' in the 1960s. It acts as a reflex therapy, and is based on the principle that different zones in the ear represent different parts of the body. Functional problems of the patient can therefore be influenced by needle stimulation of the respective zones in the ear.

Research has been carried out over the last 30 years to study the efficacy of acupuncture and auriculotherapy in the treatment of substance abuse. Unfortunately, it is difficult to define an adequate control group. Studies can only be single blinded, and the standardised point combination that would be needed for scientific studies is not available as each patient has a different disharmony pattern and therefore different point combinations will be used in each individual's treatment.

However, research studies and case reports generally support the theory that acupuncture and auriculotherapy *are* effective in the treatment of substance abuse (Rampas and Pereira 1993). As can be expected from an understanding of their working mechanisms, the effects of these treatments are more general than those of orthodox drugs. They are usually incorporated into a more conventional detoxification programme, their primary aim being to rebalance the individual's energy flows and thus stop the craving for addictive substances such as drugs, nicotine and alcohol, alleviate withdrawal symptoms, and calm, relax and energise the patient. In appropriate circumstances, they can also be used to treat the side-effects of methadone use (Shoovanasai and Visuthuimak 1975, Shakus and Smith 1979, Smith 1979, Brumbaugh 1993, Blewington et al. 1994).

The frequency of therapy sessions varies according to individual needs, but normally consists of one or two sessions a day at the beginning of the detoxification programme (plus self-massage of points), reducing to two or three times weekly as the programme progresses – the ultimate aim being for the patient to be sufficiently well-balanced to discontinue the treatments. Both therapies are considered very safe, with less than 0.1% of those treated suffering side-effects such as the formation of small haematomas, slight bleeding, local irritation or, in extremely rare cases, infection or collapse (although the latter can be avoided by treating the patient in the recommended lying position). Infections are slightly more common in long-term auriculotherapy treatments and in highly immuno-compromised patients.

Experience has shown that patients suffering from alcohol addiction usually welcome acupuncture and auriculotherapy treatments, finding them both helpful and stabilising.

Ayurveda

'Ayurveda' means the 'science of life' (*ayur* – life; *veda* – science) and is a holistic approach which has been developed in India over the past 4,000 years. It is mentioned in the *Vedas* (sacred scriptures of India), and based on the ancient wisdom of the *Rishis* (holy wise men).

The guiding principle of Ayurveda is not only healing the sick, but also the prevention of illness and preservation of life. Ayurveda works by determining the balance of the vital energies in the body, called *Tridoshas*, or three *doshas* (constitutional types), which are more commonly known by their Sanskrit names – *Vata* (air), *Pita* (fire) and *Kafha* (water). Every individual's constitution is governed by a combination of these *doshas*, although one will usually predominate. An ayurvedic practitioner, after assessing the constitution and determining the *dosha*-type, will help patients to create balance or harmony in their life by recommending changes to lifestyle, and diet, by employing relaxation methods such as meditation or yoga, and by prescribing various treatments and remedies.

Ayurveda has been effectively used in alcohol addiction to restore energy balance, strengthen the immune system and treat liver disorders. Examples of typical ayurvedic herbal remedies, including medicinal properties, uses and effects, are given below.

Mentat

Mentat is a herbal formulation comprising *Nardostachys jatamansi*, *Bacopa monnieri*, *Cantella asiatica*, *Prunus amygdalus* and *Acorus calamus*.

Jatamansi (Musk Root, *Jatamansi*). *Jata-Mansone*, an active principle of *Nardostachys jatamansi*, effects a significant reduction in hyperactivity, restlessness and aggressiveness in hyperactive children. In adults it improves intellect, memory and exerts tranquillising, anxiolytic and antidepressant properties. It also helps in the treatment of substance abuse, especially alcohol and recreational drugs.

Bacopa monnieri (Thyme leafed gratiola, *Brahmi*) is reported to improve the intellect and also acts as an anti-anxiety agent. It exhibits sedative and tranquillising properties and is used to treat restlessness in children, and various mental disorders in both adults and children.

Cantella asiatica (Indian pennywort, *Gotu-Kola*) helps improve memory, the powers of concentration and intellectual ability in children and adults. Its safe, non-analgesic action also helps in the treatment of opiate addiction.

Prunus amygdalus (Almond, *Vatada*) is reported to improve mental functions in both children and adults.

Acorus calamus (Sweetflag, *Vacha*) has been used in indigenous systems of medicine to improve memory retention and recall. It exhibits mild sedative and potent tranquillising effects. A combination of *B monnieri* and *A calamus* is of significance in the treatment of many mental ailments in children and adults.

Clinical trials conducted with Mentat have indicated that among its other great benefits, it has prevented the development of dependence on various drugs and helped in the process of withdrawal and cessation of harmful alcohol/drug use.

Liv.52

Liv.52 is a herbal formulation comprising *Capparis spinosa*, *Cichorium intybus*, *Solanum nigrum*, *Terminalia arjuna*, *Cassia occidentalis*, *Achillea mille-folium*, *Tamarix gallica* and *Mandur bhasma*.

Capparis spinosa (Capers, *Himsra*) has shown antihepatotoxic activity and has been used to treat liver ailments.

Cichorium intybus (Wild chicory, *Kasani*) is useful in the treatment of various liver disorders such as hepatitis resulting from heavy alcohol or drug use.

Solanum nigrum (Black nightshade, *Kakamachi*) has a predominant action on the liver and has shown hepatoprotective activity in cases of toxicity induced by drugs and chemicals.

Terminalia arjuna (Arjuna, *Arjun*) is a known antioxidant and hepatopro-tective, found to be effective in the treatment of cirrhosis of the liver.

Cassia occidentalis (Negro Coffee, *Kasamarda*) has a protective effect on the liver against various hepatoxins.

Achillea millefolium (Yarrow, *Biranjsipha*) is used in various hepatic disor-ders.

Mandur bhasma (Oxide of iron) is a ferroso-ferric oxide used in several debilitating ailments such as anaemia, hepatitis and spleen disorders. It is a powerful haematinic and tonic, and is valuable in the treatment of haemolytic jaundice and microcytic anaemias.

Liv.52 has been extensively studied for various hepatological malfunc-tions. A number of experimental studies conducted on liver damaged by various hepatotoxins such as CC149, mercuric chloride10, cadmium11 and ethanol, observed that Liv.52 significantly maintained biochemical parame-ters and reduced histological abnormalities induced by alcohol (Warrier 1997, Frawley 1998).

Herbal Medicine (the Western Approach)

Herbal medicine triggers the neurochemical response in the body and has three primary functions: self-healing, detoxification and nourishment. It has been used in all cultures for many centuries, and modern medicine traces its roots back to the ancient Greek philosopher Hippocrates, who wrote about plant remedies. Chinese and Egyptian records dating back over 2,000 years also refer to the healing properties of herbs.

Herbal medicine uses all parts of plants – flower, root, leaf, seed and stem – in its preparations. There are many herbal remedies on the market today; one of the most widely used being *Valeriana officinalis* or, as it is more commonly known, Valerian (Latin: 'to be well'). It is a safe and non-addictive herb which has been used as a sedative and relaxant since the time of the Roman Empire. Its key constituents comprise Volatile Oil (up to 1.4%) including Bornyl acetate, Beta-caryphyllene, Iridoids (Valpotriates), Valtrate and Isovatrate alkaloids. During the Middle Ages it was known as 'all heal', and was credited with many virtues. For example, in 1592, herbalist Fabius Calumna published a detailed treatise on herbal medicine in which he claimed to have cured his epilepsy using Valerian. It is popularly used today to treat many stress-related illnesses, including alcohol or drug dependence, as it reduces mental overactivity and nervous excitability. It offers a beneficial substitute for the traditional 'remedies' typically used by people to help them 'switch off', such as alcohol and drugs, eliciting a calming rather than directly sedative effect on the mind. Many symptoms of anxiety, including tremors, panic, palpitations and sweating, can be relieved with Valerian, which is also a useful remedy for insomnia, whether caused by anxiety, overexcitement or withdrawal symptoms.

Extensive research has been carried out in Germany and Switzerland on the therapeutic properties of Valerian. This has provided conclusive evidence that Valerian reduces nervous activity by prolonging the action of an inhibiting neurotransmitter, lowers blood pressure, and promotes and improves the quality of sleep. There are several herbal preparations that may assist in detoxification of the whole system and, especially, the liver.

Yoga and Meditation

Yoga is of ancient Indian origin, typically used as a method of self-education and self-control. Although thought by many to be either a form of gymnastic exercise or religion, it is in fact neither, being originally developed to purify and obtain control of body and mind. It consists of a number of different techniques such as body exercises (*Asanas*), breathing exercises (*Pranayana*), cleansing exercises (*Kriyas*) and deep relaxation techniques (*Samkalpa*). These form an ideal combination for the treatment of alcoholism. Yoga is usually incorporated into an addiction treatment programme because of its calming and mood-improving effects (reducing anxiety, nervousness and insomnia). It harmonises the regulative nervous system and eases the symptoms of hypersalivation (dry mouth), hyperperspiration and abdominal cramps. It improves self-image, and helps make and maintain positive changes in the individual's lifestyle. The therapeutic effects of yoga are generated through body–mind interaction. By performing body exercises in a slow, relaxed and concentrated way, the patient gradually develops more confidence in his or her body.

Yoga should be taught and practised with a well-trained teacher who is adept at adjusting the programme to individual needs. Caution should be shown when using this method of treatment with patients suffering from psychotic or borderline psychotic illnesses, as the experience can be too strong for them. A number of studies have examined the impact of yoga and meditation in relation to alcohol and other drug problems, often with positive conclusions (Benson 1969, Sharma and Shukla 1988, Shapiro 1992, Zinn et al. 1992, Telles et al. 1993, Alexander et al. 1994, Miller et al. 1995).

Reiki

'Reiki' is a Japanese word meaning 'spiritual or universal life energy'. It is another approach to 'energy work' and can best be described as a spiritual system that requires no religious belief. All that is needed by the patient is a willingness to heal. Reiki was developed in Japan from 1922 to 1926 by Dr Mikao Usui and became widely practised there at that time. From the mid-1970s it spread rapidly in the US and throughout the world. Anyone with an interest in learning Reiki can be readily taught by a 'master'.

Being essentially holistic, Reiki works at all levels of the body, mind and spirit (McKenzie 1998). It can take the form of 'hands-on' healing or be as formless as a focus of love shared across time and space. The effects of Reiki are not at all easy to quantify, but its popularity and widespread use point to its value. A skilled Reiki practitioner is able to focus upon what it is that the problem drinker/drug user truly needs – beyond the sedative effect of their current 'fix'. Reiki helps supply this need – without effort, without drama, quietly, peacefully and in the most appropriate manner for a particular person at a particular time.

It has been said that Reiki is an aspect of love. Experience with alcoholics has shown time and time again that somewhere, down at the level at which we hold our most deeply felt pain, is a 'self' which feels unloved or, worse, unlovable. It is here that Reiki may work its quiet magic, bringing about the necessary transformation at a speed that feels comfortable to the individual.

Used in conjunction with meridian therapies and a physical regime of detoxification, Reiki can offer significant support to a recovering alcohol-dependent person.

Biofeedback

Biofeedback is a non-conventional treatment which trains individuals to recognise the mental and emotional states that accompany corresponding physiological responses. With practice, these responses can be reduced as required. Electrodes, linked to a measuring device, are attached to the part of the body from which responses are being measured. Feedback is provided by sound (a tone that varies with the measurement), visually (with the movement of a needle), or by colour changes. For example, blood pressure can be recorded, muscle tension registered using an electromyograph, and changes in sweat production monitored through electrodes attached to the palms of the hands (nervous tension increases perspiration – the renowned 'sweaty palm' syndrome). Indeed, biofeedback is the science behind the lie detector employed in criminal prosecutions.

The importance of biofeedback was realised when scientists researching brainwaves discovered that students could teach themselves to shift from one brainwave frequency to another at will. In everyday waking life people are on the beta frequency, while the state of relaxed awareness is on alpha frequency. Theta frequency correlates to drowsy daydreaming, and delta is the frequency of deep sleep.

The efficacy of biofeedback training is emphasised in many studies. For example, Denny et al. (1991) studied the effect of the amount of biofeedback training received upon abstinence from alcohol. The researchers found that the frequency of sobriety for those patients who had had at least six training sessions was significantly better than those with less or no training. The effect was most prominent for those receiving the highest level of biofeedback training (more than eight sessions).

In another, randomised, study of 110 patients recruited from a five-stage worksite blood pressure screening programme, Irvine and Logan (1991) examined the efficacy of relaxation therapy as sole treatment for mild hypertension. Participants were randomised to twelve weeks of relaxation or support therapy. Outcome blood pressure assessments made by assessors who were unaware of group allocation, revealed similar decreases in both the groups at post-treatment and six-month follow-ups. Biofeedback also showed that when practitioners of transcendental meditation slipped into alpha frequency, their blood pressure was lowered. The results concluded that although a superior blood pressure effect was not associated with relaxation therapy, alcohol consumption decreased in both treatment groups, suggesting that both interventions facilitated changes directly in health risk behaviours and indirectly on blood pressure level. Later studies showed that not only could people raise or lower the temperature of their fingertips by using autogenic training (imagining their fingers as warmer or colder), but they also did so more quickly if they could monitor their progress.

A recent investigation by Sharp et al. (1997) focused on the facilitation of internal locus of control in adolescent alcoholics through a brief biofeedback-assisted autogenic relaxation training procedure. This found that the treatment group was significantly more in internal locus of control after training. They were also significantly more so than the control group post-training. The study concluded that alcoholics are significantly more external in their locus of control than 'non-alcoholics'. Autogenic relaxation facilitated through biofeedback may be an important component in therapeutic intervention for people with drinking problems.

Significant inroads into the benefits of biofeedback have been made in recent years. For example, a sophisticated mind-controlled computer programme – Relaxplus – has been developed at St Bartholomew's Hospital, London, which converts the screen image of a mermaid into an angel as an individual relaxes. In addition, the mystery of how the mind is able to overrule the involuntary workings of the autonomic nervous system is rapidly being unravelled through research into psychoneuroimmunology, the science of the mind–brain–body connection. This has obvious beneficial repercussions in the field of therapy for people with severe alcohol problems.

Hypnotherapy

The word 'hypnosis' (from the Greek root *hypnos*, meaning 'sleep') is misleading because the phenomenon to which it refers is not a form of sleep; rather, it is a complex process of attentive receptive concentration. Although peripheral awareness is reduced in both sleep and hypnosis, focal awareness, which is diffuse in sleep, is at optimal capacity during the hypnotic trance.

Originally, hypnotists believed hypnosis to be a form of sleep and relied on using authoritarian techniques for inducing a deep trance in their clients. Modern hypnotherapists now believe that the depth of trance has no bearing on the treatment and it is essential to build up a rapport with the patients in order to enable them to make changes.

Milton Erickson is widely acknowledged as a leading practitioner of medical hypnosis. Although he died in 1980, his work and examples have continued to be at the cutting edge of all hypnotic interventions for the healthier development and growth of those seeking such support. What is less known is Erickson's individual approach to psychotherapy and his early Neuro Linguistic Programming. His approach was both radical and caring and a growing reputation has seen his work subject to ever-closer scrutiny and examination (Haley 1967).

The essence of Erickson's technique was his gentle induction method whereby a client is gradually introduced to the hypnotic trance. His use of metaphor and a persistent care of language (there is no 'problem', there is only 'challenge' – no one is 'alone', they are 'independent') are now more widely understood as reframing. Erickson had a firm belief that every individual possesses an extraordinary level of personal resources which frequently goes unacknowledged and unrecognised.

The clients referred to the hypnotherapist are usually profoundly disturbed. Therapy begins with a gathering of sensory-specific information, constant reframing and an early attempt to reduce stress levels by creative visualisation and, with agreement, hypnosis.

Tasking has in one way or another long been used by hypnotherapists to restrict alcohol intake and change habits. Anyone would find it difficult to change established habits. There is evidence that individuals pass through a number of recognisable stages as they come to make up their minds about breaking a damaging habit.

In the experience of many working in the field of alcohol and drug problems, physical, psychological and social deprivation are commonplace. Many practitioners recognise the extent to which personal traumas and emotional needs drive individuals to their very limits and even to the point of self-destruction (Caprio 1985, Vandamme 1986, Hadley 1996).

It is well known that the heavy and harmful use of alcohol and other drugs may lead to physical and psychological dependence (see Chapter 2). The 'traditional' treatments of psychotherapy, counselling and detoxification have their vital roles to play. Even so, no one type of therapeutic approach works for everyone; there is clearly room for a variety of routes or approaches. However, it is emphasised, that the effectiveness of alternative approaches should be assessed. Project MATCH (described above by Nick Heather) provides a good example of such a comparative evaluation.

Hypnosis has long suffered from the suspicions of the uninformed and so its usage has been largely restricted to the prevention of smoking and a limited range of habit disorders. However, very few authoritative studies have been conducted in this field in relation to alcohol and drug dependency.

A study by Orman (1991) of a 24-year-old chemically dependent patient demonstrated the success of age regression and reframing in the treatment of such conditions. This field invites further research and courageous exploration. Once more, it is stressed that properly conducted evaluation is required.

Meridian Therapies

An interesting tool has emerged over recent years, which takes an unusual approach to dealing with alcohol and drug dependence and, indeed, a wide spectrum of ills ranging from phobias to physical ailments. TFT™ (Thought Field Therapy™) and EFT™ (Emotional Freedom Technique™) are based on two premises. The first is that all negative emotions are a result of a disruption in the body's energy system (Craig and Fowlie 1995). The second is the remarkable discovery that simply by tapping, in sequence, the originating points of some of the body's energy meridians, these disruptions can be cleared. The disappearance of the negative emotions is usually permanent.

The lines of energy are identical to the meridians described in traditional Chinese medicine (particularly acupuncture). The process is simple, easily learnt by the patient, and its effects may be dramatic.

The procedure was first discovered and taught by Callaghan (1996), who named it Thought Field Therapy™ or TFT™. Craig (Craig and Fowlie 1995) developed the process still further, simplifying an approach to mental health that was already astonishingly simple and effective. Craig also introduced some positive emotional aspects that many practitioners and students feel has considerably enhanced this whole field of research and practice. This 'enhanced' version was subsequently called 'Emotional Freedom Therapy™'.

When an individual is dependent on either a substance or an unwanted behaviour pattern, underlying this dependence – in almost all cases – is both a sense of something missing from his or her life and the presence of anxiety. More often than not, the latter derives from the former. If this missing link is not found and replaced by whatever is really wanted and needed, the addiction is likely to continue; it may sometimes alter its focus (that is, a dependence on alcohol may change to a craving for nicotine or chocolate), but the person remains dependent because the underlying cause is still there.

In addition, although a person with a severe drinking problem might clearly state his or her determination to break free from the grip of this behaviour, all too often he or she may manifest all of the traits of a person unwilling to do so. Such an individual seems to be resisting with the strength of desperation the very thing he or she says, and knows, he or she wants. This phenomenon, well known to psychologists, was identified by Callaghan (1996) and Craig (Craig and Fowlie 1995) as 'psychological reversal' (PR) and is specifically addressed in the meridian therapies and dealt with routinely as part of the treatment. While tapping the relevant points, a phrase such as 'Even though I have this craving for —— I accept myself deeply and completely', is repeated. It has been found that by holding a simple thought such as this while tapping the points which are, as it were, the gateway to the blocks or short-circuits in the energy system, the tendency to be psychologically reversed disappears. This simple process has had positive repercussions in energy work with several types of dependent behaviour. What was, in the past, often a lengthy process (the 'one step forward, two steps back' syndrome often encountered with so-called addictive personalities) can be considerably shortened by using this method.

Although the meridian therapies can frequently dispose of traumatic memories, grief, and so on, with unexpected ease and sometimes in a matter of minutes, success with dependence requires a much longer process. Traditional methods of treating alcohol problems – the Twelve-step process, hypnotherapy, aversion therapy and sometimes sheer willpower – often result in the former problem drinker turning to gambling, smoking or other problem behaviours, possibly including wife/husband/child-abuse. In these cases, it is clear that the underlying cause of dependence was not overcome, with the individual merely switching from one kind of dependent behaviour to another.

It has therefore been realised that dependent behaviour is in itself not the root problem; rather, it represents the patient's 'solution' to the underlying issue which is emotional unrest manifesting as frequent feelings of anxiety. Craig (Craig and Fowlie 1995) suggests that all dependent behaviour simply serves as 'sedatives' or 'tranquillisers' to temporarily 'medicate' this generalised anxiety. Despite the obviously negative effects of dependence upon alcohol and other substances, the patient would rather suffer these consequences than experience the seemingly ever-present anxiety.

This anxiety is not always conscious; in fact, a major contributor to dependent behaviour is often a level of anxiety that is deeply rooted in the subconscious. This explains why so many alcohol- or drug-dependent people are psychologically reversed: the dependent person's system is not giving permission to work on the problem because without the 'tranquilliser' he or she is left with a constant anxiety. In the face of this, the cure seems worse than the dependence itself.

In EFT™ the ultimate goal of all healing is personal peace. Most people have anxieties, self-doubts, and so on, and use some form of harmful behaviour (however mild) to cope with them. EFT™ is a powerful tool for neutralising the emotional drivers underlying addictive behaviour. Supported by the underlying idea, 'Even though I get drunk so often, I deeply and completely accept myself', EFT™ is used to sequentially neutralise the various levels of fear, guilt, anger and traumatic memories that undermine peace of mind. Once the generalised anxiety has lessened, the need for subduing consciousness with alcohol should fade. Having removed the psychological aspect of the addiction, there remains only the chemical part of it. Assuming that this state is reached, the meridian therapies may be effectively used to minimise cravings while the patient spends whatever time is necessary to detoxify his or her body.

RESEARCH, EFFECTIVENESS AND LIMITATIONS

More than 4,000 trials in complementary medical research have been identified by the Cochrane Collaboration. However, most of the research programmes and papers are of poor quality in comparison to those based on conventional medicine. In the UK, only 0.08% of the total research budget is being spent on complementary and alternative medicine. In the US, the Office of Alternative and Complementary Medicine within the National

Institute of Health has now become a centre in its own right. This provides both a structure and appropriate funding (US$50 million (£33 million) per annum) on research efforts. The Foundation for Integrated Medicine's report emphasises the influence of an appropriately supported national agenda for research into complementary and alternative medicine as there is a wide and growing interest in this field.

Astin (1998), in a study to investigate possible predictors of alternative health care use, concluded that a majority of alternative users appear to be choosing alternative medicine not as a result of being dissatisfied with conventional medicine but largely because they find health care alternatives to be more congruent with their own values, beliefs and philosophical orientations towards health and life. Paramore (1997) analysed data from the general probability sample (n = 3,450) of the 1994 Robert Wood Johnson Foundation Access to Care survey. The results indicate that nearly 10% of the American population, almost 25 million persons, saw a professional in 1994 for at least one of the following four therapies: chiropractic, relaxation technique, therapeutic massage or acupuncture.

Astin et al. (1998) have reported that a large number of physicians are either referring to or practising some of the more prominent and well-known forms of complementary/alternative therapy, and that many physicians believe these therapies to be useful and effective. Approximately half the respondents believed in the efficacy of acupuncture (51%), chiropractic (53%) and massage (48%), while fewer believed in the value of homeopathy (26%) and herbal approaches (13%).

Knipschild et al. (1990), in a survey among 293 GPs in The Netherlands highlights the findings that many believe in the efficacy of common alternative procedures. High scores were especially found for manual therapy, yoga, acupuncture, hot bath therapy and homeopathy. Other procedures such as iridology, faith healing and many food supplements were considered less useful. Kleijnen et al. (1991) assessed the methodological quality of 105 trails of homeopathy to ascertain the efficacy of homeopathy based on evidence from controlled trials in humans. The result showed a positive trend, regardless of the quality of the trial or the variety of homeopathy used. Overall, of the 105 trials with interpretable results, 81 trials indicated positive results whereas in 24 trials no positive effects of homeopathy were found.

Zollman and Vickens (1999) explored the factors limiting research in complementary medicine and pointed out both a lack of funding and a lack of research skills. The latter is due to there being no formal training either in the critical evaluation of existing research or in practical research. There is also a lack of academic infrastructure, for example, computer and library facilities, statistical support and university research grants, and a difficulty in undertaking and interpreting systematic reviews due to the poor quality of research.

This poor-quality research, on the one hand, and the growing demand for complementary medicine by the public, on the other, requires a true integration of complementary/alternative therapies into the mainstream of conventional medicine.

This author proposes an integrated and multifaceted approach which could be termed 'multidimensional medicine'.

THE WAY FORWARD

Dependence on alcohol or other drugs is a multidimensional problem. It is important to consider that human beings are complex creatures whose health and well-being depend on balance in all dimensions of life and existence, broadly described as the physical, behavioural, energy and vibrational aspects of their being.

These different life dimensions are, however, interdependent. This means that when an imbalance occurs in one dimension, it can affect all others. To support a return to a natural state of health and balance, it is necessary to:

- assess the client's state in various dimensions affecting his or her well-being
- treat with the appropriate healing modalities (chosen from integrated medicine) for balance in each dimension.

Multidimensional assessment should address the individual's:

- *physical well-being* – biophysical state of health and dependency on alcohol/drugs
- *behavioural well-being* – causes and effects of problematic use
- *energetic well-being* – the flow of energy as evidenced by vitality or fatigue
- *environmental well-being* – the effects of one's environment on one's well-being.

Consider the example of a client presenting with a long history of alcohol problems. We will have:

- *physical* – biochemical dependency on alcohol
- *behavioural* – psychological dependency on alcohol
- *energy* – disturbances and blockages in his or her energy field (for example, dependence may cause energy blockages in the solar plexus and heart chakra)

- *environmental* – socialisation with heavy/problem drinkers, response to music, colour, chaos at home or a generally unhealthy environment.

The multidimensional assessment should ideally be carried out by four practitioners, including a psychiatrist (for physical/psychological well-being), a psychologist/counsellor (behavioural well-being), a Reiki therapist (energetic well-being) and a social worker with a deeper understanding of the living environment of the dependent person and how it can affect his or her well-being.

The multidimensional assessment team should discuss their findings in a group and together they should frame the ideal and unique care package for the dependent/problem drinker. They should select the most suitable balance of treatment and practitioners for the complete well-being of the client, comprising conventional, complementary or alternative medicine.

Conventional therapy may, as noted above, involve detoxification, rehabilitation and counselling – addressing imbalances in the emotional, behavioural and physical dimensions only. However, all the various dimensions of the patient will be addressed by the multidimensional assessment and treatment programme. This approach may include, for example, sessions of Reiki healing, ayurveda, hypnotherapy, cognitive-behavioural therapy, music and mantra and/or conventional treatment.

In conclusion, it is likely that the interest in and demand for complementary therapies will continue to grow. Interest in the potential contribution of such approaches in relation to problems associated with alcohol and other drugs has been emphasised by the success of a conference on this topic. This event, arranged by the Addictions Forum, took place in Edinburgh in 1994. Subsequent meetings have also included sessions on complementary approaches. Interest in such approaches has become commonplace and they are increasingly being used as part of the wide range of services now available to help people to overcome problems with alcohol.

9
Evidence-Based Alcohol Education in Schools

Linda Wright

INTRODUCTION

This chapter takes a critical look at the rhetoric, common assumptions and research evidence that inform school-based alcohol education initiatives. It identifies the main evidence and theories that have guided research on alcohol education and discusses the ways they have limited past approaches to gathering evidence, and the interpretation of the evidence that has been collected. The constraints and challenges of conducting alcohol education in an evidence-based way are reviewed in the broader context of health promotion.

This chapter is written against the background of available international evidence, but the main focus of discussion is on alcohol education as practised in UK schools. The full scope of alcohol education is far broader, in terms of settings, target groups and the range of practitioners who have a role as alcohol educators (Wright 1993). There can be few people in the UK whose lives are not touched directly or indirectly by the consequences of drinking alcohol, whatever their own drinking habits may be. At the level of basic entitlements, every citizen has the right to education about alcohol. Any strategy to reduce or prevent alcohol-related harm depends on knowledgeable, skilled planners and practitioners. Within a community approach to alcohol education, many people have a potential role as alcohol educators or are in a position to promote safer drinking or prevent alcohol misuse. They range from lay people such as parents, youth leaders, young people (as peer educators), religious leaders, local politicians, licensees and bar staff, through to professional workers in education, health and social care, and those involved in the alcohol industry. While young people have received more research attention than other groups, there are many other targets and uses for alcohol education, such as professional development in health promotion, informing decision-making and service planning and supporting social policy development (Howe 1989, Wright 1993, Plant and Plant, 1997).

Schools are not the only setting for alcohol education with young people, nor, as will be argued here, are they necessarily the most appropriate or effective setting for such activities. However, most evaluation studies have focused on young people in the school setting, while work on alcohol issues with young people in informal education settings has been seriously neglected as a subject for research and evaluation (Wright 1999a). Informal educators such as youth and community workers have enormous potential as alcohol educators because of the nature of their relationship with young people. Voluntarism is a defining characteristic of informal education, and if young people do not like the alcohol education that is offered then they can 'vote with their feet' by choosing not to participate. Informal educators are also able to operate in the settings where young people choose to spend their leisure time and where they choose to consume alcohol, including street corners, bus shelters, clubs, cafes and bars. Informal education therefore offers greater opportunity to tailor the messages and methods of alcohol education to young people's cultural and drinking practices. It has been established that it is possible to enhance youth workers' competence and confidence as alcohol educators through carefully structured training based on a thorough training needs assessment (Wright 1999a).

Again, because evaluation studies have been almost exclusively focused on alcohol education aimed at school-age children, this chapter does not examine work with other groups such as parents or whole population community-based strategies in detail, although recent work suggests that such approaches have achieved promising outcomes.

Finally, it is also important to note that most of the evidence reviewed here derives from health education initiatives – planned opportunities for people to learn about alcohol and health – rather than the broader health promotion approach advocated by the World Health Organization. The content of this book reflects this broader health promotion approach, defined by the World Health Organization as 'the process of enabling people to enable people to increase control over and to improve their health' (1985: 6). Health promotion in relation to alcohol *includes* health education as well as preventive health services, community development, organisational development, healthy public policies, environmental health measures and economic, legislative and regulatory activities (Ewles and Simnett 1999).

THERE'S A LOT OF IT ABOUT

From the earliest days of public concern about alcohol-related problems in Britain, alcohol education in schools has been considered a socially desirable endeavour. As early as 1909, during the early years of state provision of education, the Board of Education issued its first syllabus for temperance education in state elementary schools. It recommended at least three lessons be given each year (more than in many modern primary schools) on eating and drinking, the effects of alcohol on the body and the evil consequences of intemperance. Since then, the priority allocated to alcohol education in schools has waxed and waned alongside general social trends in education and health. From the 1960s onwards there has been a considerable increase in alcohol education activity in schools as part of the general expansion in the personal, social and health education curriculum, and more recently, within health promotion and the new public health agenda (Wright 1999a).

The current UK government has high expectations of alcohol education as an element of health promotion in UK schools, particularly in the context of prevention of substance misuse (SOHHD 1994, DfEE 1995, 1998, SCODA 1999a, 1999b). Its commitment to tackling health inequalities (DoH 1998, NHS Executive 1999) and social exclusion, 'best value' in public services and to promoting excellence in schools (Government White Paper 1997) includes an expectation that all schools will become healthy schools. 1998 saw the introduction of a National Healthy Schools Programme in England, aiming at promoting a whole school approach to personal, social and health education and citizenship. The programme 'reflects a commitment to work across government, the private and voluntary sectors and with local agencies and the communities they serve to build sustainable health schools' (Monks and Purcell 1999: 1). This approach incorporates not only the taught curriculum but also the school organisation, development, policies, culture and environment, community involvement and partnerships with parents and carers. Part of this programme is a £2.85 million National Healthy Schools Scheme, launched in autumn 1999, to support the development of local healthy schools via accredited education and health partnerships. To achieve accreditation, local schemes are expected to provide *evidence* to demonstrate achievement of national quality standards (DfEE/DoH 1999a). Drug education (including alcohol education) is specified in the quality standards.

Many UK Drug Action Teams have chosen to include alcohol within their local action plans to tackle drug misuse, although the national strategy focuses solely on illegal drugs (Cabinet Office 1999) with a national alcohol strategy promised in the year 2000. If this national alcohol policy follows the lead taken by the national drug strategy, it will shift the emphasis from dealing with the consequences of alcohol problems to prevention and education. There will be even greater expectations of schools to deliver 'effective' alcohol education as a way of tackling heavy or inappropriate drinking.

Despite these high expectations currently placed on schools to deliver effective alcohol education (or perhaps because of them), few have attempted to look behind the alcohol education label to seriously question what is there. This lack of clarity has then been translated into assumptions that have limited the approach to gathering evidence and interpretations of the evidence that has been elicited.

EVIDENCE-BASED ALCOHOL EDUCATION

The current context for alcohol education suggests that pressures on its practitioners to deliver effective programmes and to justify the use of increasingly scarce resources have never been greater. Within the fields of health and social care in Britain, there has been a strong move towards evidence-based practice over the last five years. Alcohol education, like the broader field of health promotion, is expected to be based on sound evidence. However, the alcohol research literature does not acknowledge that evidence-based practice in health promotion is still in its infancy, not least because there is considerable debate about what this means and the best ways of achieving it. Health promoters from all disciplines are expected to practise within multiple definitions of what counts as evidence, in what contexts and for what purposes (Perkins et al. 1999).

WHAT COUNTS AS EVIDENCE?

Before considering the available evidence, it is worth considering the paradigms within which the evidence about alcohol education is collected and interpreted. Most health educators and health promoters query the specialised use of the word 'evidence' that is currently in use in clinical contexts, where the specified hierarchy of evidence derives from scientific research, relying almost exclusively on quantitative methods. This approach has underpinned much of the study of health behaviour (Milburn et al. 1995). All of the effectiveness reviews on alcohol education and most of the research studies on young people and alcohol have been conducted within this paradigm, while other forms and sources of evidence have tended to be discounted or overlooked. Academic books, reviews and articles on alcohol education have tended to treat the subject as an entirely separate phenomenon from the rest of the school curriculum, paying scant attention to the extensive body of evidence on curriculum development, teaching and learning drawn from educational research. With some notable exceptions (for example, Bagnall 1991, Coggans and Watson 1995), learning from the broader discipline of health promotion has also been discounted or overlooked. This is in marked contrast to the current Department for Education and Employment (DfEE) guidance on alcohol education as part of drug education, which recommends that it is based on broad educational principles – integration, whole school approaches and a holistic model of personal, social, health and now citizenship education (Department for Education and Employment 1998). A growing literature on the theory and practice of evidence-based health promotion now acknowledges that other research paradigms, other theories of knowledge, do exist and have important contributions to make to the understanding of alcohol education and health promotion in general (Macdonald et al. 1996, Ziglio 1997, Nutbeam 1998, Perkins et al. 1999).

The 'interpretivist' perspective offers a particularly useful additional framework for understanding and evaluating health promotion. Although still relatively uncommon in health care research, this approach has long been accepted in the social sciences and has made a substantial contribution to educational theory and practice (Reason 1994, Eisner 1997). It assumes that human behaviour, for example young people's use of alcohol, or alcohol education in schools, is viewed as being socially and culturally defined rather than objective fact. In the first example, the purpose of research is seen as exploring how young people understand and make sense of their world and the place and meaning of alcohol within it. This kind of evidence helps alcohol educators to understand why young people drink and is important in tailoring learning to their needs, motivations and interests. Research on alcohol education in schools conducted within this perspective would focus on its location, organisation and delivery in the school curriculum and its multiple interpretations by members of the school community (for example, students, staff, parents, governors). This kind of evidence would help alcohol educators to design realistic programmes tailored to the resources and culture of the school, and to increase the chances of successful programme adoption, implementation and long-term sustainability. Researchers adopting an 'interpretivist' view commonly use qualitative methods. Evaluators working with this approach use an action research approach which enables learning to be channelled into action throughout the project's life rather than waiting until the work has been completed.

The UK government's health strategy, *Our Healthier Nation* (Secretary of State for Health 1998), and the more recent Government White Paper on public health, *Saving Lives: Our Healthier Nation* (1999), both acknowledge that young people's drinking behaviour and its consequences are a complex interplay of individual, interpersonal and environmental factors, which are culturally specific (Wright 1999b). Unfortunately, despite an abundance of survey data on young people's drinking, some of which is reviewed in Chapters 4 and 5, relatively little is known about drinking in specific cultures in the UK (May 1992, Wright 1999b). There is, even now, a limited understanding about how drinking practices fit into adolescent social worlds, the meaning of drinking to different groups of young people of various ages and cultural backgrounds, the norms and rules that govern their drinking behaviour, and how these compare with adults' norms (Wright 1999b). The need to explore the place and meaning of drinking in girls' and young women's lives is a particular priority for alcohol education because it appears that some gender differences in frequency and consumption may have declined in recent years (Goddard 1997a, 1997b, M.L. Plant 1997, ONS 1998, Wright 1999b).

As Webb (1999) points out, the application of the dominant scientific approach to gathering evidence about alcohol education not only restricts the evidence that is considered, but may result in misleading judgements about what is effective and provide poor advice to policy-makers, purchasers and providers of alcohol education. For example, there is cold comfort to be derived from a recent systematic review of evaluations of 'alcohol misuse' prevention programmes for young people commissioned by the NHS Centre for Reviews and Dissemination (Foxcroft et al. 1997). In applying strict scientific study design criteria and reporting only studies achieving behavioural outcomes, the authors found that of 500 papers screened, only 33 met the inclusion criteria and most of these had some methodological shortcomings. The only advice they were able to provide was that 'the lack of reliable evidence means that no one type of prevention programme can be recommended' (Foxcroft et al. 1997: 536).

The solution, according to the authors, is better-designed evaluations of effectiveness. Whilst this is undoubtedly the case, they do not consider the possibility that a more pragmatic and inclusive approach to gathering and using evidence might also be useful. Nor do they acknowledge the likelihood that even the best-designed 'gold standard' randomised control trial is unlikely to be able to confidently attribute health outcomes (drinking behaviours) to alcohol misuse prevention inputs, because of the multiple determinants and time scales involved before some outcomes are seen.

A further shortcoming of this limited approach to gathering evidence about alcohol education has been the focus in evaluation studies on *what* rather than *how*. Even positive outcome evaluations have limited value to alcohol educators if there is insufficient information provided about the inputs, processes and methods employed to allow them to be replicated. This evidence is essential in enabling practitioners to decide whether this would be an affordable and appropriate approach to use locally in their school with their particular students. The best-designed and evaluated North American alcohol education studies involve inputs that are simply beyond the resources of schools in the UK. For example, few UK schools would be able to replicate Botvin's substance misuse prevention programme (Botvin et al. 1995a, 1995b), which involves 15 sessions and 10 boosters, even though this programme has demonstrated long-term effectiveness in terms of reduced substance use. Moreover, if it is accepted that drinking is culturally determined, practitioners will want to know whether the findings of any evaluation are transferable to the group and context in which they are working. Because of such cultural differences, the findings from the North American studies that comprise the bulk of the current evidence may not transfer to young people in the UK. Replicative studies are needed to test promising findings. Even so, it should be emphasised that the available world-wide literature provides little convincing evidence that alcohol education has succeeded in changing behaviours. There is some evidence that it may increase awareness and change attitudes, even if only briefly.

These limitations of the dominant approach to gathering evidence also contribute to the evidence–practice gap that is well-documented in the literature on professional practice in health and social care generally (Maguire 1990, Haines and Jones 1994, Blackburn et al. 1997) and in alcohol education in particular (Plant and Plant 1997). Alcohol education practitioners are only likely to use evidence if they perceive it as useful and applicable to them, in their role, context and setting. The current evidence does not adequately acknowledge the uniqueness of practice contexts or the processes of educational change. When school-based alcohol education evaluations identify positive outcomes they often apply to a set of unique conditions which are not reproducible in other schools. Although there is evidence from evaluations of North American schools programmes that high-integrity (fidelity) alcohol education programmes have more impact than low-integrity programmes (Pentz et al. 1989a, 1989b, 1990, Botvin 1990, Botvin et al. 1995a), in real life it is almost impossible to achieve an alcohol education programme that has a totally controlled set of inputs, processes and outputs. White and Pitts (1997) point out that ensuring programmes are delivered as intended is also very expensive, because they require highly detailed teaching materials and either external staff or intensive teacher preparation to ensure committed programme leaders.

In relation to the process of change, the alcohol treatment field has embraced the stages of change model (Prochaska and DiClemente 1992) as a useful way of understanding the process of individual behaviour change. Health promotion has utilised this model as a framework for promoting individual lifestyle changes and has even attempted to extend it to population-level interventions, despite concerns about equity (Whitehead 1997). Yet among the alcohol and drug research community and commissioners and planners of alcohol education interventions, there is little recognition of alcohol education being a process of educational change. The reviewers of alcohol and drug education evaluation studies have noted this lack of attention paid to recording and measuring programme implementation (Kinder et al. 1980, Schaps et al. 1981, Goodstadt 1986, 1989, Moskowitz 1989, Dorn and Murji 1992).

There is extensive empirical evidence that educational change is indeed a process with several identifiable stages, from dissemination and adoption through implementation to institutionalisation and ultimately outcomes (Fullan 1991). Each stage has its own dynamics, enabling and limiting factors and progression through the stages is measured in years rather than months. This time frame is consistently ignored by planners or commissioners of school-based alcohol education and by programme evaluators, with an expectation that a new school alcohol education programme can move from adoption to successful outcomes within one school year. Research studies on dissemination and implementation in health care are still relatively rare, but there is useful literature on the features of successful implementation of educational change (Fullan 1991) and a small body of evidence on implementation of health/alcohol education in schools (see review by Dobson and Wright 1995). There is also a growing literature on effective health promotion in schools (Denman 1994, Moon et al. 1999a, 1999b), and on health promotion and young people in other settings (Aggleton 1996).

Box 9.1 summarises the research findings on factors contributing to the successful implementation of alcohol education in schools. Each of the factors has some empirical support. The model is adapted from a study by TACADE of effective implementation of drug education in schools in five European Countries (Dobson and Wright 1995). While these factors provide a framework for facilitating programme implementation, further research is required to establish the interfactoral relationships and their relative importance.

The traditional view of what counts as evidence has provided practitioners in Britain with relatively little useful information to inform the planning, delivery and evaluation of alcohol education programmes. The 'quiet methodological revolution' that has taken place in evaluation studies (Denzin and Lincoln 1994) has been largely ignored by the alcohol research world. A more pluralistic and pragmatic approach to evidence gathering is urgently needed, particularly in Britain. Alcohol researchers and practitioners could learn much from the growing literature on mixed methodologies that acknowledge evidence from both the scientific-empiricist and the qualitative–interpretative traditions (Wright 1999c). Adoption of these approaches does not imply that interest in outcomes is abandoned or that quantitative data is not collected; it merely acknowledges that a whole range of different forms of evidence can inform the multifaceted nature of alcohol education.

Box 9.1:
Factors enabling successful implementation of alcohol education in schools.

School Climate
- There is a culture of innovation within the school
- The school principal actively supports the programme
- The staff have good working relationships
- The school is politically stable

Curriculum
- The degree of change required for the implementation of the programme relates to the culture of innovation
- Alcohol education is not presented as an isolated programme, but within a whole school approach to health
- The school has an established personal, social and health education programme
- Alcohol education is included in the school development plan
- There is a whole school approach to teaching and learning styles

Socio-political context
- The government encourages alcohol education
- The school is required by law to provide alcohol education
- The school programme is supported by the local community
- The school is close to its community
- Quality working relationships exist with community agencies
- Advice is available to parents

Need and priority
- The school sees a need for an alcohol education programme
- The programme meets the school's needs
- The school sees alcohol education as a high priority
- The students want an alcohol education programme

Students
- The students identify with the school
- The students want an alcohol education programme

Resources
- Relevant teaching materials are available
- Practical support is available locally
- Financial support is available
- Time is available
- Counselling is available
- Space is available for seeing students

Teachers
- There is a committed and efficient coordinator
- In-service training for teachers is provided
- The teachers are willing to change their approach
- The teachers feel confident to provide alcohol education
- The teachers have counselling skills
- Alcohol education is included in teachers' job descriptions
- Alcohol education is included in the teacher appraisal scheme

Programme characteristics
- The programme has clear goals
- Student learning outcomes are specified
- All or most of the programme is delivered
- The programme is delivered as planned
- The programme is successful at an early stage
- The programme includes effective and ongoing monitoring and evaluation
- Teaching methods and activities in the programme are specified
- The programme has high visibility
- The programme has been evaluated

Source: Adapted with permission from a model developed by TACADE in B.E. Dobson and L. Wright (1995), *A Consultative Project on Effective Implementation of Drug Education in Five European Countries*, Salford: TACADE.

WHAT ARE THE CRITERIA FOR SUCCESS?

The published effectiveness reviews on alcohol and drug education are strongly dominated by evaluations and interventions from the US, many of which have assumed that the sole legitimate purpose of alcohol education is to prevent young people from drinking or to delay the onset of drinking until at least the age of 21.

There are a number of difficulties in applying these assumptions to the UK and to other countries where adolescent drinking is the norm. The first relates to philosophical basis for alcohol *education* interventions. In contrast to the medical model of alcohol education, with its specific behavioural goals (stopping or reducing drinking) and the outcome criteria set for success in evaluation studies, education is primarily concerned with rationality and freedom of choice (Hirst 1969). Within an educational approach, therefore, the primary goal of alcohol education is to facilitate informed and rational decision-making, irrespective of the ultimate decision that is made.

This fundamental difference between educational and medical models of health education helps to explain the logical inconsistencies revealed by effectiveness reviews of alcohol education programmes. Their almost exclusive focus on the goal of preventing or reducing alcohol use among young people has meant that other goals and sound educational achievements have been overlooked. Thus early effectiveness reviews of alcohol education revealed that it was possible to increase students' knowledge about alcohol, but dismissed this approach because it was not also accompanied by a reduction in drinking (Kinder et al. 1980, Schaps et al. 1981). Similarly, programmes that have aimed to develop self-esteem or change alcohol-related attitudes and values were again judged as ineffective because they did not achieve changes in alcohol use among young people (Hansen et al. 1998). Educationalists would argue that increasing knowledge, developing self-esteem and challenging anti-social attitudes and values are legitimate learning goals in their own right and essential in developing informed choice.

Perhaps the most important problem with applying such limited behavioural criteria is that it simply sets alcohol education up to fail. In the UK, young people are socialised into a society in which drinking alcohol is an integral part of the social and leisure activities of over 90% of adults (Wright 1999b). During their mid-teens drinking alcohol becomes the norm for the peer group; long before the age of 18, when they can legally buy alcohol or drink it in a licensed bar, the majority of young people in all areas of the UK, as in many other countries, are drinking on a regular basis (Miller and Plant 1996, Hibell et al. 1997, Plant and Miller 2000). As noted in Chapter 4, between the ages of 16 and 18 most young people in the UK rapidly acquire adult drinking habits, in terms of drinking prevalence, consumption levels and settings for drinking (Wright 1999b).

Over the last 10–15 years there has been a dramatic increase in the recreational use of illicit drugs by young people, as part of some major changes in youth culture in Britain. As Brain and Parker (1997) observe, young people in the 1990s purchase and consume leisure, rather than create it for themselves. Intoxicating substances including both alcohol and illicit drugs are purchased alongside clothing, fast food and thrill rides as part of hedonistic consumerism. Over the last decade, the beverage alcohol industry has successfully responded to social and economic changes that produced a decline in traditional patterns of male, working-class beer consumption by targeting this new market of young consumers. The industry has diversified and repackaged alcoholic beverages to match desired youth lifestyles, and increased their strength in a direct attempt to appeal to a new generation of psychoactive consumers (Brain 1998).

Given the importance of drinking in youth culture and its emphasis in most adults' social lives, it is hardly surprising that schoolchildren in the UK have little interest either in waiting until they are older before they start to drink, or in stopping drinking altogether. Young adults are the population group least likely to be non-drinkers (ONS 1998). Compared to adults, young people are more tolerant of drunkenness and less likely to support public policy measures which would affect their own drinking behaviour, such as increased prices or stricter controls on sales, advertising or taxation (MORI 1994).

Against this tide of social norms supporting drinking by young people in Britain, is it reasonable to expect alcohol education programmes to reduce or defer alcohol consumption? As Aldridge et al. argue in relation to young people's drug use: 'it is simply unrealistic to rely on health education messages to challenge what are major changes in youth culture in general and in consumption in particular' (1998: 171).

Recent commentators on the role of alcohol education in preventing alcohol misuse have all reached similar conclusions – that it is unreasonable to rely solely on alcohol education to achieve major changes in social behaviour (Keeling 1994, Plant and Plant 1997, Leigh 1999).

A more realistic approach would be to base the criteria by which school-based alcohol education is judged to have 'worked' on what schools can reasonably be expected to achieve, as educational institutions. This position is endorsed by the UK government's Advisory Council on the Misuse of Drugs (1993), which states that 'the aim of drug education is to enable pupils to make healthy informed choices', and more recent guidance issued by national bodies such as the DfEE (1995, 1998), OFSTED (1997) and the government's Healthy Schools Programme (DfEE/DoH 1999b).

Evaluators' preoccupations with young people's alcohol consumption have left a considerable evidence gap in school-based alcohol education in Britain. The gap is a pretty fundamental one. It is concerned with the dearth of useful and relevant findings to inform teaching and learning in relation to developing young people's alcohol-related knowledge, attitudes, values and skills

EVIDENCE ABOUT THE BASIS FOR ACTION: ASSUMPTIONS ABOUT YOUNG PEOPLE'S DRINKING

While the nature of evidence-based alcohol education is undoubtedly a highly contested area, one area of common ground is acknowledgement that working in an evidence-based way is an attitude of mind, similar to 'research-mindedness', of repeatedly asking: 'How do we know? Who says so?' When the rationale for alcohol education is questioned in this way, it exposes a plethora of common practices and assumptions about youthful drinking which have become accepted on the basis of little or no evidence. Six of the more important assumptions are challenged here:

1. Young people should not drink
2. Young people's drinking is deviant
3. Young people drink to help them to cope with problems
4. Young people will get into trouble through drink
5. Young people are pressured into drinking by their peers
6. 'Batch management': all young people are the same.

Young People Should Not Drink

One important factor which has been found to inhibit youth workers from enacting their important role in alcohol education in informal settings is their concern that they should not be seen to approve of 'underage' drinking (Wright 1999a). Similar constraints are even more likely to apply in formal educational settings that are sensitive to the views of parents and governors. Alcohol education aimed at adults is based on harm-reduction principles, accepting that drinking is both pleasurable and risky. Public education campaigns in the UK have emphasised weekly sensible/low-risk drinking levels, knowing the amount of alcohol in different drinks and other strategies to minimise harm. There is much more ambivalence about adopting a harm-reduction approach with young people, apart from with certain high-risk groups such as alcohol-related offenders (McMurran and Hollin 1993). Adults' moral disapproval of young people's drinking has prevented researchers from asking useful questions and has framed the way evidence is interpreted (Dorn 1983, Wright 1999b). For example, compared to the wealth of data on young people's alcohol consumption, which has been collected over many years, the evidence on the place and meaning of drinking in young people's lives is relatively recent and patchy – because, after all, they should not be drinking at all, should they?

Young People's Drinking is Deviant

Many research studies have focused on the problems related to young people's drinking and have labelled young drinkers as deviant. This is a particularly dominant paradigm in North American studies, where the predominant assumption is that *any* use of alcohol by young people is problematic. Drinking under the age of 21 is actually illegal in the US, whereas in the UK the situation is quite different and in some ways more ambiguous. In fact it is legal for people in the UK to consume alcohol (but not on licensed premises) from the age of five! There are legal restrictions on buying alcohol and on where young people can drink (that is, not on licensed premises or in public places with local by-law restrictions) but drinking *per se* is not illegal for young people in the UK.

Recently, British researchers have challenged this perspective, arguing that adolescent drinking in Britain is essentially normal behaviour, which is part of the process of socialisation and reflects adult norms and drinking practices within the wider cultural setting (Sharp and Lowe 1989, May 1992, Lowe et al. 1993, Parker 1995). As noted in Chapter 4, in the UK, alcohol consumption begins at ages 8–12, with virtually all 12–14-year-olds having had some experience of drinking. However, the majority of young teenagers (11–16) do not drink regularly, and most of those who do drink, consume only small amounts. As Sharp and Lowe have remarked, seeing youthful drinking as inevitably problematic 'runs the risk of turning what is essentially normal behaviour into something deviant' (1989: 305).

Young People Drink to Help Them to Cope with Problems

Theories seeking to explain why young people drink are important in informing alcohol education strategies, because assumptions about cause will determine views about responses and solutions. Many of the causal hypotheses derived from analytical studies have used frameworks which define young people's drinking as pathological in some way, by examining personality traits, peer-group pressure and relationships with other problem behaviours such as family dysfunction or delinquency. Referring to young people in the UK, Sharp and Lowe point out that these ideas about cause run the risk of turning what is essentially a normal part of adolescent socialisation into something deviant:

> It is highly unlikely that over 90 per cent of the 16-year-old population are victims of poor parents, pressurising peers and inadequate personalities. The way forward seems to lie in understanding what drinking means to a young person and how these meanings are propagated. (1989: 305)

British analytical studies of young people's drinking are relatively rare and a large proportion of the available evidence is derived from North American research. The large cultural differences that exist between young drinkers in the UK and the US mean that the results of North American studies must be treated with caution in other settings. In particular, North American classifications of young 'heavy drinkers' or young 'problem drinkers' may not be appropriate to young people in the UK or in other countries.

Four theoretical models predominate in analytical studies of young drinkers:

- problem behaviour theory
- social learning theory
- reasoned action/planned behaviour theory
- social/environmental influences.

However, it should be noted that the lack of British analytical studies means that there is insufficient direct evidence to support any one theory in preference to another, or to enable a convincing synthesis of several differing perspectives.

The Jessors' *problem behaviour theory* (Jessor and Jessor 1977) is an individually based, psychological perspective. It argues that certain individuals are predisposed to adopt a range of problem behaviours, such as heavy drinking, because they have particular personalities and beliefs and behave in ways which are approved of by others who are important to them. On the basis of longitudinal studies in the US, Jessor and colleagues have reported that adolescent problem behaviours are interrelated (Donovan and Jessor 1978, Jessor et al. 1980, Jessor et al. 1991). Similar clusters of problem behaviours have been observed in Sweden, where a longitudinal study found that early social and behavioural factors, substance misuse and risky use of alcohol were all predictors for both drink driving and public drunkenness (Karlsson and Romelsjö 1997). The Jessors' argument, which in the UK is supported, subject to a number of pragmatic modifications, by Plant and Plant (1992), Miller and Plant (1999a) and Turtle et al. (1997) is that there are organised patterns of adolescent risk-taking behaviours and that such risk-taking is part of adolescent lifestyles. The evidence that heavy drinking is associated with other risky behaviour such as illicit drug use or unsafe sexual practices, implies a need for health education programmes which adopt a broad lifestyle approach rather than focusing solely on drinking behaviour.

Within the British context, problem-behaviour theory has been criticised on two counts. First, as previously discussed, it implies that young people's drinking is deviant (Sharp and Lowe 1989). Second, it fails to take into account the influence that the drinking environment has on young people's drinking (Knibbe et al. 1991)

Social learning theory proposes that drinking alcohol is learned behaviour. According to Maloff et al. (1979), children learn 'cultural recipes' which explain how to use alcohol (and other substances) to obtain desired results. Cultural recipes also describe where, when, how much and what type of alcohol consumption is socially sanctioned. Children and young people learn these recipes through the *modelling* and *reinforcement* of people who are significant to them, especially family and peers (Bandura 1977). A considerable body of empirical evidence supports this theory, in relation to the development of drinking attitudes and behaviour and the context of family life and peer influence.

The *theory of reasoned action* (Fishbein and Ajzen 1975, Ajzen and Maddon 1986) argues that people's behaviour can be accurately predicted by their stated *intention* to act in a certain way. Behavioural intentions are considered to be a product of an individual's beliefs, attitudes, evaluations of the consequences of a course of action, perceived social norms and perceived drinking skills. The influence of the drinking environment is assumed to be expressed through these variables. Applied to young people's alcohol consumption, this theory suggests that their actual drinking behaviour can be predicted by asking young people what they would do (including how much they would drink) in certain situations. There is some empirical support for this model in relation to a variety of behaviours including smoking and drinking (Ajzen and Fishbein 1980, Sutton 1987).

General objections to this model are that the causal relationships between attitudes, norms, self-efficacy and behaviour are rarely proven and that it excludes a person's experience, that is, his or her current and past behaviour. In relation to young drinkers, MacAndrew and Edgerton (1969) pose a more fundamental objection – that it assumes that young people feel obliged to act in accordance with the beliefs and norms about drinking alcohol. From a cross-cultural perspective, they argue that the settings for drinking in Western cultures can be characterised as 'time out', or granting permission to ignore the normal social rules of behaviour. Thus they suggest that the model may not take into account the degree to which young people, when drinking outside of the home environment, feel free to behave in ways which are inconsistent with their attitudes, beliefs and norms. MacAndrew and Edgerton's argument is also supported by Traeen and Kvalem's (1996) analysis of the function of alcohol in young people's sexual behaviour.

Social and environmental influences may be important in explaining young people's drinking behaviour. Supporters of this perspective do not suggest that such influences account for all variations in young people's drinking behaviour. They argue that the context and settings in which young people drink alcohol and the physical and social environment in which young people live have a greater significance than is acknowledged within the models described above. A growing body of evidence is accumulating to support this view. For example, a longitudinal study of influences on the drinking of 15-year-old New Zealanders found that situational characteristics, such as drinking location, who was present and time of day, explained a large amount of the variation in the amount of alcohol consumed (Connolly et al. 1992).

An observational study of 16–20-year-olds in The Netherlands found that the drinking situation is a particularly important influence on young men's drinking (Van de Goor et al. 1990). This study found that young men tended to drink faster when music was played more loudly and when they were part of an all-male group. In contrast, only the group influenced young women's drinking rates. Young women drank faster when drinks were bought in 'rounds' and when there was more movement in and out of the drinking group. A follow-up study (Knibbe et al. 1991) set out to test whether the amount young people drank in public places, such as bars and discos, was due to reasoned behaviour or related to the situation. They found that for young men, the drinking situation contributed more to variations in consumption than their alcohol-specific beliefs, norms and self-efficacy. Frequency of visiting pubs, clubs, and so on, was the most important factor for young men. Group pressure to drink and size of the drinking group were also important. For young women, perceptions that they could control their consumption when they were in different moods (that is, when they felt tense, angry, cheerful, and so on) and social norms were the factors most strongly correlated with consumption levels. This study also found that young people's perceived skills in being able to control their drinking in different drinking situations (such as when expected to buy a round, when offered a drink) contributed little to actually controlling consumption, when group pressure was experienced.

Despite the fact that most of young people's drinking (and that of adults) takes place during their leisure time, relatively little research has been done on defining the relationships between drinking and leisure. Kunz's review (1997) of the (mainly North American) literature found that most studies focused on special populations, for example, college athletes, limiting the degree to which findings could be generalised. Drinking patterns were crudely measured in leisure surveys, while leisure questions in alcohol surveys were equally unsophisticated, as found in Hendry et al.'s work (1993) on young people's leisure and lifestyles in the UK. To inform health promotion interventions, it would seem important to understand more about the leisure contexts that support both safe and risky drinking behaviour among young people.

These findings have important implications for alcohol education and point to the need for similar studies to examine the influence of context and settings on the drinking behaviour of young people in Britain. British studies rarely make these variables the central focus of interest. For example, Shepherd and Brinkley's study (1996) of young males injured in urban city-centre violence found that all injuries took place within one postal code area and at least 85% of assaults took place in a bar or shortly after leaving one. The authors tentatively suggest that the settings for drinking might be appropriate targets for health promotion interventions. If social settings *do* have the degree of influence on young people's drinking behaviour that is suggested, then, as Knibbe et al. (1991) point out, educational interventions which are mainly aimed at changing individual attitudes and norms are unlikely to achieve a relevant change in consumption levels. Interventions which seek to develop individual self-efficacy in teaching skills to deal with different situations might help, but these results suggest that effective interventions will also need to directly target and change the settings and environments where young people drink. These conclusions support the view that school-based alcohol education needs to be part of a multi-stranded, community-wide, health promotion intervention.

The theories described above are largely derived from research within a scientific–positivist paradigm. Research conducted within an 'interpretivist' philosophy lends further support to the view that the *social contexts* for young people's drinking are an important key to understanding alcohol's place and meaning. However, as young people's social worlds are diverse and local, care must be taken in extrapolating conclusions from these studies to young people in general. The recent UK studies available to date (for example, Gofton 1990, Tierney et al. 1991, Parker 1996, Brain and Parker 1997, Pavis et al. 1997) are by no means comprehensive. Interpretations of young people's drinking can also be drawn from qualitative studies of other aspects of young people's health behaviour, such as Backett and Davison's work (1992) on the meaning of health and illness in different cultural settings, Hirst's study (1994) of young people's sexual risk-taking and Hirst and McCamley-Finney's study (1994) of young people's illicit drug use in Sheffield.

Some key themes emerge from these studies, many of which complement and reinforce understandings derived from descriptive surveys and analytical studies:

- *Drinking is functional*
  There is some evidence that among young people, heavier drinkers are more likely to drink alcohol as a coping strategy, or to escape from problems or stress (Turtle et al. 1997, Mathrani 1998). However, most young people use alcohol because they perceive it to meet other needs, particularly facilitating social interaction and altering mood (Dorn 1983, Gofton 1990, Foxcroft and Lowe 1993). In the 11–16 age group, descriptive studies have found that the more young people drink, the more likely they are to hold positive attitudes to alcohol and to particularly value the social benefits attached to drinking (Davies and Stacey 1972, Aitken 1978, Plant et al. 1985, M.A. Plant et al. 1990b, HEA/MORI 1992, Turtle et al. 1997).
- *Drinking as hedonism*
  Pleasure seeking and having a good time are features of young people's use of alcohol.
- *Drinking to get drunk*
  In considering young people's motivations for drinking, few alcohol education programmes acknowledge that young people deliberately drink to get drunk. Young people in the UK, especially heavier drinkers, admit to drinking 'to get drunk' and, compared to adults, are more tolerant of drunkenness. They consciously plan to 'binge' drink on certain occasions and perceive that their friends approve of this practice (Gofton 1990, Lewthwaite 1990, Gillespie et al. 1991, Brain and Parker 1997, Fox 1997, Mathrani 1998). Lending support to the above conclusions about the importance of intoxication to young people, it appears that binge drinking is common to young people in other parts of the

industrialised world, for example, Western and some parts of Eastern Europe, the US and Canada, Australia and New Zealand (Harford and Grant 1987, Gillespie et al. 1991, Knibbe et al. 1991, Hibell et al. 1997).

Acknowledgement of the importance of intoxication for young people's drinking would enhance alcohol educators' credibility in the eyes of young people and would allow academics to ask more useful questions such as those asked by Gillespie et al. (1991). This Australian study found that young people do not consider the more serious consequences of binge drinking (drinking a lot on one occasion) to be likely outcomes; while they believe they have the skills to control their drinking, they may not apply them in binge-drinking situations. However, we currently have little information about social norms for drunken behaviour among young people in the UK. Little is known about the behavioural self-control strategies young people adopt. Such information would be invaluable in planning alcohol education programmes that are credible to young people.

* *Drinking as consumerism*
  Young people, including younger teenagers, purchase and evaluate alcohol using the same sort of criteria as they would apply to any other consumer goods: flavour, value for money to achieve a buzz, selection of drinks and drinking styles which fit the image, style and fashion of youth culture (Gofton 1990, Coffield and Gofton 1994, Brain and Parker 1997).

* *Drinking as part of leisure*
  Drinking alcohol is an integral part of young people's (and adults') leisure activities. Brain and Parker (1997) observe that young people in the 1990s purchase and consume leisure rather than create it for themselves. There are abundant leisure choices to be purchased, including fast food, cinemas, go-karting, amusement parks and thrill rides. Intoxicating substances (illicit drugs and alcohol) are purchased and consumed within this framework.

* *Drinking combined with illicit drug use*
  One of the biggest current changes to youth culture is the increasing normalisation of illicit drug use. Alcohol is evaluated and used within an ever-expanding repertoire of mind-altering substances (Hirst and McCamley-Finney 1994, Parker and Measham 1994).

* *The importance of the drinking environment*
  The setting and group(s) in which young people drink are important mediators of drinking behaviour and its outcomes. The dynamic interaction between the individual and the group are gender-, age- and culture-specific. Young people behave in different ways when drinking, according to the drinking environment (Burns 1980, Van de Goor et al. 1990, Connolly et al. 1992, Fox 1997, Mathrani 1998).

- *The importance of boundaries*

  In addition to group norms and dynamics, the amount of parental control, unsupervised time, spending power, school, tertiary education, sports, hobbies and employment, all regulate young people's use of alcohol. Young people whose lives have fewer boundaries will consequently have fewer boundaries to their drinking. For example, studies in the north-west of England (Brain and Parker 1997) and in Germany (Alheit 1994) have found that young people who are unemployed or excluded from school have been observed to use alcohol to fill time and add structure and meaning to their day.

Young People will get into Trouble through Drink

The assumption that drinking alcohol increases the likelihood that young people will harm themselves or others is an important part of the rationale for alcohol education. For example, there may be concern that by drinking, young people risk serious illness or becoming dependent on alcohol. However, youthful drinking behaviour is *not* a good predictor of alcohol-related illness or physical dependence in later life (Plant et al. 1985, Fillmore 1988, Sharp and Lowe 1989). The alcohol-related harm experienced by young people, such as accidents, violence and crime, is related to intoxication and episodic drunkenness (binge drinking) rather than alcohol dependence or chronic heavy drinking. Cancers, heart disease, liver cirrhosis and other health consequences of chronic heavy drinking are rarely seen in young drinkers.

Concern about producing a nation of 'young alcoholics' is therefore not a reasonable justification for alcohol education targeted at young people. However, there is ample evidence that youthful drinking is associated with a wide range of risks and harms, although establishing causal relationships between drinking and specific risks is often problematic. For example, it is commonly believed that young people get involved in crime as a result of drinking alcohol. Parker observes that this is one of the central tenets of current political discourse on law and order, which 'requires youth, alcohol and offending to be inseparably handcuffed' (1996: 282).

Recent British and international studies have confirmed that unravelling cause and effect in the relationship between young people's drinking and crime is not as straightforward as it seems (Collins 1982, Tuck 1989, Marsh and Fox-Kibby 1992, Parker 1996), finding evidence to support all three principal relationships – drinking causes crime, crime causes drinking and drinking and crime share common causes (Fergusson et al. 1996). Laboratory experiments show that anti-social behaviour, particularly aggression, increases with increased doses of alcohol. There are many studies that find that heavy drinking by young people and offending behaviour have shared antecedents, including family life, use of other drugs, intelligence and early behavioural tendencies. There is also evidence that anti-social behaviour may lead to heavy or inappropriate drinking. On balance, recent longitu-dinal studies have found that young people's drinking and offending share common causes, rather than that drinking causes crime (Raskin White et al. 1993, Fergusson et al. 1996). Even in drink-defined offences such as alcohol-impaired driving and drunkenness, early social, family and behavioural factors and use of other drugs have been identified as contributing to these crimes, in addition to drinking alcohol (Karlsson and Romelsjö 1997).

As recently noted (Alcohol Concern 1996), whatever the connections between alcohol use by young people and crime, it is important to remember that:

- most young people over the age of 16 drink alcohol and do not commit criminal offences
- alcohol-using offenders do not commit crimes every time they drink.

Careful examination of the relationships between alcohol and other risks, such as violence, illicit drug use or sexual risk-taking, reveals similar complexities which are rarely acknowledged in alcohol education programmes (Wright 1999b). Teaching resources and teacher in-service training materials such as TACADE's *Alcohol Education: Issues for the '90s* (TACADE 1992) represent alcohol risks as a set of alarming statistics. Moreover, the harms related to young people's own drinking, especially anti-social behaviour, are the main focus of media attention and public anxiety, and this individualistic focus is reflected in published alcohol education materials and in school programmes (Wright 1991). The harm that young people experience due to adults' drinking, particularly that of parents, is less acknowledged, and is rarely featured in alcohol education programmes. Indeed, until very recently, the impact of family life on young people's drinking has tended to be overlooked in school-based alcohol education, despite the existence of a well-researched evidence base (Lowe et al. 1993) and current DfEE guidelines (1998) that drug education programmes should involve parents.

Young People are Pressured into Drinking by their Peers

Peer-group pressure is frequently given as an explanation for adolescent drinking. Cross-sectional studies consistently show that young people who drink tend to have friends who drink, while those who do not drink tend to have friends who also do not drink (Iannotti et al. 1996). Although there have been few longitudinal studies which might shed light on the direction of the influence, researchers have overwhelmingly chosen to interpret the association as evidence to support the notion of peer-group influence. Davies (1992b), May (1993) and Coggans and McKellar (1994) suggest that this is because alternative explanations do not accord with the prevailing moral disapproval of young people's drinking. It is more comfortable to interpret this evidence as young people being led astray by others than to consider the possibility of peer association – that young people might enjoy drinking alcohol and choose to associate with others who hold the same views. The latter peer-association explanation is supported by a North-American four-year longitudinal study which found that perceived friends' substance use (alcohol, tobacco and marijuana) is more likely to be a *product* of an adolescent's previous substance use than a precursor of subsequent use (Iannotti et al. 1996).

Young people are active players in social relationships. They choose to drink in certain ways because this behaviour meets (or they believe it to meet) their needs. There is considerable evidence from ethnographic studies in Britain and elsewhere to support the view that adolescent drinking is socially organised and subject to a set of 'rules' which regulate and structure drinking behaviour within a specific situation (Dorn 1983, Glassner and Loughlin 1987, Dean 1990, Gofton 1990, Wylie and Casswell 1991, McDonald 1994, Pavis et al. 1997). There is a dynamic relationship between individual self-determination and social group influences – in managing their social worlds, young people actively influence the rules and norms set by the groups to which they belong (Wright 1999b). These studies also identify the friendship group(s) in which young people do their drinking as the focus of this dynamic, rather than the wider group of schoolmates or other peers (Gofton 1990, Brain and Parker 1997, Fox 1997).

The qualitative studies also indicate that different groups of young people have very different drinking cultures, as contrasted by observations of young city-centre pub-users in the north-east (Gofton 1990), Asian young women in Bedford (Wright and Buczkiewicz 1995), 14–15-year-olds and young street-drinkers in the north-west (Newcombe et al. 1995, Brain and Parker 1997). Furthermore, few young people are members of only one drinking group and they will move into other group settings as they mature. The social context for drinking has an impact on their drinking behaviour, so that a group will drink in different ways depending on the circumstances and environment (Burns 1980, Knibbe et al. 1991).

These conclusions have important implications for health promotion and alcohol education. If peer pressure is an inadequate explanation of young people's drinking, it follows that programmes based on resistance to peer pressure will have little success; their evaluation to date would seem to confirm this, though some success has been found in relation to smoking (Flay 1985, Plant and Plant 1999).

The finding that friendship groupings rather than classmates or general 'peers' are the focus for social influences on young people's drinking poses logistical problems for classroom work on alcohol education. It suggests that, where practicable, alcohol education involving group work should utilise friendship groupings rather than the more usual random allocations or groups based on academic ability. It also reinforces the potential for alcohol education within informal settings, particularly detached youth work, based on engagement with friendship groupings of young people who drink together, on their own territory, wherever that may be – street corners, bus shelters, playing fields, launderettes or licensed premises (Wright 1999a).

'Batch Management': All Young People are the Same

Guidance notes issued with published alcohol education materials for use in schools usually include fine words about acknowledging differences between pupils and ensuring that the material meets individual learning needs. However, in practice, there will always be some element of 'batch management' in classroom teaching. The resources to provide individually tailored learning programmes to each individual in a class of 30 will always be limited. This applies even within core academic subject areas such as Maths or English where a teacher will have, through routine testing and appraisal, a great deal of information about individual skill and performance levels. Equivalent information about pupil performance in relation to alcohol, in terms of alcohol-related knowledge, attitudes and behaviour, is not necessarily even collected by schools. To inform the alcohol education programme, a conscientious teacher may be able to collect basic health-related behaviour details for the class or year group, for example, by using the instruments produced by the University of Exeter Schools Health Education Unit (Balding 1999), or to pre-test knowledge or attitudes, but this type of evidence may not be sufficient to tailor a programme to pupils' needs. Classroom teachers have limited opportunities to discover what drinking alcohol means to their pupils, in terms of its place in their social worlds; worlds which are outside the classroom, take place in friendship groups rather than age or academic ability and, for younger pupils, may be conducted entirely outside of adult supervision.

Discussion of these assumptions illustrates how the complex realities of young people's lives are not being acknowledged in alcohol education programmes (Wright 1999b). Similar criticisms have been levelled at health promotion initiatives in general (Smith and Harding 1989, Hirst 1994). My recent literature review of what young people in Britain know, think and do about alcohol (Wright 1999b) found that young people's drinking is frequently presented as a set of worrying statistics of harm. Alcohol education is normally commissioned, planned and conducted by adult professionals, based on their notions of what young people need. A more comprehensive approach to needs assessment, involving collaboration between school staff, health services, alcohol agencies and researchers, should include an assessment of young people's felt needs and an acknowledgement of these complexities. This evidence would enable schools to move forward from the stereotypical assumptions discussed above to deliver a curriculum that is more closely aligned to the realities of young people's drinking. The use of active participatory learning methods and peer-led initiatives will encourage young people to relate their learning about alcohol to their lives outside the classroom. School programmes also need to move beyond their traditional focus on individuals to include approaches that acknowledge and address the social, environmental and situational factors that shape young people's drinking.

ALCOHOL EDUCATION METHODS AND APPROACHES

The limited assumptions used in gathering evidence, the almost exclusive focus on behavioural outcomes as success criteria and the stereotypical assumptions made about young people's drinking have in turn restricted the framework for applying the evidence to alcohol education practice. Approaches are judged to 'work' only if they result in reductions in alcohol consumption. Their application to UK settings is further limited by the fact that the available evidence is heavily dominated by North American studies with few published accounts of alcohol education outcome evaluations conducted in Britain and so the question of transferability applies, as discussed above. Foxcroft et al.'s effectiveness review (1997) found only two British studies which met their rigorous inclusion criteria, while White and Pitts (1997) included only one study in their wider review of health promotion with young people for the prevention of 'substance misuse'.

In contrast, a plethora of educational materials exist. Ten years ago Swadi (1989) reviewed 108 drug education resources used in England and Wales. At that time most were found to employ only factual information, despite recommendations by the DfEE that alcohol and drug education, as part of personal, social and health education, should involve attitude and values clarification, cognitive and life skills, as well as seeking to increase knowledge. As Plant and Plant (1997) point out, only a tiny proportion of these materials have been evaluated, at least in terms of published evidence.

Given the major limitations in the evidence base, it is hardly surprising that it yields meagre pickings for alcohol educators in the UK. Early evaluations revealed that school programmes that focused on alcohol or other drugs were less effective than person-focused approaches (De Haes and Schuurman 1975, Kinder et al. 1980). Fear arousal or scare tactics were found to be ineffective, largely due to their lack of credibility with the target audience who found the images and messages inconsistent with their own experience of alcohol (De Haes and Schuurman 1975, Dorn and Murji 1992). Participatory learning techniques were found to be superior to formal teaching styles in facilitating attitude and values clarification (De Haes and Schuurman 1975).

After researchers dismissed the fear appeals and information-based programmes of the mid-1960s and 1970s and the affective focused programmes in the mid-1970s and 1980s as ineffective in changing young people's drinking or drug use (Randall and Wong 1976, Kinder et al. 1980, Battjes 1985, Moskowitz 1989), North American schools seized on positive evaluations of the social influences approach (Tobler 1986, Botvin and Botvin 1992, Plant and Plant 1999). Since the mid-1980s, social skills training programmes have been the predominant approach to alcohol and drug education in North American schools. These programmes are of two basic types. The first focuses mainly on developing the skills to resist peer pressure and establishing conservative norms, and the second on developing a repertoire of social and life skills such as decision-making, assertiveness, communication and coping skills.

Proponents of these approaches maintain that they are the only school-based strategies of proven effectiveness in reducing adolescent drug use (Botvin and Botvin 1992). However, when Gorman (1996) reviewed the published evaluations of these programmes in relation to *alcohol* (as opposed to use of tobacco, cannabis or other drugs), he found that the majority of studies had little or no impact on young people's drinking behaviour. As already discussed, similar dismal conclusions have been reached by British reviewers (Foxcroft et al. 1997, White and Pitts 1997).

These conclusions are consequences of simplistic thinking about the nature and causes of adolescent drinking. As Gorman (1996) points out, social skills programmes attempt to influence a very narrow range of factors that influence young people's drinking. In focusing on interpersonal factors, they ignore intrapersonal factors and the economic, cultural and environmental influences that shape young people's lives. Developing young people's social skills is a legitimate and appropriate element of schooling, but few teachers in Britain would be naive enough to expect that even the most socially competent adolescents will necessarily choose to be non-drinkers.

OTHER APPROACHES

During the last decade, several new approaches to alcohol education have been tried. None have been thoroughly evaluated in UK contexts. The best that can be concluded on the basis of the current evidence is that they have some promise, but more process and outcome evaluation is required to establish their value to schools in the UK.

Several North American studies have found that young people's drinking habits are more closely related to their perceptions about their friends' drinking than to objective measures or self-reports of friends' actual drinking (Wilks et al. 1989, Iannotti and Bush 1992, Iannotti et al. 1996). These findings have informed a promising approach to alcohol education in the US. Approaches based on *correcting perceived social norms* have succeeded in modifying the attitudes and drinking behaviour of college students in the US (Perkins 1995), but this approach has yet to be evaluated in British schools or colleges. It involves re-presenting data to give a more positive message. For example, referring to UK data on young teenagers, the accurate statement that 'virtually all 12–14-year-olds have some experience of alcohol' can equally accurately be re-presented as 'the majority of 12–14-year-olds do not drink regularly and most consume only very small amounts' (Wright 1999b).

Peer-led approaches to school-based alcohol education are currently fashionable, based on assumptions that peer interactions are important in shaping young people's drinking and that young people will have greater credibility than teachers in leading alcohol education sessions in schools. There is some evidence to support peer-led approaches, although this is again largely drawn from evaluations of drug education programmes rather than alcohol and derives from studies outside of the UK. These differences are important, because regular illegal drug use, though increasing, is still only practised by a minority of young people in Britain, while the majority of school leavers drink alcohol regularly. Two meta-analyses of drug prevention programmes conclude that peer-led programmes have positive effects, although the two studies disagree about their impact. Tobler's analysis (1986) of 143 adolescent drug prevention programmes representing five approaches concluded that peer programmes showed greater effects than knowledge and/or affective approaches in terms of changes in knowledge, attitudes and life skills, as well as the more restrictive drug-use criteria. A later, more rigorous, meta-analysis by Bangert-Drowns (1988) identified positive effects on attitudes and knowledge but not on drug use. Bangert-Drowns also concluded that group discussion was particularly effective when peer leaders were used. Botvin (1990) cautions that selection of peer leaders is important, suggesting that leaders should be credible to 'high-risk' individuals, good communicators and hold 'responsible attitudes'. Others have found that it is the peer leaders who gain the most in terms of knowledge, self-esteem and attitudes to school (Resnick and Gibbs 1988).

Milburn's review (1996) of published work on peer education in general and on sexual health promotion in particular, identified inherent problems with the practical application of this approach. She found that the work is extremely diverse in aims, methods, findings and levels of evaluation. In

232 The Alcohol Report

accord with the criticisms made here, she observes that the theoretical background is underdeveloped. She also identifies ethical issues about the imposition of adult agendas on young people, definitional differences in deciding who is a 'peer' and operational differences in peer-educator recruitment, timing and inputs. Consequently, as has already been noted in relation to other approaches, there is currently insufficient evidence to guide schools wishing to set up peer-education programmes.

The promotion of *alternatives* to illicit drug use and anti-social behaviours such as car crime is currently popular with agencies working with high-risk groups such as young offenders. The potential success of this approach rests on its ability to provide appealing alternative activities to young people that meet the same or similar needs as the high-risk behaviour. Application of this approach to alcohol education in school settings means the extension of school's traditional classroom role into young people's leisure time, and into the domain of community and youth work and local social and leisure provision for young people. Because the rules of engagement in informal education (for example, voluntarism) are fundamentally different from formal education, informal alcohol education has its own paradigms, theory and practice (Wright 1999a) which are not discussed here. However school-based alcohol programmes within a wider interagency initiative could make healthy choices easier for young people by involvement in developing the local provision of alternatives that are not centred on drinking alcohol.

Integrating the school-based alcohol education initiative into a broader community intervention to prevent alcohol misuse has achieved some positive evaluations in the US (Kumpher 1997, Windle 1999) and this approach is central to the British Government's drug misuse prevention strategy (Home Office Drugs Prevention Initiative 1998). It has not yet been systematically evaluated in the UK.

CONCLUSIONS: THERE IS A BABY IN THE BATH WATER

There are two main groups of prevention strategies that may reduce alcohol consumption: individual-based strategies such as alcohol education (as currently practised in Britain), and population-based strategies addressing the drinking context and environment, or controls on availability, marketing and price. In reviewing the evidence to support each type of approach, Leigh (1999) suggests that where the benefits of changing behaviour are substantial and immediate and the costs are modest, education *may* be the most efficient approach. The arguments presented in this chapter suggest that when these two criteria are applied to young people in the UK, the limitations of much of our current school-based alcohol education programmes are immediately exposed.

Referring to the situation in the US, Leigh (1999) questions whose interests alcohol education programmes are serving, suggesting that as an individual-based strategy, alcohol education is actively supported by the alcohol industry to divert attention from more effective population-based strategies. Similar comments can be applied to the activities of some beverage alcohol companies in the UK in relation to terms of reference of the Portman Group, which includes, as one of its three main aims, the reduction of alcohol misuse through *educational programmes and practical initiatives* (Portman Group/HEA 1992).

The current government emphasis on interagency working and 'joined-up' thinking acknowledges that complex issues like youthful drinking require complex solutions. It is not a question of *either* alcohol education *or* population-based strategies – both are needed and both should be part of a broader strategy to tackle alcohol-related problems across the whole population.

As Plant and Plant point out (1997), young people have a moral right to be educated about alcohol as part of their experience of schooling. Schools, as instruments of education and as agents for change, have been given a responsibility for becoming healthy schools, not only for their pupils but for the wider community. Having virtually emptied the alcohol education bath of its evidence bathwater and scrubbed down its walls, it is important not to throw these babies out with the bathwater. There is an urgent need to redefine the rationale for school-based alcohol education as part of a broader health promotion strategy to define the kinds of research and evaluation evidence that will usefully inform it and to fund the kinds of work that will gather it.

Based on the arguments and evidence presented here, Box 9.2 proposes a new framework for school-based alcohol education. It suggests a more pragmatic and inclusive approach to gathering and using research evidence to inform school-based alcohol education programmes. It takes a more realistic view of what educational programmes can legitimately be expected to achieve on their own or as part of a wider community-based health promotion initiative. It acknowledges the place of alcohol in the lives of young people in the UK. It moves away from the individualistic model of health education to view health as a social product (Naidoo and Wills 1994) and alcohol education as a political issue (Bagnall 1991).

In Britain throughout the 1990s, public and political concern about the increased use of illegal drugs by young people has very effectively diverted attention from the problems associated with youthful drinking. The priority given to tackling illegal drug use has driven funding, policies, interventions and research. The need to develop a more useful evidence base for school-based *alcohol* education continues to be overlooked. The issues raised here invite practitioners and researchers alike to reflect on their approach to alcohol education. Is it really evidence-based? And if not, why not?

Box 9.2: A new framework for evidence-based alcohol education in schools

The evidence base
- Acknowledges the contributions of different research paradigms including scientific-positivism and interpretivism
- Utilises evidence from the wider fields of health promotion and educational research
- Gathers evidence on process as well as outcomes
- Acknowledges the process of educational change; gathers evidence to inform the effective dissemination, adoption, implementation and continuation of alcohol education, as well as measuring outcomes
- Gathers evidence about place and meaning of young people's drinking as well as data on drinking behaviour

Programme planning and implementation
- Bases programme planning and implementation on the available evidence, taking into account the uniqueness of the practice context (see Box 9.1)
- Bases programme on high-quality evidence-based needs assessment, including young people's own felt and self-assessed need as well as professionally defined needs
- Sets clearly defined and realistic educational objectives
- Builds in developmental research, process and post-implementation evaluation into the programme and shares the findings with others
- Integrates alcohol education into a broader programme of personal, social, health and citizenship education
- Integrates alcohol education into a healthy schools approach
- Integrates the school programme into a local community-based alcohol misuse prevention initiative
- Moves beyond individually focused interventions to acknowledge social, economic and environmental factors that shape young people's drinking. Supports local interagency intiatives to address these factors
- Involves parents and carers

Content and Delivery
- Selects content and delivery methods appropriate to the learning objectives
- Avoids the use of fear appeals and scare tactics
- Provides accurate, credible, balanced information relevant to young people's needs
- Acknowledges the place and meaning of drinking alcohol in young people's lives at different ages and stages in development and prepares them to minimise the associated risks and harms.
- Adopts a broad lifestyles approach
- Uses active participatory learning methods

10
Summary and Conclusions

Martin Plant and Douglas Cameron

New books about alcohol appear at frequent intervals. Because of the rate at which the available literature expands, most have a fairly short shelf-life before being dated or superseded. This book, doubtless, will prove to be no exception to this rule. Even so, it is hoped that the information presented above will provide an overview of a number of key areas that will have some value for a few years. Unless one has nothing else to do, it is doubtful that anybody can grasp more than a fraction of what has been written about this topic. It is hoped that the preceding nine chapters have provided a window into some of the many possible views related to the production, use and consequences of the consumption of beverage alcohol.

As noted in Chapter 1, this book is in some ways a successor to an earlier text, *Drinking and Problem Drinking*, published nearly 20 years ago (Plant 1982). A lot has changed in the 'alcohol field' since then and a comparison of the two works would simply serve to emphasise how much more evidence is available now than in the past. Because of this, it is probably easier to provide an 'evidence-based' balanced picture of some aspects of alcohol and its use now than ever before. But perhaps what is most alarming, or reassuring (depending upon one's philosophical position), is that there is now less certainty than ever before. Yesterday's truths are today's travesties, and some of the views expressed in this book by its various contributors will no doubt appear conspicuously flawed in another couple of decades, if not much sooner. For example, the current substantial body of evidence showing a low level alcohol consumption to have a cardio-protective effect has recently been questioned (Fillmore 2000).

It does seem still irrefutable that very heavy levels of alcohol consumption are bad for you. But even in this strong correlation, the role of Hepatitis C on Hepatic cirrhosis mortality rates, for so long seen as the most robust indicator of levels of alcohol-related harm related to gross consumption, has yet to be satisfactorily disentangled. The interesting emerging paradigm showing that particular patterns of alcohol use, not gross per capita consumption, are better predictors of alcohol problems, merits more attention. As shown by some of the evidence cited above, drinking patterns wax and wane, both for communities and for individuals. The relationship between alcohol consumption and its consequences is complex, since various sub-groups of people drink with different patterns, and the latter influence the types of consequences that ensue from drinking (Grant and Litvak 1998).

Concern about the adverse effects of heavy and inappropriate drinking has led to a considerable number of attempts to curb levels of alcohol-related problems. There are two distinct and valid traditions in relation to such alcohol control polices. One of these emphasises the importance of reducing per capita alcohol consumption. The second, described in some detail above, does not, but seeks to target and reduce specific adverse effects. The maxim of this approach is 'avoid problems when you drink'. Yet one of the purposes behind the consumption of beverage alcohol is to enhance the possibility of risk-taking within socially-prescribed limits. Totally safe drinking may well not be worth the candle. Similarly, although superficially utopian, would we really want to consume an alcoholic beverage which carried with it a zero risk of a hangover, whatever the dose?

Alcohol education has clearly not emerged as a panacea for alcohol problems. Even so, alcohol education has obvious importance and it is right that both the young and others, should be provided with accurate information about alcohol. Health promotion is a key element in the battery of policies that are required in order to reconcile the popularity and potential for harm of alcohol, with the need to check its ill effects and to respond constructively to its associated problems. It is hoped that this book provides a realistic, practical and helpful guide for teachers and others entrusted with the task of educating young people about drinking.

People drink in different ways at different stages in their lives, so the distinction between those who are 'problem drinkers' and those who are not is neither clear-cut nor permanent. As previously emphasised by Cameron (1995), many of those who do experience 'alcohol problems' seek help from agencies to get them through the bad times. Many such people will survive and many simply cut down or give up their harmful drinking 'spontaneously'; that is, without any therapeutic intervention. Absolutist positions about the effectiveness of various treatment approaches for those with alcohol problems are now untenable in the face of evidence such as that provided by the Project MATCH Research Group (1997a). There is certainly no suggestion that any specific approach has a unique or unassailable pre-eminence in terms of its impact. This suggests that looking at alternative treatment approaches and ideologies may be worthwhile, for many do show a high level of customer acceptance and satisfaction. Nevertheless, it is critical that even if alcohol intervention systems do no good, they should do no harm – they should not make matters worse for the presenting drinker. The case for that for both conventional and alternative therapies is yet to be established beyond reasonable doubt. What is the impact upon an individual's identity of being 'a treatment failure'? It is probably time that we seek consistency in the messages delivered by the various agencies involved in this 'alcohol business':

> The general population, and 'early problem drinkers', and 'alcoholics' and 'unmotivated skid row drunks' can all be helped using the same set of beliefs and strategies. The health education and promotion messages are the same as the minimal intervention messages. And they are the same as the treatment messages. (Cameron 1997: 246)

Klaus Mäkelä, a well-known researcher, once wrote (to paraphrase) that we drink alcohol because it is good for us, and study it because it is bad for us. This aptly sums up the major paradox and reality of beverage alcohol. Its consumption is enduringly popular; and so too (inevitably?) the problems associated with it are widespread. It has been a recurring theme throughout this book that most of those who drink, mainly do so without problems and simply enjoy alcohol as a facet of their social lives. The 'downside' of this equation is that many people suffer from their own use of alcohol, or from that of other people.

What is to be done about this? At the time of writing, political concern, in Britain anyway, is much more focused on illicit drugs than on alcohol, even though the latter involves far more people and much higher rates of problems. Alcohol is simply not viewed as being 'sexy', or as politically important. This could be very depressing. Many of those working in the 'alcohol field' are underpaid, undervalued and insecure. Moreover, as experience shows, responses to alcohol problems may be inadequate, short-lived, half-hearted and underfunded. Sadly, they are usually all of these things.

Even so, it should be acknowledged that many people are strongly committed to making things better. In communities all over the world, people are working together to prevent or reduce levels of alcohol problems and to support and aid those who are harmed by the adverse effects of somebody's drinking. As a corollary of this activity, the 'alcohol literature' keeps on growing and evidence keeps on accumulating. This has added greatly to our knowledge about most aspects of alcohol. It has also undermined some old beliefs and assumptions.

The most obvious way forward is to build an armoury of 'effective' responses designed to prevent, reduce and manage alcohol problems within their midst, wherever they occur. As related by the preceding chapters, there are examples of 'good practice' in many areas of concern. Some of these may be utilisable in many settings. Others may not always be appropriate. The choice of policies should be influenced by whether or not they are socially or politically acceptable/appropriate; whether or not they can demonstrate a tangible, positive impact, and whether this impact can be sustained.

Bibliography

The following references were invaluable in the writing of this book. Many, though not all, have been cited directly in the text. It is hoped that this bibliography will be helpful to those wishing to read further.

Aase, J.M. (1994) 'Clinical recognition of FAS: Difficulties of detection and diagnosis', *Alcohol Health and Research World* 18: 5–9.

Aase, M.M., Jones K.L. and Clarren S.K. (1995) 'Do we need the term "FAE"?', *Pediatrics* 95: 428–30.

Abel, E.L. (1991) *Fetal Alcohol Syndrome*, Medical Economics Books New Jersey: Oradell.

Abel, E.L. (1998) *The Fetal Alcohol Abuse Syndrome*, New York: Plenum Press.

Adams, W.L., Garry, P.J. and Rhyne, T. et al. (1990) 'Alcohol intake in the healthy elderly', *Journal of the American Geriatric Society* 38: 211–16.

Adams, W.L. and Smith Cox, N. (1995) 'Epidemiology of problem drinking among elderly people', *International Journal of the Addictions* 30: 1693–716.

Advisory Council on the Misuse of Drugs (1993) *Drug Education in Schools: The Need for a New Impetus*, London: HMSO.

Aggleton, P. (1996) *Health Promotion and Young People*, London: Health Education Authority.

Aguirre-Molina, M. and Van Ness, E. (1991) *Communities Take Charge! A Manual for the Prevention of Alcohol and Other Drug Problems Among Youth*, Piscataway, NJ, University of Medicine and Dentistry of New Jersey – Robert Wood Johnson Medical School, Dept. of Environmental and Community Medicine, Division of Consumer Health Education.

Aitken, P.P. (1978) *Ten to Fourteen Year Olds and Alcohol*, Edinburgh: HMSO.

Ajzen, I. and Fishbein, M. (1980) *Understanding Attitudes and Predicting Social Behaviour*, New York: Prentice Hall.

Ajzen, I. and Maddon, J.T. (1986) 'Prediction of goal directed behaviour: attitudes, intentions and perceived behavioural control', *Journal of Experimental Social Research* 22: 453–74.

Alcohol Concern (1996) *Alcohol and Crime: Information Pack*, London: Alcohol Concern.

Alcoholics Anonymous (1955) *The Story of How Many Thousands of Men and Women Have Recovered from Alcoholism*, 2nd edition, New York: AA World Services.

Alcoholics Anonymous World Services (1980) *Alcoholics Anonymous*, New York: AA World Services.

Aldridge, J., Measham F. and Parker, H. (1998) 'Rethinking young people's drug use', *Health Education* 5: 64–172.

Alexander C.N., Robinson, D. and Rainforth, M. (1994) 'Treating alcoholic, nicotine and drug abuse through TM: A review and statistical meta-analysis', *Alcoholism Treatment Quarterly* 11: 11–84.

Alheit, P. (1994) *Taking the Knocks*, London: Cassell.

Ametrano, I.M. (1992) 'An evaluation of the effectiveness of a substance abuse prevention program', *Journal of College Student Development* 33: 507–15.

Anderson, K. (1995) *Young People and Alcohol, Drugs and Tobacco*, Copenhagen, World Health Organization Regional Publications European Series No. 66.

Anderson, K. and Plant, M.A. (1996) 'Abstaining and carousing: Substance use among adolescents in the Western Isles of Scotland', *Drug and Alcohol Dependence* 41: 189–96.

Anderson, K., Plant, M.A. and Plant, M.L. (1998) 'Associations between drinking, smoking and illicit drug use among adolescents in the Western Isles of Scotland', *Journal of Substance Misuse* 3: 13–20.

Anderson, P., Cremona, A., Paton, A., Turner, C. and Wallace, P. (1993) 'The risk of alcohol', *Addiction* 88: 1493–508.

Anderson, P. and Scott, E. (1992) 'The effect of general practitioner's advice to heavy drinking men', *British Journal of Addiction* 87: 891–900.

Annis, H.M. and Chan, D. (1983) 'The differential treatment model: empirical evidence from a personality typology', *Criminal Justice and Behavior* 10: 159–73.

Archer, J. (ed.) (1994) *Male Violence*, London: Routledge.

Arellano, C.M. (1996) 'Child maltreatment and substance use: A review of the literature', *Substance Use and Misuse* 31: 927–35.

Arnold, M.J. and Laidler, T.J. (1994) *Situational and Environmental Factors in Alcohol-Related Violence (Vol. 7)*, Canberra: Government Publishing Services, Australia.

Astin, J.A. (1998) 'Why patients use alternative medicine: Results of a national study', *Journal of the American Medical Association* 279: 1548–53.

Astin, J.A. et al. (1998) 'A review of the incorporation of complementary and alternative medicine by mainstream physicians', *Archives of Internal Medicine* 152: 2303.

Atkinson, R.M. (1994) 'Late onset problem drinking in older adults', *International Journal of Geriatric Psychiatry* 9: 321–6.

Babcock, R.F. (1966) *The Zoning Game*, Madison, WI: University of Wisconsin Press.

Babor, T.F., Ritson, E.B. and Hodgson, R.J. (1986) 'Alcohol-related problems in the primary health care setting: a review of early intervention strategies', *British Journal of Addiction* 81: 23–46.

Backett, K. and Davison, C. (1992) 'Rational or reasonable? Perceptions of health at different stages of life', *Health Education Journal* 51: 55–9.

Baer, J., Marlatt, A., Kivlahan, D., Fromme, K., Larimer, M. and Williams, E. (1992) 'An experimental test of three methods of alcohol risk reduction with young adults', *Journal of Clinical and Consulting Psychology* 60: 974–9.

Bagnall, G. (1987) 'Alcohol education and its evaluation – some key issues', *Health Education Journal* 46: 162–5.

Bagnall, G. (1991) *Educating Young Drinkers*, London: Tavistock/Routledge.

Bagnall, G. and Plant, M.A. (1991) 'AIDS risk, alcohol and illicit drug use amongst young adults in areas of high and low rates of HIV infection', *AIDS Care* 3: 355–61.

Bailey, J. (1995) 'An Evaluation of Compulsory Breath Testing in New Zealand', in Kloeden, C.N. and McLean A.J. (eds) *Alcohol, Drugs and Traffic Safety, Volume 2*, Australia: NHMRC Road Accident Research Unit, 834–9.

Bailey, W.J. (1990) 'Affecting alcohol and other drug use via large lecture drug education course: The Indiana University experience', *The Eta Sigma Gamma* 22: 23–26.

Baillie, R. (1996) 'Determining the effects of media portrayals of alcohol: Going beyond short term influence', *Alcohol and Alcoholism* 31: 235–42.

Balding, J.W. (1999) *Young People in 1998*, Exeter: University of Exeter, Schools Health Education Unit.

Bandura, A. (1969) *Principles of Behavior Modification*, New York: Holt.

Bandura, A. (1977) *Social Learning Theory*, Englewood Cliffs, NJ: Prentice Hall.

Bandura, A. (1978) '"Self Efficacy": Toward a unifying theory of behavioral change', *Psychology Review* 84: 191–215.

Bandy, P. and President, P.A. (1983) 'Recent literature on drug abuse and prevention and mass media, focusing on youth, parents, women and the elderly', *Journal of Drug Education* 13: 255–71.

Bangert-Drowns, R. (1988) 'The effects of school-based substance abuse education: a meta analysis', *Journal of Drug Education* 18: 243–64.

Barber, J.G., Bradshaw, R. and Walsh, C. (1989) 'Reducing alcohol consumption through television advertising', *Journal of Consulting and Clinical Psychology* 57: 613–8.

Bass, K. (1996) (Program Director, Community Coalition for Substance Abuse Prevention and Treatment, Los Angeles, CA), 'Community organizing/mobilization as a method of addressing alcohol problems', Presentation at the Alcohol Policy Ten Conference, 4–8 May, Toronto: Addiction Research Foundation.

Bateson, G. (1997) *Cybernetics of the Self: A Theory of Alcoholism in Steps to an Ecology of Mind*, New York: Ballantine Books.

Baton, L. and Atherton, H. (1995) *A Report on Older People's Attitudes Towards Alcohol*, Epsom: Crossbow Research.

Battjes, R.J. (1985) 'Prevention of adolescent drug abuse', *International Journal of the Addictions* 20: 1113–34.

Bauman, K.E. and Ennett, S.T. (1996) 'On the importance of peer influence for adolescent drug use: commonly neglected considerations', *Addiction* 91: 185–98.

Baum-Baicker, C. (1985) 'The psychological benefits of moderate alcohol consumption: a review of the literature', *Drug and Alcohol Dependence* 15: 305–22.

Beachamp, D.E. (1980) *Beyond Alcoholism: Alcohol and Public Health Policy*, Philadelphia, PA: Temple University Press.

Beck, A.T., Wright, A.T., Newman, C.F. and Liese, B.S. (1993) *Cognitive Therapy of Substance Abuse*, New York: Guilford.

Beck, A.Y., Rush, A.J., Shaw, B.F. and Emery, G. (1979) *Cognitive Therapy of Depression*, New York: Guilford.

Becker, G. and Murphy, K. (1988) 'A theory of rational addiction', *Journal of Political Economy* 96: 675–700.

Becker, M., Warr-Leeper G.A. and Leeper H.A. (1990) 'Fetal Alcohol Syndrome: A description of oral motor articularity, short-term memory, grammatical and semantic disabilities', *Journal of Communication Disorders* 23: 97–124.

Beecher, L. (1826) *Six Sermons on the Nature, Occasions, Signs, Evils and Remedy of Intemperance*, Boston, MA: T.R. Marvin.

Beirness, D.J., Simpson, H.M., Mayhew, D.R. and Wilson, R.J. (1993) 'Canadian trends in drinking driver fatalities', in Utzelmann, H.D., Berghaus, G. and Kroj, G. (eds), *Alcohol, Drugs and Traffic Safety*, Rheinland GmbH, Koln: Verlag TUV, 1062–7.

Benham, K. (1983) *San Francisco Alcohol Fact Book*, San Francisco, CA: Trauma Center Foundation, San Francisco Prevention Project, November.

Bennett, N., Jarvis, L., Rowlands, O., Singleton, N. and Haselden, L. (1996) *Living in Britain Results From the 1994 General Household Survey*, London: HMSO.

Bennie, C. (1987) 'The Study of 102 General Practitioners in Forth Valley Health Board: Their Attitude Towards Alcohol-Related Problems in Terms of Role Security and Therapeutic Commitment'. Unpublished postgraduate thesis, Paisley College of Technology (now the University of Paisley).

Bennie, C. (1992) 'Home detoxification service for problem drinkers: a pilot study', *Alcoholism: The Quarterly Newsletter for Medical and Allied Professions* 1: 1–3.

Bennie, C. (1997) 'A comparison of home detoxification and minimal intervention strategies for problem drinkers', *Alcohol and Alcoholism* 33: 157–63.

Bennie, C. (1999) Personal communication.

Benson, H. (1969) 'Yoga for drug abuse', *New England Journal of Medicine* 281: 1133.

Beresford, T. and Gomberg, E. (eds) *Alcohol and Ageing*, New York: Oxford University Press.

Beresford, T.P. and Lucey, M.R. (1995) 'Ethanol metabolism and intoxication in the elderly', in Beresford, T.P. and Gomberg, E.S. (eds) (1995) *Alcohol and Ageing*, New York: Oxford University Press.

Berger, D.E. and Marelich, W.D. (1997) 'Legal and social control of alcohol-impaired driving in California: 1983–1994', *Journal of Studies on Alcohol* 58: 518–23.

Bergman, B. and Brismar, B. (1994) 'Characteristics of violent alcoholics', *Alcohol and Alcoholism* 29: 451–7.

Berridge, V. (1989) 'History and addiction control: The case of alcohol', in Robinson, D., Maynard, A. and Chester, R. (eds) *Controlling Legal Addictions*, London: Macmillan.

Berridge, V. (1998) *Opium and the People*, London: Free Association Books.

Bien, T.H., Miller, W.R. and Boroughs, J.M. (1993a) 'Motivational interviewing with outpatients', *Behavioural and Cognitive Psychotherapy* 21: 347–56.

Bien, T.H., Miller, W.R. and Tonigan, J. (1993b) 'Brief interventions for alcohol problems: a review', *Addiction* 88: 315–36.

Blackburn, C., Graham, H. and Scullion, P. (1997) 'Evaluation of disseminating research on women's smoking to health practitioners', *Health Education Journal* 56: 113–24.

Blewington V., Smith, M. and Clipton, D. (1994) 'Acupuncture as a detoxification treatment: An analysis of controlled research', *Journal of Substance Abuse Treatments* 11: 289–307.

Bloomfield, K.M., Ahlström, S., Allamaini, A., Choquet, M., Cipriani, F., Gmel, G., Jacquat, B., Knibbe, R., Kubicka, L., Lecomte, T., Miller, P., Plant, M.L. and Spak, F. (1999) *Alcohol Consumption and Alcohol Problems among Women in European Countries*, Berlin: Free University of Berlin.

Bongers, I., van de Goor, I., Van Oers, H. and Garretsen, H. (1998) 'Gender differences in alcohol-related problems: controlling for drinking behaviour', *Addiction* 93: 411–21.

Boothman, D. (1979) 'A study of patterns of drinking in patients attending seven general practitioners', *Health Bulletin* 37: 51–5.

Boots, K., and Midford, R. (1998) 'From resentment to enthusiasm: how a university initiated alcohol harm reduction research project evolved into Western Australia's largest regional community drug service team'. Paper presented at the Kettil Bruun Society's 4th Symposium on Community Action research and the Prevention of Alcohol and Other Drug Problems, Russell, New Zealand.

Botvin, G.J. (1985a) 'The life skills training program as a health promotion strategy: theoretical issues and empirical findings', *Special Services in the Schools* 1: 9–23.

Botvin, G.J. (1985b) 'Prevention of adolescent substance abuse through the development of personal and social competence', in Glynn, T.J., Lenkfeld, C.G. and Ludford, J.P. (eds) *Preventing Social Problems Through Life Skills Training*, Seattle, WA: University of Washington Press.

Botvin, G.J. (1990) 'Substance abuse prevention: theory, practice and effectiveness', in Tonry, M. and Wilson, J.Q. (eds) *Drugs and Crime*, Chicago, IL: University of Chicago Press.

Botvin, G.J., Baker, E., Dusenbury, L., Botvin, E.M. and Diaz, T. (1995a) 'Long term follow-ups of a randomised drug abuse preventional trial', *Journal of the American Medical Association* 273: 1106–12.

Botvin, G.J., Baker, E., Filazzola, A.D. and Botvin, E.M. (1995b) 'A cognitive-behavioural approach to substance abuse prevention: a one-year follow up. *Addictive Behaviours* 15: 47–63.

Botvin, G.J. and Botvin, E.M. (1992) 'School-based and community-based prevention approaches', in Lowinson, J., Ruiz, P. and Millman, R. (eds) *Substance Abuse: A Comprehensive Textbook*, Philadelphia, PA: Williams and Wilkins, 910–27.

Bradford, N. (1996) *The Hamlyn Encyclopaedia of Complementary Health*, London: Hamlyn.

Brain, K. (1998) 'The emergence of the post-modern alcohol order', Keynote speech, 11th International Conference on Alcohol, Liverpool.

Brain, K. and Parker, H. (1997) *Drinking with Design: Alcopops, Designer Drinks and Youth Culture*, London: Portman Group.

Brewers and Licensed Retailers Association (BLRA) (1994, 1995 and 1996) Memoranda to HM Treasury on beer duty.

Brewers and Licensed Retailers Association (BLRA) (1995) *Statistical Handbook*, London, BLRA.

Brewers and Licensed Retailers Association (BLRA) (1997) *Statistical Handbook*, London: BLRA.

Brewers and Licensed Retailers Association (BLRA) (1998) *Statistical Handbook*, London: BLRA.

Brewers and Licensed Retailers Association (BLRA) (1999) *Statistical Handbook*, London: BLRA.

British Medical Association (BMA) (1993) *Complementary Medicine: New Approaches to Good Practice*, Oxford: Oxford University Press.

Brower, K.J., Mudd, S., Blow, F.C., Young, J.P. and Hill, E.M. (1994) 'Severity and treatment of alcohol withdrawal in elderly versus younger patients', *Alcoholism, Clinical and Experimental Research* 18: 196–201.

Brown, J.M. and Miller, W.R. (1993) 'Impact of motivational interviewing on participation and outcome in residential alcoholism treatment', *Psychology of Addictive Behaviors* 7: 211–18.

Brumbaugh, A.G. (1993) 'Acupuncture: new perspectives in chemical dependency treatments', *Journal of Substance Abuse Treatments* 10: 35–43.

Bruun, K., Edwards, G., Lumio, M., Mäkelä, K., Pan, L., Popham, R., Room, R., Schmidt, W., Skog, Ø-J., Sulkunen, P. and Österberg, E. (1975) *Alcohol Control Policies in Public Health Perspective*, Helsinki: Finnish Foundation for Alcohol Studies.

Buck, D., Godfrey, C. and Richardson, G. (1994) *Should Cross-Border Shopping Affect Tax Policy?* York: YARTC Occasional Paper 6, Centre for Health Economics, University of York.

Buning, E. (1993) Comments at workshop on defining harm reduction, *Fifth International Conference on the Reduction of Alcohol Related Harm*, Toronto, Canada, March.

Burns, L. (1980) 'Getting rowdy with the boys', *Journal of Drug Issues* 10: 273–86.

Burns, L. Flaherty, B., Ireland, S. and Frances, M. (1995) 'Policing pubs: what happens to crime?', *Drug and Alcohol Review* 14: 369–75.

Cabinet Office (1999) *Tackling Drugs to Build a Better Britain*, London: The Stationery Office.

Cahalan, D. (1970) *Problem Drinkers: A National Survey*, San Francisco, CA: Jossey-Bass, Inc.

Cahalan, D. and Cisin, A. (1968) 'American drinking practices: Summary of findings from a national probability sample', *Quarterly Journal of Studies on Alcohol* 29: 139–51.

Cahalan, D., Cisin, I.H. and Crossley, H.M. (1969) *American Drinking Practices: A National Study of Drinking Behavior and Attitudes*, New Brunswick, NJ: Rutgers Center of Alcohol Studies.

Callaghan, R.J. (1996) *Thought Field Therapy™ Trauma and Treatment*, California: Indian Wells.

Camberwell Council on Alcoholism (1980) *Women and Alcohol*, London: Tavistock.

Cameron, D. (1983) 'Self-management of relapse prevention', in Curson, D., Rankin, H. and Shepherd, E. (eds) *Relapse in Alcoholism*, Northampton: ACIS.

Cameron, D. (1985) 'Why alcohol dependence – and why now?', in Heather, N., Robertson, I. and Davies, P. (eds) on behalf of the New Directions in the Study of Alcohol, *Crucial Issues in Dependence, Treatment and Prevention*, London: Croom Helm.

Cameron, D. (1995) *Liberating Solutions to Alcohol Problems: Treating Problem Drinkers Without Saying 'No'*, Northvale, NJ: Jason Aronson Inc.

Cameron, D. (1997) 'Keeping the customer satisfied: harm minimisation in clinical practice', in Plant, M.A., Single, E. and Stockwell, T. (eds) *Alcohol: Minimising the Harm: What Works?* London: Free Association Books, 233–47.

Cameron, D. (2000) 'Alcohol use – a perspective', in Cooper, D.B. (ed.) *Alcohol Use: The Handbook*, Oxford: Radcliffe Medical.

Canadian Brewers Association (1997) *Alcohol Beverage Taxation and Control Policies*, Canada: CBA.

Caprio, F.S. (1985) *Better Health with Self-Hypnosis*, London: Parker Publishing.

Carruthers, S.J. and Binns, C.W. (1987) 'The standard drink and alcohol consumption', *Drug and Alcohol Review* 11: 363–70.

Cartwright, A.K.J. (1977) 'The effect of role insecurity on the therapeutic commitment of alcoholism counsellors', London: Maudsley Alcohol Pilot Project.

Cartwright, A.K.J. (1980) 'The attitude of helping agents towards the alcoholic client: the influence of experience, support, training and self-esteem', *British Journal of Addiction* 75: 413–31.

Casswell, S., Gilmore, L., Maguire, V. and Ransome, R. (1989) 'Changes in public support for alcohol policies following a community-based campaign', *British Journal of Addiction* 84: 515–22.

Casswell, S., Gilmore, L., Silva, P. and Brasch, P. (1983) 'Early experiences with alcohol: a survey of an eight and nine year old sample', *New Zealand Medical Journal* 96: 1001–3.

Cavallo F., Russo R. and Zotti C. (1995) 'Moderate alcohol consumption and spontaneous abortion', *Alcohol and Alcoholism* 30: 195–201.

Cavan, S. (1966) *Liquor License: An Ethnography of Bar Behavior*, Chicago, IL: Aldine.

Chaney, E.F., O'Leary, M.R. and Marlatt, G.A. (1978) 'Skill training with alcoholics', *Journal of Consulting and Clinical Psychology* 46: 1092–104.

Chandler Coutts, M., Graham, K., Braun, K. and Wells, S. (forthcoming), 'Preliminary evaluation of a training program for bar staff on preventing aggression in bars', *Journal of Drug Education*.

Chapman, P.H. and Huygens, I. (1988) 'An evaluation of three treatment programmes for alcoholism: an experimental study with 6 and 18 month follow-up', *British Journal of Addiction* 83: 67–81.

Chen, W. and Dosch, M. (1987) 'Comparison of drinking attitudes and behaviors between participating and non-participating students in a voluntary alcohol education program', *Journal of Alcohol and Drug Education* 32: 7–13.

Chen, W., Dosch, M. and Cychosz, C. (1982) 'The impact of a voluntary educational program – Tip it Lightly, Alcohol Awareness Week – On the drinking attitudes and behaviors of college students', *Journal of Drug Education* 12: 125–35.

Chick J., Lloyd, G. and Crombie, E. (1985) 'Counselling problem drinkers in medical wards: a controlled study', *British Medical Journal* 290: 965–7.

Christensen, E. (1995) 'Families in distress: the development of children growing up with alcohol and violence', *Arctic Medical Journal* 54, Supplement 1: 53–9.

Cisler, R., Holder, H.D., Longabaugh, R., Stout, R.L. and Zweben, A. (1998) 'Actual and estimated replication costs for alcohol treatment modalities: case study from Project MATCH', *Journal of Studies on Alcohol* 50: 503–12.

Clement, S. (1984) Working With Alcohol-Related Problems: General Practitioners, Salford Community Alcohol Team Project: Unpublished manuscript.

Clement, S. (1986) 'The identification of alcohol-related problems by general practitioners', *British Journal of Addiction* 81: 257–64.

Coffield, F.J. and Gofton, L. (1994) *Drugs and Young People*, London: Institute for Public Policy Research.

Coggans, N. and McKellar, S. (1994) 'Drug use amongst peers: peer pressure or peer preference', *Drugs: Education, Prevention and Policy* 1: 15–25.

Coggans, N. and Watson, J. (1995) *Drug Education: Approaches, Effectiveness and Implications for Delivery*, Edinburgh: Health Education Board for Scotland.

Collins, D.J. and Lapsley, H.M. (1991) *Estimating the Economic Costs of Drug Abuse in Australia*, Canberra: Commonwealth Department of Community Services and Health.

Collins, D.J. and Lapsley, H.M. (1996) *The Social Costs of Drug Abuse in Australia in 1988 and 1992*, Canberra: Commonwealth Department of Human Services and Health.

Collins, J.J. Jnr. (ed.) (1982) *Drinking and Crime*, London: Tavistock.

Collins, M.N., Burns, T., Van Den Berk, P.A.H. and Tubman, G.F. (1990) 'A structured programme for out-patient alcohol detoxification', *British Journal of Psychiatry* 156: 871–4.

Connolly, G.M., Casswell, S., Stewart, J. and Silva, P. (1992) 'Drinking context and other influences on the drinking of 15 year old New Zealanders', *British Journal of Addiction* 87: 1029–36.

Conyne, R.K. (1984) 'Primary prevention through a campus alcohol education project', *The Personnel and Guidance Journal*, May: 524–8.

Cook, P.J. (1981) 'The effect of liquor taxes on drinking cirrhosis and auto fatalities', in Moore, M. and Gerstein, D. (eds) *Alcohol and Public Policy: Beyond the Shadow of Prohibition*, Washington, DC: National Academy of Sciences, 255–85.

Cook, P.J. and Moore, M. (1993a) 'Drinking and schooling', *Journal of Health Economics* 12: 411–429.

Cook, P.J. and Moore, M. (1993b) 'Taxation of alcoholic beverages', in Hilton, M.E. and Bloss, G. (eds) *Economics and the Prevention of Alcohol-Related Problems*, National Institute on Alcohol Abuse and Alcoholism Research Monograph 25, Rockville, MD: US Department of Health and Human Services, 33–58.

Cook, P.J., and Moore, M.F. (1993c) 'Violence reduction through restrictions on alcohol availability', *Alcohol Health and Research World* 117: 151–6.

Cook, P.J. and Tauchen, G. (1982) 'The effect of taxes on heavy drinking', *Bell Journal of Economics* 13: 379–90.

Cooper, D.B. (1994) *Alcohol Home Detoxification and Assessment*, Oxford: Radcliffe Medical Press.

Craig, G. and Fowlie, A. (1995) *Emotional Freedom Techniques™ The Manual*, California: The Sea Ranch, 2nd edition, 1997.

Craig, J. (1997) *Almost Adult*. NISRA Occasional Paper 3, Belfast: Northern Ireland Statistics and Research Agency.

Crain, M., Deaton, T., Holcombe, R. and Tollison, R. (1977) 'Rational choice and the taxation of sin', *Journal of Public Economics* 8: 239–45.

Cummings, C., Gordon, J.R. and Marlatt, G.A. (1980) 'Relapse: strategies of prevention and prediction,' in Miller W.R. (ed.) *The Addictive Behaviors*, Oxford: Pergamon.

Currie, C., Hurrelmann, K., Settertobulte, W., Smith, R. and Todd, J. (eds) (2000) *Health and Health Behaviour among Young People*, Copenhagen: World Health Organization.

Davies, J.B. (1992a) *The Myth of Addiction*, Reading: Harwood.

Davies, J.B. (1992b) 'Peer group influence and youthful alcohol consumption: an opinion', in Addictions Forum Conference Report, 'Alcohol and Young People: Learning to Cope', 7 October.

Davies, J.B. and Stacey, B. (1972) *Teenagers and Alcohol: A Developmental Study in Glasgow*, London: HMSO.

Davis, D. (1994) *Reaching Out to Children with FAS/FAE*, West Nyack, New York: The Center for Applied Research in Education.

Davis, J.E. and Reynolds, N.C. (1990) 'Alcohol use among college students: responses to raising the purchase age', *Journal of American College Health* 38: 263–9.

Dean, A. (1990) 'Culture and community: Drink and soft drugs in Hebridean youth culture', *Sociological Review* 38: 517–63.

De Haes, W.F.M. (1987) 'Looking for effective drug education programmes: 15 years' exploration of the effects of different drug education programmes', *Health Education: Theory and Practice* 2: 433–8.

De Haes, W.F.M. and Schuurman, J.H. (1975) 'Results of an evaluation study of three drug education methods', *International Journal of Health Education* 18: 1–16.

DeJong, W. and Wallack, L. (1992) 'The role of designated driver programs in the prevention of alcohol-impaired driving: a critical reassessment', *Health Education Quarterly* 19: 429–42.

Denman, S. (1994) 'Do schools provide an opportunity for meeting the Health of the Nation targets?', *Journal of Public Health Medicine* 10: 219–22.

Denny, M.R., Baugh, J.L. and Hardt, H.D. (1991) 'Sobriety outcome after alcoholism treatment with biofeedback participation: A pilot inpatient study', *International Journal of Addictions* 26: 335–41.

Denzin. N. and Lincoln, Y. (1994) *Handbook of Qualitative Research*. London: Sage.

Department for Education and Employment (DfEE) (1995) *Drug Prevention and Schools Circular 4/95*, London: DfEE.

Department for Education and Employment (DfEE) (1998) *Protecting Young People: Good Practice in Drug Education in Schools and the Youth Service*, London: DfEE.

Department for Education and Employment/Department of Health (DfEE/DoH) (1999a) *Healthy Schools: What it is and How it Will Work*. Guidance issued to Local Healthy Schools Co-ordinators, August, London: DfEE/DoH.

Department for Education and Employment/Department of Health (DfEE/DoH) (1999b) *The National Healthy Schools Scheme*, London: The Stationery Office.

Department of Health (DoH) (1995) *Sensible Drinking: The Report of an Inter-Departmental Working Group*, London: DoH.

Department of Health (DoH) (1998) *Independent Inquiry into Inequalities in Health*, London: The Stationery Office.

Department of Health (DoH) (1999) Personal communication.

Department of Transport (DoT) (1990) *Blood Alcohol Levels in Fatalities in Great Britain 1988*, Transport and Road Research Laboratory (UK).

Dight, S. (1976) *Scottish Drinking Habits*, London: HMSO.
Dobson, B.E. and Wright, L. (1995) *A Consultative Project on Effective Implementation of Drug Education in Five European Countries*, Salford: TACADE.
Donovan, C. and McEwan, R. (1994) 'A review of the literature examining the relationship between alcohol use and HIV-related sexual risk taking in young people', *Addiction* 90: 319–28.
Donovan, D. and Mattson, M. (eds) (1994) 'Alcoholism treatment matching research: methodologic and clinical approaches', *Journal of Studies on Alcohol*, Supplement 12.
Donovan, J.E. and Jessor, R. (1978) 'Adolescent problem drinking: psychosocial correlates in a national sample study', *Journal of Studies on Alcohol* 39: 1506–24.
Dorn, N. (1983) *Alcohol, Youth and the State*, Oxford: Croom Helm.
Dorn, N. and Murji, K. (1992) *Drug Prevention: A Review of the English Language Literature*, Research Monograph 5, London: ISDD.
Dorn, N. and South, N. (1983) *Message in a Bottle: Theoretical Overview and Annotated Bibliography on the Mass Media and Alcohol*, Aldershot: Gower.
Douglas, R. (1986) 'Alcohol management policies for recreation departments: development and implementation of the Thunder Bay model', in Giesbrecht, N. and Cox, R. (eds) *Prevention and the environment*, Toronto: Addiction Research Foundation.
Douglas, R.R. (1990) 'Formulating alcohol policies for community recreation facilities: tactics and problems', in Giesbrecht, N., Conley, P., Denniston, R.W., Gliksman, L., Holder, H., Pederson, A., Room, R. and Shain, M. (eds) *Research, Action, and the Community: Experience in the Prevention of Alcohol and Other Drug Problems*, Rockville, MD: US Department of Health and Human Services OSAP Prevention Monograph 4: 61–7.
Douglas, R., Wagenaar, A. and Barkey, P. (1979) *Alcohol Availability, Consumption, and the Incidence of Alcohol-Related Social and Health Problems in Michigan*, Highway Safety Research Institute, University of Michigan, Ann Arbor, MI: US Department of Commerce, National Technical Information Service, May.
Drever, F. (ed.) (1995) *Occupational Health: Decennial Supplement*, London: HMSO.
Drewery J. and Rae J.B. (1969) 'A group comparison of alcoholic and non-alcoholic marriages using the interpersonal perception technique', *British Journal of Psychiatry* 115: 287–300.
D'Zurilla, J.J. and Goldfried, M.R. (1971) 'Problem solving and behaviour modification', *Journal of Abnormal Psychology* 78: 107–26.
Edwards, G., Anderson, P., Babor, T., Casswell, S., Ferrence, R., Giesbrecht, N., Godfrey, C., Holder, H., Lemmens, P., Mäkelä, K., Midanik, L., Norström, T., Österberg, E., Romelsjö, A., Room, R., Simpura, J. and Skog, Ø-J. (1994) *Alcohol Policy and the Public Good*, Oxford: Oxford University Press.
Edwards G. and Gross, M.M. (1976) 'Alcohol Dependence: provisional description of a clinical syndrome', *British Medical Journal* 1: 1058–61.
Edwards, G., Orford, J., Egert, S., Guthrie, S., Mitcheson, M.N., Oppenheimer, E. and Taylor, C. (1977) 'Alcoholism: a controlled trial of treatment and advice', *Journal of Studies on Alcohol* 38: 1004–31.
Eisenberg, D.M. et al. (1998) 'Trends in alternative medicine use in the United States, 1990–1997: Results of a follow up national survey', *Journal of the American Medical Association* 280 : 1569–75
Eisner, E.W. (1997) *The Enlightened Eye: Qualitative Inquiry and the Enhancement of Educational Practice*, New York: Merril.
Elkind, D. (1967) 'Egocentrism in adolescence', *Child Development* 30: 1025–34.
Elkind, D. (1984) 'Teenage thinking: implications for health care', *Paediatric Nursing* 10: 383–5.

Elkind, D. (1985) 'Cognitive development and adolescent disabilities', *Journal of Adolescent Health Care*, 6: 84–9.

English, D., Holman, D., Milne, E., Winter, M., Hulse, G., Codde, G., Bower, C., Corti, B., De Klerk, C., Lewin, G., Knuiman, M., Kurinczuk, J. and Ryan, G. (1995) *The Quantification of Drug Caused Morbidity and Mortality in Australia, 1992*, Canberra: Commonwealth Department of Human Services and Health.

Engs, R. (1977) 'Let's look before we leap: the cognitive and behavioral evaluation of a university alcohol education program', *Journal of Alcohol and Drug Education* 22: 39–45.

Engs, R.G. and Hanson, D.J. (1986) 'Age-specific alcohol prohibition and college students' drinking problems', *Psychological Reports* 59: 979–84.

Engs, R.G. and Hanson, D.J. (1988) 'University students' drinking patterns and problems: Examining the effects of raising the purchase age', *Public Health Reports* 103: 667–73.

Engs, R. and Mulhall, P. (1981) 'Again – let's look before we leap: the effects of physical activity on smoking and drinking patterns', *Journal of Alcohol and Drug Education* 26: 65–74.

Erickson, P.G., Riley, D.M., Cheung, Y.W. and O'Hare, P. (eds) (1997) *Harm Reduction: A New Direction for Drug Policies and Programs*, Toronto: University of Toronto Press.

Ernst, E. (2000) 'Prevalence of use of complementary/alternative medicine: a systematic review', *Bulletin of the World Health Organization* 78: 252–7.

Evans, L. (1991) *Traffic Safety and the Driver*, New York: Van Nostrand Reinhold.

Ewles, L. and Simnett, I. (1999) *Promoting Health*, Edinburgh: Bailliere Tindall.

Fazey, C. (1977) *The Aetiology of Psychoactive Substance Use*, Paris: UNESCO.

Fergusson, D.M., Lynskey, M.T. and Horwood, L.J. (1996) 'Alcohol misuse and juvenile offending in adolescence', *Addiction* 91: 483–94.

Fichter, M.M., Glynn, S.M., Weyerer, S., Liberman, R.P. and Frick, U. (1997) 'Family climate and expressed emotion in the course of alcoholism', *Family Process* 36: 203–21.

Fillmore, K.M. (1987) 'Women's drinking across the life course as compared to men's', *British Journal of Addiction*, 82: 801–11.

Fillmore, K.M. (1988) *Alcohol Use Across the Life Course: A Critical Review of Seventy Years of International Longitudinal Research*, Toronto: Addiction Research Foundation.

Fillmore, K.M. (2000) 'Is alcohol really good for your heart?', *Addiction* 95: 173–74.

Finkelstein, N. (1993) 'Treatment programming for alcohol and drug-dependent pregnant women', *Journal of Drug Issues* 28: 1275–309.

Finkelstein, N. (1994) 'Treatment issues for alcohol and drug-dependent and parenting women', *Health and Social Work* 19: 7–15.

Finlay D.G. (1978) 'Alcoholism and systems theory: building a better mousetrap', *Psychiatry* 41: 272–8.

Finnegan L.P. (1994) 'Perinatal morbidity and mortality in substance using families: effects and intervention strategies', *Bulletin on Narcotics* 46: 19–43.

Fishbein, M. and Ajzen, I. (1975) *Belief, Attitude, Intention and Behaviour: An Introduction to Theory and Research*, Reading, MA: Addison Wesley.

Flay, B.R. (1985) 'What do we know about the social influences approach to smoking prevention? Review and recommendations', in Bell, C. et al. (eds) *Prevention Research: Deterring Drug Abuse among Children and Adolescents*. NIDA Research Monograph 63: Washington, DC: NIDA, 67–112.

Flynn, C. and Brown, W. (1991) 'The effects of a mandatory alcohol education program on college student problem drinkers', *Journal of Alcohol and Drug Education* 37: 15–24.

Foon, A.E. (1988) 'The effectiveness of drinking-driving treatment programs: a critical review', *International Journal of the Addictions* 23: 151–74.

Fossey, E. (1994) *Growing Up With Alcohol*, London, Tavistock/Routledge.

Foster, K., Wilmot, A. and Dobbs, J. (1990) *General Household Survey 1988*, London: HMSO.

Fox, K. (1997) *Taskforce on Underage Alcohol Misuse. Report on the Under-18 Panel Meetings*, London: Portman Group.

Fox, K., Merrill, J., Chang, H. and Califano, J. (1995) 'Estimating the costs of substance abuse to the Medicaid hospital care program', *American Journal of Public Health* 85: 48–54.

Foxcroft, D., Lister-Sharp, D. and Lowe, G. (1997) 'Alcohol misuse prevention for young people: a systematic review reveals methodological concerns and lack of reliable evidence of effectiveness', *Addiction* 92: 531–7.

Foxcroft, D.R. and Lowe, G. (1993) 'Self attributions for alcohol use on older teenagers', *Addiction Research* 1: 1–9.

Frawley, D. (1998) *Ayurveda and the Mind*, Delhi: Motilal Banarsidas.

Fullan, M.G. (1991) *The New Meaning of Educational Change*, London: Cassell.

Gaines A.D. (1992) 'From DSM-I to III-R; voices of self, mastery and the other: a cultural constructivist reading of U.S. psychiatric classification', *Social Science and Medicine* 35: 3–24.

Garafas, G. (1995) *The Effects of Regulation on the Price of Beer in the UK Beer Industry*, Oxford: Regulatory Policy Institute.

Garmonsway, G.N. and Simpson, J. (1965) *The Penguin English Dictionary*, Harmondsworth: Penguin, 236.

Garretsen, H., Bongers, I. and Van Oers, H. (2000) Personal communication.

Garvin, R.B., Alcorn, J.D. and Faulkner, K.K. (1990) 'Behavioral strategies for alcohol abuse prevention with high risk college males', *Journal of Alcohol and Drug Education* 36: 23–34.

Gay, J., Minelli, M., Tripp, D. and Keilitz, D. (1990) 'Alcohol and the athlete: a university's response', *Journal of Alcohol and Drug Education* 35: 81–6.

Geller, E., and Kalsher, M. (1990) 'Environmental determinants of party drinking', *Environment and Behavior* 22: 74–90.

Geller, E., Russ, N. and Delphos, W. (1987) 'Does server intervention make a difference?' *Alcohol Health and Research World* 11: 64–9.

German National Statistical Office (1999) *Annual Statistical Review*, Germany: National Statistical Office.

Gerson, L.W. and Preston, D.A. (1979) 'Alcohol consumption and the incidence of violent crime', *Journal on Studies of Alcohol* 41: 307–12.

Gerstein, D. and Green, L. (eds) (1993) *Preventing Drug Abuse, What Do We Know?* Washington, DC: National Academy Press.

Gibbs, J. and Bennett, S. (1990) *Together We Can Reduce the Risks*, Seattle, WA: Seattle Health Education Foundation.

Giesbrecht, N., Gonzalez, R., Grant, M., Österberg, E., Room, R., Rootman, I. and Towle, L. (1989) *Drinking and Casualties: Accidents, Poisonings and Violence in International Perspective*, London: Tavistock/Routledge.

Gillespie, A., Davey, J., Sheenan, M. and Stedson, D. (1991) 'Thrills without spills. The Educational implications of research into adolescent binge drinking for a school based intervention', *Drug Education Journal of Australia* 5: 121–12.

Gin and Vodka Association (various years) Submissions on excise duty and in particular its 1998 memorandum.

Glassner, B. and Loughlin, J. (1987) *Drugs in Adolescent Worlds: Burnouts to Straights*, Basingstoke: Macmillan.

Gliksman, L. (1986) 'Alcohol management policies for municipal recreation departments: an evaluation of the Thunder Bay model', in Giesbrecht, N. and Cox, A. (eds) *Prevention and the Environment*, Toronto: Addiction Research Foundation, 198–204.

Gliksman, L., Douglas, R.R., Rylett, M. and Narbonne-Fortin, C. (1995) 'Reducing problems through municipal alcohol policies: the Canadian experiment in Ontario', *Drugs: Education, Prevention and Policy* 2: 105–18.

Gliksman, L., Douglas, R.R., Thomson, M., Moffat, K., Smythe, C. and Caverson, R. (1990) 'Promoting municipal alcohol policies: an evaluation of a campaign', *Contemporary Drug Problems* 17: 391–420.

Gliksman, L., McKenzie, D., Single, E., Douglas, R., Brunet, S. and Moffatt, K. (1993) 'The role of alcohol providers in prevention: an evaluation of a server intervention program', *Addiction* 88: 1189–97.

Goddard, E. (1977) *Young Teenagers and Alcohol in 1996. Volume 2 Scotland*, London: Office for National Statistics.

Goddard, E. (1986) *Drinking and Attitudes to Licensing in Scotland*, London: HMSO.

Goddard, E. (1991) *Drinking in England and Wales in the late 1980s*, London: HMSO.

Goddard, E. (1996) *Teenage Drinking in 1994*, London: Office of Population Censuses and Surveys.

Goddard, E. (1997a) *Young Teenagers and Alcohol in 1996. Volume 1. England*, London: Office for National Statistics.

Goddard, E. (1997b) *Young Teenagers and Alcohol in 1996. Volume 2. Scotland*, London: Office for National Statistics.

Goddard, E. (1999) *Drinking: Adults' Behaviour and Knowledge in 1998*, London: Office for National Statistics.

Goddard, E. and Higgins, V. (1999a) *Smoking, Drinking and Drug Use among Young Teenagers in 1998, Volume 1: England*, London: Office for National Statistics.

Goddard, E. and Higgins, V. (1999b) *Smoking, Drinking and Drug Use among Young Teenagers in 1998, Volume 2: Scotland*, London: Office for National Statistics.

Godfrey, C. (1989) 'Factors influencing the consumption of alcohol and tobacco: the use and abuse of economic models', *British Journal of Addiction* 84: 1123–8.

Godfrey, C. (1994) 'Economic influences on change in population and personal substance behaviour', in Edwards, G. and Lader, M. (eds) *Addiction: Processes of Change*, Oxford: Oxford Medical Publication, Oxford University Press, 163–87.

Gofton, L. (1990) 'On the town: drink and the new lawlessness', *Youth and Policy* 29: 33–9.

Goldstein, P.J. (1979) *Prostitution and Drugs*, Lexington, MA: Lexington Books.

Gomberg, E.S. (1982) *Alcohol Use and Alcohol Problems among the Elderly*, Alcohol and Health Monograph 4 (Special Population Issues). Rockville, MD: NIAAA: DHHS, 263–90.

Gonzalez, G. (1982) 'Alcohol education can prevent alcohol problems: A summary of some unique research findings', *Journal of Alcohol and Drug Education* 27: 2–12.

Gonzalez, G. (1991) 'Five-year changes in alcohol knowledge, consumption and problems among students exposed to a campus-wide alcohol awareness program and a rise in the legal drinking age', *Journal of Alcohol and Drug Education* 37: 81–91.

Goode, E. (1972) *Drugs in American Society*, New York: Alfred A. Knopf.

Goodstadt, M. (1986) 'School-based drug education in North America. What is wrong? What can be done?', *Journal of School Health* 56: 278–81.

Goodstadt, M. (1989) 'Substance abuse curricula vs school drug policies', *Journal of School Health* 59: 246–50.

Gordis, E. and Fuller, R. (1999) 'Project MATCH', *Addiction* 94: 57–9.

Gorman, D.M. (1996) 'Do school-based skills training programs prevent alcohol use among young people', *Addiction Research* 4: 191–210.

Gossop, M., Powis, B., Griffiths, P. and Strang, J. (1994) 'Sexual behaviour and its relationship to drug-taking amongst prostitutes in South London', *Addiction* 89: 961–70.

Gossop, M. et al. (1999) *NTORS: Two Year Outcomes: The National Treatment Outcome Research Study*, London: DoH.

Gottesfield, Z. and Abel, E.L. (1991) 'Maternal and paternal use: effects on the immune system of the offspring', *Life Science* 48: 1–8.

Government White Paper (1997) *Excellence in Schools*, London: HMSO.

Government White Paper (1999) *Saving Lives: Our Healthier Nation*, London: HMSO.

Graham, K. (1985) 'Determinants of heavy drinking and drinking problems: the contribution of the bar environment', in Single, E. and Storm, T. (eds) *Public Drinking and Public Policy*, Toronto: Addiction Research Foundation, 71–84.

Graham, K. (1986) 'Identifying and measuring alcohol abuse among the elderly: serious problems with existing instrumentation', *Journal of Studies on Alcohol* 47: 322–6.

Graham, K. and Chandler Coutts, M. (forthcoming) 'Community action research: who does what to whom and why? Lessons learned from local prevention efforts (International Experiences)', *Substance Use and Misuse*.

Graham, K. and Homel, R. (1997) 'Creating safer bars', in Plant, M.A., Single, E. and Stockwell, T. (eds) *Alcohol: Minimising the Harm: What works?*, London: Free Association Books, 171–92.

Graham, K., LaRocque, L., Yetman, R., Ross, T. J. and Guistra, E. (1980) 'Aggression and barroom environments', *Journal of Studies on Alcohol* 41: 277–92.

Graham, K., West, P. and Wells, S. (forthcoming), 'Evaluating theories of alcohol-related aggression using observations of young adults in bars', *Addiction* (accepted subject to revisions).

Grant, M. (1986) 'Comparative analysis of the impact of alcohol education in North America and Western Europe', in Babor, T. (ed.) *Alcohol and Culture-Comparative Perspectives from Europe and North America*, New York: New York Academy of Sciences, 198–210.

Grant, M. (ed.) (1998) *Alcohol and Emerging Markets: Patterns, Problems and Responses*, International Center for Alcohol Policies Series on Alcohol in Society, Philadephia, PA: Brunner/Mazel.

Grant, M. and Litvak, J. (eds) (1998) *Drinking Patterns and Their Consequences*, International Center for Alcohol Policies Series on Alcohol in Society, Philadelphia, PA: Brunner/Mazel.

Grant, M. and Ritson, E.B. (1983) *The Prevention Debate*, London: Croom Helm.

Graves, K.L. (1993) 'An evaluation of the alcohol warning label: a comparison of the United States and Ontario, Canada between 1990 and 1991', *Journal of Public Policy and Marketing* 12: 19–29.

Green, L. (1979) 'National policy in the promotion of health', *International Journal of Health Education* 22: 161–8.

Greenfield, S. (1997) *The Human Brain*, London: Weidenfeld and Nicholson.

Greenfield, T.K. (1994) 'Improving causal inference from naturalistic designs: self-selection and other issues in evaluating alcohol control policies', *Applied Behavioral Science Review* 2: 45–61.

Greenfield, T.K. (1997) 'Warning labels: evidence on harm reduction from long-term American surveys', in Plant, M.A., Single, E. and Stockwell, T. (eds) *Alcohol: Minimising the Harm: What Works?*, London: Free Association Books, 105–25.

Greenfield, T.K., Graves, K.L. and Kaskutas, L.A. (1993) 'Alcohol warning labels for prevention: national survey findings', *Alcohol, Health and Research World* 17: 67–75.

Greenfield, T.K. and Kaskutas, L.A. (1993) 'Early impacts of alcoholic beverage warning labels: national study findings relevant to drinking and driving behavior', *Safety Science* 16: 689–707.

Grossman, M., Chaloupka, F.J., Saffer, H. and Laixuthai, A. (1993) *Effects of Alcohol Price Policy on Youth*, Cambridge, MA, National Bureau of Economic Research Working Paper 4385.

Grossman, S., Canterbury, R.J., Lloyd, E. and McDowell, M. (1994) 'A model approach to peer-based alcohol and other drug prevention in a college population', *Journal of Alcohol and Drug Education* 39: 50–61.

Grube, J.W. (1997) 'Preventing sales of alcohol to minors: results from a community trial', *Addiction 92*, Supplement 2: S251–S260.

Gruenewald, P.J. (1993) 'Alcohol problems and the control of availability: theoretical and empirical issues', in Hilton, H.E. and Bliss, G. (eds) *Economics and the Prevention of Alcohol-Related Problems*, NIAAA Research Monograph 25, DHHS Publication No. (NIH) 93–3513. Washington, DC: US Government Printing Office.

Gruenewald, P.J., Ponicki, W.R. and Holder, H.D. (1993) 'The relationship of outlet densities to alcohol consumption: a time-series cross-sectional analysis', *Alcoholism: Clinical and Experimental Research* 17: 38–47.

Guydish, J. and Greenfield, T. (1990) 'Alcohol-related cognitions: do they predict treatment outcome?', *Addictive Behaviors* 15: 423–30.

Hadley, J. (1996) *Hypnosis for Change*, Oakland, CA: New Harbinger Publications.

Haines, A. and Jones, R. (1994) 'Implementing findings of research', *British Medical Journal* 308: 1488–92.

Haley, J. (ed.) (1967) *Advanced Techniques of Hypnosis and Therapy: Selected Papers of Milton H. Erickson, MD*, New York: Grune and Stratton.

Halmesmäki, E., Välimäki, M. and Roine, R. (1989) 'Maternal and paternal alcohol consumption and miscarriage', *British Journal of Obstetrics and Gynaecology* 96: 188–91.

Hamilton, C.J. and Collins, J.J. Jnr (1982) 'The role of alcohol in wife beating and child abuse: a review of the literature', in Collins, J.J. Jnr (ed.) *Drinking and Crime*, London: Tavistock, 253–87.

Hammer, T. and Vaglum, P. (1989) 'The increase in alcohol consumption in women: a phenomenon related to accessiblity or stress? A general population study', *British Journal of Addiction* 84: 767–75.

Hampton, R.L., Gullotta, T.P., Adams, G.R., Potter, E.H. and Weissberg, R.P. (eds) (1993) *Family Violence: Prevention and Treatment*, London: Sage.

Hanninen, V. and Koski-Jannes, A. (1999) 'Narratives of recovery from addictive behaviours', *Addiction* 94: 1837–48

Hansen, W.B. (1992) 'School-based substance abuse prevention: a review of the state of the art in curriculum, 1980–1990', *Health Education Research* 7: 403–30.

Hansen, W.B., Johnson, C.A., Flay, B.R., Graham, J.W. and Sobol, J. (1998) 'Affective and social influences and approaches to the prevention of multiple substance abuse among 7th grade students: results from Project SMART', *Preventive Medicine* 17: 135–54.

Harbison, J. and Haire, T. (1980) *Drinking in Northern Ireland*, Belfast: Social Research Division, Public Policy Unit, Department of Finance.

Harding, J.R., and Wittman, F.D. (1995) 'ASIPS and community-level prevention planning using police incident data with a GIS', Paper presented at the Annual Conference of the Urban and Regional Information Systems Association, 16–20 July, San Antonio, TX; Berkeley, CA: CLEW Associates, July.

Harford, T.C. and Grant, B. (1987) 'Psychosocial factors in adolescent drinking contexts', *Journal of Studies on Alcohol* 48: 551–7.

Harlap, S., Shiono P.H. and Ramecharan S. (1979) 'Alcohol and spontaneous abortion', *American Journal of Epidemiology* 110: 372.

Harre, R. (1979) *Social Being*, Oxford: Blackwell.

Harre, R. (1986) *Social Construction of Emotions*, Oxford: Blackwell.

Hauge, R. (1999) 'The public health perspective and the transformation of Norwegian alcohol policy', Paper presented at the 25th Annual Alcohol Epidemiology Symposium, Kettil Bruun Society, Montreal.

Hauritz, M., Homel, R., McIllwain, G., Burrows, T. and Townsley, M. (forthcoming) 'Reducing violence in licensed venues through community safety action projects: The Queensland experience', *Contemporary Drug Problems.*

Hawkins, J.D., Catalano, R.F. and Miller, J.Y. (1992) 'Risk and protective factors for alcohol and other drug problems in adolescence and early adulthood: Implications for substance abuse prevention', *Psychological Bulletin* 112:1.

Hawks, D., Lang, E., Stockwell, T., Rydon, P. and Lockwood, A. (1993) 'Public support for the prevention of alcohol-related problems', *Drug and Alcohol Review* 12: 243–50.

Hawthorne, G. (1996) 'The social impact of Life Education: estimates drug use prevalence among Victorian primary school students and the statewide effect of the Life Education programme', *Addiction* 91: 1151–60

Hawthorne, G., Garrard, J. and Dunt, D. (1995) 'Does Life Education's drug education program have a public health benefit?', *Addiction* 90: 205–16.

Hayashida, M., Alterman, A.I. and McLellan, T. (1989) 'Comparative effectiveness and costs of in-patient and out-patient detoxification of patients with mild to moderate alcohol withdrawal syndrome', *New England Journal of Medicine* 320: 358–65.

Hays, R.D. and Ellikson, P.L. (1990) How generalizable are adolescents' beliefs about pro-drug pressures and resistance self-efficacy?', *Journal of Applied Social Psychology* 20: 321–40.

Health Education Authority (HEA)/MORI (1992) *Tomorrow's Young Adults*, London: HEA.

Health Education Board for Scotland (HEBS) (1994) *That's the Limit: A Guide to Sensible Drinking*, Edinburgh: HEBS.

Heath, D. (ed.) (1995) *International Handbook on Alcohol and Culture*, Westport, CT: Greenwood Press.

Heather, N. (1986) 'Minimal treatment intervention for problem drinkers', in Edwards, G. (ed.) *Current Issues in Clinical Psychology*, London: Plenum Press.

Heather, N. (1994) 'Weakness of will: a suitable topic for scientific study?', *Addiction Research* 2: 135–9.

Heather, N. (1995) *Treatment Approaches to Alcohol Problems* (WHO Regional Publications, European Series No. 65), Copenhagen: World Health Organization.

Heather, N., Campion, P. D., Neville, R. G. and MacCabe, D. (1987) 'Evaluation of a controlled drinking minimal intervention for problem drinkers in general practice', *Journal of the Royal College of General Practice* 37: 356–62.

Heather, N. and Robertson, I. (1997) *Problem Drinking*, 3rd edition, Oxford: Oxford University Press.

Heather, N. and Tebbutt, J. (eds) (1989) *The Effectiveness of Treatment for Drug and Alcohol Problems: An Overview*, NCADA Monograph Series No. 11, Canberra: Australian Government Printing Service.

Hendry, L.B., Shucksmith, J., Love, J.G. and Glendinning, A. (1993) *Young People's Leisure and Lifestyles*, London: Routledge.

Hennessy, M. and Seltz, R.F. (1990) 'The situational riskiness of alcoholic beverages', *Journal of Studies on Alcohol* 51: 422–7.

Hester, R.K. and Miller, W.R. (eds) (1995) *Handbook of Alcoholism Treatment Approaches: Effective Alternatives*, Needham Heights, MA: Allyn and Bacon.

Hibell, B., Andersson, B., Bjarnason, T., Kokkevi, A., Morgan, M. and Narusk, A. (1997) *The 1995 ESPAD Report: Alcohol and Other Drug Use among Students in 26 European Countries*, Stockholm: Swedish Council for Information on Alcohol and Other Drugs.

Hilton, M.E. and Kaskutas, L.A. (1991) 'Public support for warning labels on alcoholic beverage containers', *British Journal of Addiction* 86: 1323–33.

Hinderliter, S.A. and Zelenak, J.P. (1993) 'A simple method to identify alcohol and other drug use in pregnant adults in a pre-natal care setting', *Journal of Perinatology* 13: 93–102.

Hingson, R., Berson, J. and Dowley, K. (1997) 'Interventions to reduce college student drinking and related health and social problems,' in Plant, M.A., Single, E. and Stockwell, T. (eds) *Alcohol: Minimising the Harm: What Works?*, London: Free Association Books.

Hingson, R., Strunin, L., Berlin, B. and Heeren, T. (1990) 'Beliefs about AIDS, use of alcohol, drugs and unprotected sex among Massachusetts adolescents', *American Journal of Public Health* 80: 295–9.

Hirst, J. (1994) *Not in Front of the Grown Ups*, Sheffield: Sheffield Hallam University, Pavic Publications.

Hirst, J. and McCamley-Finney, A (1994*) The Place and Meaning of Drugs in Young People's Lives*, Sheffield: Sheffield Hallam University, Health Research Unit.

Hirst, P. (1969) 'The logic of the curriculum', *Journal of Curriculum Studies* 1: 142

Hitao, G. (1994) *How to Prevent Alcohol Problems in Cities: An Evaluation of the Community Prevention Planning Demonstration Project, June 1990–September 1993*, Berkley, CA: Institute for the Study of Social Change, University of California, Berkeley, January.

Holder, H.D., Longbaugh, T., Miller, W.R. and Rubonis, A.V. (1991) 'The cost effectiveness of treatment for alcoholism. A first approximation', *Journal of Studies on Alcohol* 52: 517–40.

Holder, H.D., and Moore, R.S. (forthcoming) 'Institutionalization of community action projects to reduce alcohol use problems: systematic facilitators', *Substance Use and Misuse*.

Holder, H.D., Saltz, R.F., Grube, J. W., Voas, R.B., Gruenewald, P.J. and Treno, A.J. (1997) 'A community prevention trial to reduce alcohol-involved accidental injury and death: overview', *Addiction* 92, Supplement 2: S155–S171.

Holder, H. and Wagenaar, A. (1994) 'Mandated server training and reduced alcohol-involved traffic crashes: a time-series analysis of the of the Oregon experience', *Accident Analysis and Prevention* 26: 89–97.

Holmila, M. (ed.) (1997) *Community Prevention of Alcohol Problems*, London: Macmillan.

Holmila, M. (forthcoming) 'The Finnish case. Community prevention in a time of rapid change in national and international trade', *Substance Use and Misuse*.

Home Office Drugs Prevention Initiative (1998) *Developing Local Drugs Prevention Strategies*, London: The Stationery Office.

Homel, R., Carseldine, D. and Kearns, I. (1988) 'Drink-driving countermeasures in Australia', *Alcohol, Drugs, and Driving* 4: 113–44.

Homel, R. and Clark, J. (1994) 'The prediction and prevention of violence in pubs and clubs', in Clark, R.V. (ed.) *Crime Prevention Studies*, Volume 3, Monsey, NY: Criminal Justice Press, 1–4.

Homel, R., Hauritz, M., Wortley, R., Clark, J. and Carvolth, R. (1994). *The Impact of the Surfers Paradise Safety Action Project*, Queensland: Centre for Crime Policy and Public Safety, School of Justice Administration, Griffith University.

Homel, R., Hauritz, M., Wortley, R., McIlwaine, G. and Carvolth, R. (1997) 'Preventing alcohol-related crime through community action: The Surfers Paradise Safety Action Project', *Crime Prevention Studies* 7: 35–90.

Homel, R., McKay, P. and Henstridge, J. (1995) 'The impact on accidents of random breath testing in New South Wales: 1982–1992', in Kloeden, C.N. and McLean, A.J. (eds) *Alcohol, Drugs and Traffic Safety, Volume 2*, Australia: NHMRC Road Accident Research Unit, 849–55.

Homel, R., Tomsen, S. and Thommeny, J. (1992) 'Public drinking and violence: not just an alcohol problem', *Journal of Drug Issues* 22: 679–97.

Hore, B.D. and Plant, M.A. (eds) (1981) *Alcohol Problems in Employment*, London, Croom Helm.

Howard-Pitney, B., Johnson, M.D., Altman, D., Hopkins, R. and Hammond, N. (1991) 'Responsible alcohol service: a study of server, manager, and environmental impact', *American Journal of Public Health* 81: 197–9.

Howe, B. (1989) *Alcohol Education: A Handbook for Health and Welfare Professionals*, London: Routledge.

Hughes, S.P. and Dodder, R.A. (1986) 'Raising the legal minimum drinking age: short-term effects with college student samples', *Journal of Drug Issues* 16: 609–20.

Humphreys, K. and Moos, R.H. (1996) 'Reduced substance abuse-related health care costs among voluntary participants in Alcoholics Anonymous', *Psychiatric Services* 47: 709–13.

Hutcheson, G., Henderson, M. and Davies, J. (1995) *Alcohol in the Workplace*, Employment No. 59 Research Series, London: DfEE.

Iannotti, R.J. and Bush, P.J. (1992) 'Perceived use, actual friends' use of alcohol, cigarettes, marijuana and cocaine: which has the most influence?', *Journal of Youth and Adolescence* 21. 373–89.

Iannotti, R.J., Bush, P.J and Weinfurt, K.P. (1996) 'Perception of friends' use of alcohol, cigarettes and marijuana among urban schoolchildren: a longitudinal analysis', *Addictive Behaviours* 21: 615–32.

Institute of Medicine (IoM) (1990) *Broadening the Base of Treatment for Alcohol Problems*, Washington, DC: National Academy Press.

Institute of Medicine (IoM) (1996) *Fetal Alcohol Syndrome*, Washington, DC: National Academy Press.

Ireland, C.S. and Thommeny, J.L. (1993) 'The crime cocktail: licensed premises, alcohol and street offences', *Drug and Alcohol Review* 12: 143–50.

Irvine, M.J. and Logan, A.G. (1991) 'Relaxation therapy as sole treatment for mild hypertension', *Psychosomatic Medicine* 53: 587–97.

Jahoda, G. and Cramond, J. (1972) *Children and Alcohol: A Developmental Study in Glasgow*, London: HMSO.

Janz, N.K. and Becker, M.H. (1984) 'The Health Belief Model, a decade later', *Health Education Quarterly* 11: 1–47.

Jarvis, T.J., Tebbutt, J. and Mattick, R.P. (1995) *Treatment Approaches for Alcohol and Drug Dependence: An Introductory Guide*, Chichester: John Wiley and Sons.

Jasinki, J.L. and Williams, L.M. (eds) (1998) *Partner Violence*, London: Sage.

Jeffs, B. and Saunders, B. (1983) 'Minimising alcohol-related offences by enforcement of the existing licensing legislation', *British Journal of Addiction* 78: 67–78.

Jessor, R., Chase, J.A. and Donovan, J.E. (1980) 'Psychosocial correlates of marijuana use and problem drinking: a national sample of adolescents', *American Journal of Public Health* 70: 604–13.

Jessor, R., Donovan, J.E. and Costa, F.M. (1991) *Beyond Adolescence*, Cambridge: Cambridge University Press.

256 The Alcohol Report

Jessor, R. and Jessor, S.L. (1977) *Problem Behaviour and Psychosocial Development: A Longitudinal Study of Youth*, New York: Academic Press.

Jobst, K.A. (1998) 'Toward integrated healthcare: practical and philosophical issues at the heart of the integration of biomedical, complementary and alternative medicines', *Journal of Alternative and Complementary Medicine* 4: 123–6.

Jones K.L. and Smith D.W. (1973) 'Recognition of the Fetal Alcohol Syndrome in early infancy', *Lancet* 2: 999–1001.

Kadden, R.P., Carroll, K., Donovan, D. et al. (1992) *Cognitive-Behavioral Coping Skills Therapy: A Clinical Research Guide for Therapists Treating Individuals with Alcohol Abuse and Dependence*, Project MATCH Monograph Series, vol. 3, DHHS Pub. No. (ADM) 92–1895, Washington, DC: Department of Health and Human Services.

Kalb, M. (1975) 'The myth of alcoholism prevention', *Preventive Medicine* 4: 404–16.

Karlsson, G. and Romelsjö, A. (1997) 'A longitudinal study of social, psychological and behavioural factors associated with drunken driving and public drunkenness', *Addiction* 92: 447–57.

Kaskutas, L.A. (1993a) 'Differential perceptions of alcohol policy effectiveness', *Journal of Public Health Policy* 14: 415–36.

Kaskutas, L.A. (1993b) 'Changes in public attitudes toward alcohol control policies since the warning label mandate of 1988', *Journal of Public Policy and Marketing* 12: 30–7.

Kaskutas, L.A. (1995) 'Interpretations of risk: the use of scientific information in the development of the alcohol warning label policy', *International Journal of the Addictions* 30: 1519–48.

Kaskutas, L.A. and Graves, K. (1994) 'Relationship between cumulative exposure to health messages and awareness and behavior-related drinking during pregnancy', *American Journal of Health Promotion* 9: 115–24.

Keeling, R.P. (1994) 'Changing the context: the power in prevention: alcohol awareness, caring and community', *Journal of American College Health* 42: 243–7.

Kilpatrick, D.G., Edmonds, C.N. and Seymour, A.K. (1992) *Rape in America: A Report to the Nation*, Arlington, VA: National Victim Center.

Kinder, B.N., Pape, N.E. and Walfish, S. (1980) 'Drug and alcohol education programmes: a review of outcome studies', *International Journal of the Addictions* 15: 1035–54.

King, M.B. (1986a) 'At risk drinking among general practice attenders: validation of the CAGE Questionnaire', *Psychological Medicine* 16: 213–17.

King, M.B. (1986b) 'At risk drinking among general practice attenders: prevalence, characteristics and alcohol related problems', *British Journal of Psychiatry* 148: 533–40.

Kivlahan, D., Marlatt, A., Fromme, K., Coppel, D. and Williams, E. (1990) 'Secondary prevention with college drinkers: evaluation of an alcohol skills training program', *Journal of Clinical and Consulting Psychology*, 58: 805–10.

Klassen, A. and Wilsnack, S.C. (1986) 'Sexual experiences and drinking among women in a US national survey', *Archives of Sexual Behavior* 15: 363–92.

Kleijnen, J. et al. (1991) 'Clinical trials of homeopathy', *British Medical Journal* 302: 316–23.

Kline, R.B. and Canter, W.A. (1994) 'Can education programs affect teenage drinking? A multivariate perspective', *Journal of Drug Education* 24: 139–49.

Knibbe, R.A., Oostveen, T. and van De Goor, I. (1991) 'Young people's alcohol consumption in public places: reasoned behaviour or related to the situation?', *British Journal of Addiction* 86: 1425–33.

Knipschild, P. et al. (1990) 'Belief in the efficacy of alternative medicine among general practitioners in the Netherlands', *Social Science and Medicine* 31: 625–6.

Kolata, G.B. (1981) 'Fetal alcohol advisory debate', *Science* 214: 642–5.

Kooler, J.M. and Bruvold, W.H. (1992) 'Evaluation of an educational intervention upon knowledge, attitudes and behavior concerning drinking/drugged driving', *Journal of Drug Education* 2: 87–100.

Kraft, D.P. (1988) 'The prevention and treatment of alcohol problems on a college campus', *Journal of Alcohol and Drug Education* 34: 37–51.

Kreitman, N. (1986) 'Alcohol consumption and the preventive paradox', *British Journal of Addiction* 81: 353–63.

Kristenson, H. and Hood, B. (1984) 'The impact of alcohol on health in the general population: a review with particular reference to experience in Malmo', *British Journal of Addiction* 79: 134–45.

Kumpher, K. (1997) 'What Works in the Prevention of Drug Abuse: Individual School and Family Approaches', in *Youth Substance Abuse Prevention Initiative: Resource papers* 69–106. Washington: US Department of Health and Human Services, Substance Abuse and Mental Health Services Administration.

Kunz, J.L. (1997) 'Associating leisure with drinking: current research and future directions', *Drug and Alcohol Review* 16: 69–76.

Lang E. (1991) 'Server intervention: what chance in Australia?', *Drug and Alcohol Review* 10: 381–93.

Lang, E., and Rumbold, G. (1997) 'The effectiveness of community-based interventions to reduce violence in and around licensed premises: a comparison of three Australian models', *Contemporary Drug Problems* 24: 805–26.

Lang, E., Stockwell, T. and Lo, S.K. (1990) *Drinking Locations of Drink-Driving Offenders in the Perth Metropolitan Area*, Technical Report prepared for the Western Australian Police Department, Bentley, Western Australia: National Centre for Research into the Prevention of Drug Abuse.

Lang, E., Stockwell, T., Rydon, P. and Beel, A. (1996) 'The use of pseudo-patrons to assess compliance with licensing laws regarding under-age drinking', *Australian and New Zealand Journal of Public Health* 20: 296–300.

Lang, E., Stockwell, T., Rydon, P. and Gamble, C. (1992) *Drinking Settings, Alcohol-Related Harm and Support for Prevention Policies. Results of a Survey of Persons Residing in the Perth Metropolitan Area*. Technical Report, National Centre for Research into the Prevention of Drug Abuse, Division of Health Sciences, Bentley, Western Australia: Curtin University of Technology.

La Rosa, J.H. (1990) 'Executive women and health: perceptions and practices', *American Journal of Public Health* 80: 1450–4.

Leather, P. and Lawrence, C. (1995) 'Perceiving pub violence: the symbolic influence of social and environmental factors', *British Journal of Social Psychology* 34: 395–407.

Ledermann, S. (1956) *Alcool, Alcoolism, Alcoolisation*, Volume 1, Paris: Presses Universitaires de France.

Leedham, W. and Godfrey, C. (1990) 'Tax policy and budget decisions', in Tether, P. and Maynard, A. (eds) *Preventing Alcohol and Tobacco Problems*, Aldershot: Avebury, 96–116.

Lehto, J. and Moskalewicz, J. (1994) *Alcohol Policy During Extensive Socio-Economic Change*, Copenhagen: World Health Organization.

Leigh, B. (1990a) 'The relationship of substance use during sex to high risk behaviour', *Journal of Sex Research* 27: 199–213.

Leigh,B. (1990b) 'The relationship of sex-related alcohol expectancies to alcohol consumption and sexual behaviour', *British Journal of Addiction* 85: 919–28.

Leigh, B.C. (1999) 'Peril, chance, adventure: concepts of risk, alcohol use and risky behaviour in young adults', *Addiction* 94: 371–83.

Lemmens, P. (1994) 'The alcohol content of self-report "standard drinks"', *Addiction* 89: 593–602.

Lemoine, P. (1994) 'An historical note about the fetal alcohol syndrome', *Addiction* 89: 1021–3.

Lemoine, P., Harronsseau H., Borteyru J.P. and Menuet J.C. (1968) 'Les enfants de parents alcooliques: anomalies observées a propros 127 cas', *Ouest Médicale* 25: 476–82.

Leung, S.F. and Phelps, C.E. (1993) 'My kingdom for a drink? A review of estimates of the price sensitivity of demand for alcoholic beverages', in Hilton, M.E. and Bloss, G. (eds) *Economics and the Prevention of Alcohol-Related Problems*, National Institute on Alcohol Abuse and Alcoholism Research Monograph 25, Rockville, MD: US Department of Health and Human Services, 1–31.

Levenson, M.R. and Spiro, A. (1996) 'Age, cohort and period effects in alcohol consumption and problem drinking in middle-aged and older men', Paper presented at 22nd Annual Alcohol Epidemiology Symposium of the Kettil Bruun Society meeting, Edinburgh.

Lewthwaite, P. (1990) *Young People's Heath Choices Project*, Durham: Durham Health Authority.

Lindstrom, L. (1992) *Managing Alcoholism: Matching Clients to Treatments*, Oxford: Oxford University Press.

Linqvist, P. (1991) 'Homicides committed by abusers of alcohol and illicit drugs', *British Journal of Addiction* 86: 321–6.

Lister-Sharp, D. (1994) 'Underage drinking in the United Kingdom since 1970: public policy, the law and adolescent drinking behaviour', *Alcohol and Alcoholism* 29: 555–63.

Longabaugh, R., Wirtz, P.W., Zweben, A. and Stout, R.L. (1998) 'Network support for drinking, Alcoholics Anonymous and long-term matching effects', *Addiction* 93: 1313–33.

Loretto, W. (1994) 'Youthful drinking in Northern Ireland and Scotland: preliminary results from a comparative study', *Drugs: Education, Prevention and Policy* 1: 143–52.

Lowe, G., Foxcroft, D.R. and Sibley, D. (1993) *Adolescent Drinking and Family Life*, Reading: Harwood Academic.

McAlistair, A., Perry, C., Killen, J., Simkard, L.A. and Maudsy, N. (1981) 'Pilot study of smoking, alcohol and drug abuse prevention', *American Journal of Public Health* 70: 719–25.

MacAndrew, C. and Edgerton, R.B. (1969) *Drunken Comportment: A Social Explanation*, Chicago, IL: Aldine.

MacCall, C.A. (1998) '"Alcopop" use in Scottish bars: a pilot study', *Journal of Substance Misuse* 3: 21–9.

McCarty, D., Poore, M., Mills, K. and Morrison, S. (1983) 'Direct-mail techniques and the prevention of alcohol-related problems among college students', *Journal of Studies on Alcohol* 44: 162–70.

McCord, W. and McCord, J. (1960*) Origins of Alcoholism*, Stanford: Stanford University Press.

McCreight, B. (1997) *Recognizing and Managing Children With Fetal Alcohol Syndrome/Fetal Alcohol Effects: A Guidebook*, Washington, DC: CWLA Press.

Macdonald, G. Veen, C. and Tones, K. (1996) 'Evidence for success in health promotion: suggestions for improvement', *Health Education Research: Theory and Practice* 11: 367–76.

Macdonald, I. (ed.) (1999) *Health Issues Related to Alcohol*, London: Blackwell.

McDonald, M. (ed.) (1994) *Gender, Drink and Drugs*, Oxford: Berg.

McGovern, P.E., Glucker, D.L. and Exner, L. (1996) 'Neolithic resinated wine', *Nature* 381: 480–1.

McKay, J.R. and McLellan, A.T. (1998) 'Deciding where to start: working with polydrug individuals', in Miller, W.R. and Heather, N. (eds) *Treating Addictive Behaviors* (2nd edition), New York: Plenum.

McKechnie, R.J. (1989) *Drinking Attitudes, Knowledge and Behaviour in Dumfries and Galloway*, Dumfries: Report for Dumfries and Galloway Health Board.

McKechnie, R.J. (forthcoming) 'Drinking as skill', *Addiction Research*.

McKechnie, R., Cameron, D., Cameron, I.A. and Drewery, J. (1977) 'Teenage drinking in South West Scotland', *British Journal of Addiction* 72: 287–95.

McKenzie, E. (1998) *Healing Reiki*, London: Hamlyn.

McKillip, J., Lockhart, D., Eckert, P. and Phillips, J. (1985) 'Evaluation of a responsive alcohol use media campaign on a college campus', *Journal of Alcohol and Drug Education* 30: 88–97.

MacKinnon, D.P., Pentz, M.A. and Stacy, A.W. (1993) 'The alcohol warning label and adolescents: the first year', *American Journal of Public Health* 83: 585–7.

McKirnan, D.J. and Peterson, P.L. (1989) 'Alcohol and drug use among homosexual men and women: epidemiology and population characteristics', *Addictive Behaviors* 14: 545–53.

McKnight, A.J. (1991) 'Factors influencing the effectiveness of server-intervention education', *Journal of Studies on Alcohol* 52: 389–97.

McLean, S., Wood, L.J., Davidson, J., Montgomery, I.M. and Jones, M.E. (1994a) 'Alcohol consumption and driving intentions amongst hotel patrons', *Drug and Alcohol Review* 12: 23–6.

McLean, S., Wood, L.J., Davidson, J., Montgomery, I.M. and Jones, M.E. (1994b) 'Promotion of responsible drinking in hotels', *Drug and Alcohol Review* 13: 247–56.

McLeod, E. (1982) *Women Working: Prostitution Now*, London: Croom Helm.

McMurran, M. and Hollin, C. (1993) *Young Offenders and Alcohol-Related Crime*, Chichester: John Wiley.

Madden, S., Plant, M.A., Bennie, C. and Plant, M.L (2000) 'Home detoxification for problem drinkers: a female-friendly approach?', *Journal of Substance Use* 5: 106–11.

Maguire, J.H. (1990) 'Putting nursing research findings into practice: research utilisation as an aspect of the management of change', *Journal of Advanced Nursing* 16: 614–20.

Mäkelä, K. and Mustonen, H. (1988) 'Positive and negative experiences related to drinking as a function of annual alcohol intake', *British Journal of Addiction* 83: 403–8.

Mäkelä, K., Österberg, E. and Sulkunen, P. (1983) 'Drink in Finland: increasing alcohol availability in a monopoly state', in Single, E., Morgan, P. and deLint, J. (eds) *Alcohol, Society and the State, vol. 2: The Social History of Control Policy in Seven Countries*, Toronto: Addiction Research Foundation, 31–60.

Mäkelä, P., Valkonen, T. and Poikolainen, K. (1997) 'Estimated numbers of deaths from coronary heart disease "caused" and "prevented" by alcohol: an example from Finland', *Journal of Studies on Alcohol* 58: 455–63.

Maloff, D., Becker, H.S., Fonaroff, A. and Rodin, J. (1979) 'Informal social controls and their influences on substance misuse', *Journal of Drug Issues* 9: 161–84.

Mann, R.E., Smart, R.G., Anglin. L. and Rush, B.R. (1988) 'Are decreases in liver cirrhosis rates a result of increased treatment for alcoholism?', *British Journal of Addiction* 83: 683–8.

Manning, W.G., Blumberg, L. and Moulton, L.H. (1995) 'The demand for alcohol: the differential response to price', *Journal of Health Economics* 14: 123–48.

Marlatt, G.A. and Gordon, J. (eds) (1985) *Relapse Prevention: Maintenance Strategies in the Treatment of Addictive Behaviours*, New York: Guilford.

Marmot, M. (1996) 'A not-so-sensible drinks policy', *Lancet* 346: 1643–4.

Marsh, A., Dobbs, J. and White, A. (1986) *Adolescent Drinking*, London: HMSO.

Marsh, P. and Fox-Kibby, K. (1992) *Drinking and Public Disorder*, London: Portman Group.

Mathijssen, R. and Wesemann, P. (1993) 'The role of police enforcement in the decrease of DWI in the Netherlands, 1983–1991', in Utzelmann, H.D., Berghaus, G. and Kroj, G. (eds) *Alcohol, Drugs and Traffic Safety*, Rheinland G, Koln: Verlag TUV, 1216–22.

Mathrani, S. (1998) *Young Drinkers: A Qualitative Study*, Report to the Health Education Authority (HEA), based on research by Research Works Ltd, London: HEA.

Mattick, R.P. and Jarvis, T. (1993) *An Outline for the Management of Alcohol Problems: Quality Assurance Project*, National Drug Strategy Monograph Series No. 20, Canberra: Australian Government Publishing Service.

Mattson, M.E. and Allen, J.P. (1991) 'Research on matching alcoholic patients to treatments; findings, issues and implications', *Journal of Addictive Diseases* 11: 33–49.

May, C. (1991) 'Research on alcohol education for young people: a critical review of the literature', *Health Education Journal* 50: 195–9.

May, C. (1992) 'A burning issue? Adolescent alcohol use in Britain 1970–1991', *Alcohol and Alcoholism* 27: 109–15.

May, C. (1993) 'Resistance to peer group pressure: an inadequate basis for alcohol education', *Health Education Research* 8: 159–65.

MCM Research (1993) *Keeping the Peace: A Guide to the Prevention of Alcohol-Related Disorder*, London: Portman Group.

Medical Council on Alcoholism (MCA) (2000) (http://www.medicouncilalcoh.demon.co.uk), London: MCA.

Meichenbaum, D. (1977) *Cognitive Behavior Modification*, New York: Plenum.

Midanik, L. (1982a) 'The validity of self-reported alcohol consumption and alcohol problems', *British Journal of Addiction*, 77: 357–82.

Midanik, L. (1982b) 'Over reports of recent alcohol consumption in a clinical population: a validity study', *Drug and Alcohol Dependence* 9: 101–10.

Midanik, L. (1995) 'Alcohol consumption and social consequences, dependence, and positive benefits in general population surveys', in Edwards, G., Anderson, P., Babor, T., Casswell, S., Ferrence, T., Giesbrecht, N., Godfrey, C., Holder, H., Lemmens, P., Mäkelä, K., Midanik, L., Norström, T., Österberg, E., Romelsjö, A., Room, R., Simpura, J. and Skog, Ø-J. *Alcohol Policy and the Public Good*, Oxford: Oxford University Press.

Midford, R. (1993) 'Decriminalisation of public drunkenness in Western Australia; the process explained', *Australian Journal of Social Issues* 28: 62–78.

Midford, R., Boots, K., Masters, L. and Chikritzhs, T. (1998) 'Time series analysis of outcome measures from a community alcohol harm reduction project in Australia', Paper presented at the Kettil Bruun Society's 4th Symposium on Community Action research and the Prevention of Alcohol and Other Drug Problems, Russell, New Zealand.

Milburn, K.M. (1996) *Peer Education: Young People and Sexual Health: A Critical Review*, Health Education Board for Scotland (HEBS) Working Paper No. 2, Edinburgh: HEBS.

Milburn, K., Fraser, E., Secker, J. and Pavis, S. (1995) 'Combining methods in health promotion research: some considerations about appropriate use', *Health Education Journal* 54: 3347–56.

Miller, J.J., Fletcher, K. and Kabat-Zinn, J. (1995) 'Ten-year follow-up and clinical implications of a mindfulness meditation-based stress reduction intervention in the treatment of anxiety disorders', *General Hospital Psychiatry* 17: 192–200.

Miller, P. (1997) 'Family structure, personality, drinking, smoking and illicit drug use: a study of UK teenagers', *Drug and Alcohol Dependence* 45: 121–9.

Miller, P. and Plant, M.A. (1996) 'Drinking, smoking and illicit drug use among 15 and 16 year olds in the United Kingdom', *British Medical Journal* 313: 394–7.

Miller, P. and Plant, M.A. (1999a) 'Truancy, perceived school performance, family structure, lifestyle, alcohol, cigarettes and illicit drugs: a study of UK teenagers', *Alcohol and Alcoholism* 34; 886–93.

Miller, P. and Plant, M.A. (1999b) 'Use and perceived ease of obtaining illicit drugs amongst teenagers in urban, suburban and rural schools: a UK study', *Journal of Substance Use* 4: 24–8.

Miller, P. and Plant, M.A. (2000a) *Drinking, Smoking and Illicit Drug Use Amongst 15 and 16 Year Old School Students in Northern Ireland, A Report for the Department of Health and Social Services, Belfast*, Edinburgh: Alcohol and Health Research Centre.

Miller, P. and Plant, M.A. (2000b) 'Drinking and smoking among 15 and 16 year olds in the UK', *Journal of Substance Use* (forthcoming).

Miller, W.R. (1983) 'Motivational interviewing with problem drinkers', *Behavioural Psychotherapy* 11: 147–72.

Miller, W.R., Andrews, N.R., Wilbourne, P. and Bennett, M.E. (1998) 'A wealth of alternatives: effective treatments for alcohol problems', in Miller, W.R. and Heather, N. (eds) *Treating Addictive Behaviors*, 2nd edition, New York: Plenum, 203–16.

Miller, W.R., Benefield, R.G. and Tonigan, J.S. (1993) 'Enhancing motivation for change in problem drinking: a controlled comparison of two therapist styles', *Journal of Consulting and Clinical Psychology* 61: 455–61.

Miller, W.R. and Hester, R. (1980) 'Treating the problem drinker – modern approaches', in Miller, W.R. (ed.) *The Addictive Behaviours*, New York: Pergamon.

Miller, W.R. and Rollnick, S. (1991) *Motivational Interviewing: Preparing People to Change Addictive Behavior*, New York: Guilford.

Miller, W.R., Sovereign, R.G. and Krege, B. (1988) 'Motivational interviewing with problem drinkers: II. The Drinker's Check-up as a preventive intervention', *Behavioral Psychotherapy* 16: 251–68.

Miller, W.R., Zweben, A., DiClemente, C. and Rychtarik, R. (1992) *Motivational Enhancement Therapy: A Clinical Research Guide for Therapists Treating Individuals with Alcohol Abuse and Dependence*, Project MATCH Monograph Series, vol. 2, DHHS Pub. No. (ADM) 92–1894, Washington, DC: Department of Health and Human Services.

Monks, J. and Purcell, L. (1999) 'The National Healthy Schools Programme', *Healthy Schools Newsletter* Edition 3, London: HEA.

Monti, P.M., Abrams, D.B., Binkoff, J.A. et al. (1990) 'Communication skills training, with family and cognitive behavioral mood management training for alcoholics', *Journal of Studies on Alcohol* 51: 263–70.

Monti, P.M., Abrams, D.B., Kadden, R.M. and Cooney, N.L. (1989) *Treating Alcohol Dependence: A Coping Skills Training Guide*, New York: Guilford.

Moon, A.M., Mullee, M.A., Rogers, L., Thompson, R.L., Speller, V. and Roderick, P. (1999a) 'Helping schools to become health promoting environments – an evaluation of the Wessex Healthy Schools Award', *Health Promotion International* 14(2): 111–22.

Moon, A.M., Mullee, M.A., Rogers, L., Thompson, R.L., Speller, V. and Roderick, P. (1999b) 'Health-related research and evaluation in schools' *Health Education* 1: 27–34.

Moore, M. and Cook, P.J. (1995) *Habit and Hetrogeneity in the Youthful Demand for Alcohol*, Cambridge, MA: National Bureau of Economic Research Working Paper 5152.

Moore, M.H. and Gerstein, D.H. (eds) (1981) *Alcohol and Public Policy: Beyond the Shadow of Prohibition*, Washington, DC: National Academy Press.

Morgan, P. (1980) 'The state as mediator: alcohol problem management in the post-war period', *Contemporary Drug Problems*, Spring, 9: 107–40.

Morgan Thomas, R. (1990) 'AIDS risks, alcohol, drugs and the sex industry: a Scottish study', in Plant, M.A. (ed.) *AIDS, Drugs and Prostitution*, London: Tavistock/Routledge, 88–108.

Morgan Thomas, R., Plant, M.A. and Plant, M.L. (1989) 'Risks of AIDS among workers in the "sex industry"; some initial results from a Scottish study', *British Medical Journal* 299: 148–9.

MORI (1994) *Attitudes of the General Public Towards Policy Issues on Alcohol*, London: Unpublished report for the HEA.

Morrison, C.L., Ruben, S.M. and Wakefield, D. (1994) 'Female street prostitution in Liverpool', *AIDS* 8: 1194–5.

Morse B.A. (1993) 'Information processing', in Klienfeld, J. and Wescott, S. (eds) *Fantastic Antione Succeeds!: Experiences in Educating Children with Fetal Alcohol Syndrome*, Anchorage, Alaska: University of Alaska Press.

Moser, J. (1980) *Prevention of Alcohol-Related Problems: An International Review of Preventive Measures, Policies and Programs*, Toronto: World Health Organization.

Mosher, J.M. (1984) 'The impact of legal provisions on barroom behavior: toward an alcohol-problems prevention policy', *Alcohol* 1: 205–11.

Moskowitz, J. (1989) 'The primary prevention of alcohol problems: a critical review of the research literature', *Journal of Studies on Alcohol* 50: 54–88.

Mulford, H.A. (1977) 'Stages in the alcoholic process: towards a cumulative nonsequential index', *Journal of studies on Alcohol* 38: 563–83.

Mulford, H.A. (1994) 'What if alcoholism had not been invented? The dynamics of American alcohol mythology', *Addiction* 89: 517–20.

Murray, A. (1991) *Drinking Reasonably and Moderately with Self Control (DRAMS) Breaking the Habit: Coming Off*, Edinburgh: HEBS.

Musto, D. (1997) 'Alcohol control in historical perspective', in Plant, M.A., Single, E. and Stockwell, T. (eds) *Alcohol: Minimising the Harm: What Works?*, London: Free Association Books, 10–28.

Myers, T. (1986) 'An analysis of context and alcohol consumption in a group of criminal events', *Alcohol and Alcoholism*, 21: 389–95.

Naidoo, J. and Wills, J (1994) *Health Promotion: Foundations for Practice*, London: Bailliere Tindall.

Newcombe, R., Measham, F. and Parker, H. (1995) 'A Survey of drinking and deviant behaviour among 14–15 year olds in North West England', *Addiction Research* 2: 319–41.

Newman, I.M., Anderson, C.S. and Farrell, K.A. (1992) 'Role rehearsal and efficacy: two 15–month evaluations of a ninth-grade alcohol education program', *Journal of Drug Education* 22: 55–67.

NHS Executive (NHSE) (1999) *Saving Lives: Our Healthier Nation*, London: NHSE.

Nowinski, J., Baker, S. and Carroll, K. (1992) *Twelve Step Facilitation Therapy: A Clinical Research Guide for Therapists Treating Individuals with Alcohol Abuse and Dependence*, Project MATCH Monograph Series, vol. 1, DHHS Pub. No. (ADM) 92–1893, Washington, DC: Department of Health and Human Services.

NTC Publications (1999) *Compilation of Drink Industry Statistics*, Henley-on-Thames: NTC.

Nutbeam, D. (1998) 'Evaluating health promotion: progress, problems and solutions', *Health Promotion International* 13: 27–44.

Nutt, D. (1999) 'Alcohol and the brain: pharmacological insights for psychiatrists', *British Journal of Psychiatry* 175: 114–19.

O'Connor, J. and Saunders, W.M. (1992) 'Drug education: an appraisal of popular prevention', *International Journal of the Addictions*, 27: 165–83.

O'Donnell, M. (1985) 'Research on drinking locations of alcohol-impaired drivers: implications for prevention policies', *Journal of Public Health Policy* 6: 510–25.

Oei, T.P.S. and Jackson, P. (1980) 'Long-term effects of group and individual social skills training with alcoholics', *Addictive Behaviors* 5: 129–36.

Office for National Statistics (ONS) publications: *National Incomes Blue Book, Employment Trends, Consumer Trends, Annual Abstract of Statistics* and *Monthly Digest of Statistics*.

Office for National Statistics (ONS) (1998) *The 1996 General Household Survey*, London: HMSO.

Office of Standards in Education (OFSTED) (1997) *Drug Education in Schools*, London: HMSO.

Office of Population Censuses and Surveys (OPCS) (1995) *The Prevalence of Psychiatric Morbidity Among Adults Living in Private Households*, London: HMSO.

O'Hare, P.A., Newcombe, R., Matthews, A., Boning, E.C. and Druelser, E. (eds) (1992) *The Reduction of Drug-Related Harm*, London: Tavistock/Routledge.

O'Malley, P.M. and Wagenaar, A.C. (1991) 'Effects of minimum drinking age laws on alcohol use, related behaviors and traffic crash involvement among American youth, 1976–1987', *Journal of Studies on Alcohol* 52: 478–91.

O'Malley, S.S., Jaffe, A.J., Chang, G., Schottenfeld, R.S., Meyer, R.E. and Roundsaville, B. (1992). 'Naltrexone and coping skills therapy for alcohol dependence: a controlled study', *Archives of General Psychiatry* 49: 881–7.

Orford, J. (1985) *Excessive Appetites: A Psychological View of Addictions*, London: John Wiley.

Orford, J. and Edwards, G. (1977) *Alcoholism: A Comparison of Treatment and Advice With a Study of the Influence of Marriage*, Oxford: Oxford University Press.

Orman, D.J. (1991) 'Reframing of an addiction via hypnotherapy: a case presentation', *American Journal of Clinical Hypnosis* 33: 263–71.

Osservatorio Permanente Sui Giovani e L'Alcool (1998) *The Italians and Alcohol*, Rome: Osservatorio Permanente Sui Giovani e L'Alcool.

Österberg, E. (1995) 'Do alcohol prices affect consumption and related problems?', in Holder, H. and Edwards, G. (eds) *Alcohol and Public Policy: Evidence and Issues*, Oxford: Oxford University Press, 145–63.

Ouimette, P.C., Finney, J.W. and Moos, R.H. (1997) 'Twelve-step and cognitive-behavioral treatment for substance abuse: a comparison of treatment effectiveness', *Journal of Consulting and Clinical Psychology* 65: 230–40.

Owen, R. (1995) 'A comment on "just say 'no' to alcohol abuse and misuse"', *Addiction* 90: 133–4.

Paramore, L.C. (1997) 'Use of alternative therapies: estimates from 1994 Robert Wood Foundation National Access to Care Survey', *Journal of Pain Symptoms Management* 13: 83–9.

Parazzini F., Tozzi L., Chatenoud L. et al. (1994) 'Alcohol and risk of spontaneous abortions', *Human Reproduction* 9: 1950–3.

Parker, D., Wolz, M. and Harford, T. (1978) 'The prevention of alcoholism: an empirical report on the effects of outlet availability', *Alcoholism: Clinical and Experimental Research* 2: 339–43.

Parker, H. (1995) 'Youth Culture and the Changing Patterns of Drinking by Young People', Paper presented at Conference, 14 December 1995, *Alcohol and the Young*, London: National Childrens Bureau/Royal College of Physicians.

Parker, H. (1996) 'Young adult offenders, alcohol and criminological cul-de-sacs', *British Journal of Criminology* 36: 282–98.

Parker, H. and Measham, F. (1994) 'Pick 'n' mix. Changing patterns of illicit drug use amongst 1990's adolescents', *Drugs, Education, Prevention and Policy* 1: 5–13.

Parker, R.N. (1993) 'The effects of context on alcohol and violence', *Alcohol Health and Research World* 17: 117–22.

Parker, R.N. and Rebhun, L.A. (1995) *Alcohol and Homicide: A Deadly Combination of Two American Traditions*, New York: State University of New York Press.

Pavis, S., Cunningham-Burleys, S. and Amos, A. (1997) 'Alcohol consumption and young people: exploring meaning and social context', *Health Education Research* 12: 311–22.

Peele, S. (1997) 'Utilizing culture and behavior in epidemiological models of alcohol consumption and consequences for Western countries', *Alcohol and Alcoholism* 32: 51–64.

Peele, S. and Grant, M. (eds) (1999) *Alcohol and Pleasure: A Health Perspective*, Philadelphia, PA: Taylor and Francis.

Pentz, M.A. (1985) 'Social competence skills and self-efficacy as determinants of substance abuse in adolescence', in Schiffman, M. and Wills, T.A. (eds) *Coping With Substance Use*, New York: Academic Press.

Pentz, M.A., Dwyer, J.H., Mackinnon, D.P., Flay, B.R. and Hansen, W.B. (1989a) 'A multicommunity trial for primary prevention of adolescent drug abuse: effects on drug use prevalence', *Journal of the American Medical Association* 261: 3259–66.

Pentz, M.A., Johnson, C.A., Dwyer, J.H., MacKinnon, D.M., Hansen, W.B. and Flay, B.R. (1989b) 'A comprehensive community approach to adolescent drug abuse prevention: effects on cardiovascular disease risk behaviours', *Annals of Medicine* 21: 219–22.

Pentz, M.A., Trebow, E.A., Hansen, W.B., MacKinnon, D.M., Dwyer, J.H., Johnson, C.A., Flay, B.R., Daniels, S. and Cormack, C. (1990) 'Effects of program implementation on adolescent drug use behaviour: the Midwestern Prevention Project', *Evaluation Review* 14: 264–89.

Perkins, E.R., Simnett, I. and Wright, L. (eds) (1999) *Evidence-Based Health Promotion*, Chichester: John Wiley.

Perkins, H.W. (1995) 'Viewing the glass more empty than full', *Catalyst* 3: 2.

Pernanen, K. (1991) *Alcohol in Human Violence*, New York: Guilford Press.

Pittman, D. and Raskin White, H. (eds) *Society, Culture and Drinking Patterns Re-examined*, New Brunswick, NJ: Rutgers Center of Alcohol Studies.

Plant, E.J. and Plant, M.A. (1999) 'Primary prevention for young children: a comment on the UK government's ten year drug strategy', *International Journal of Drug Policy* (forthcoming).

Plant, M.A. (1979) *Drinking Careers: Occupations, Drinking Habits and Drinking Problems*, London: Tavistock.

Plant, M.A. (ed.) (1982) *Drinking and Problem Drinking*, London: Junction Books.

Plant, M.A. (ed.) (1992) *AIDS, Drugs and Prostitution*, London: Tavistock/Routledge.

Plant, M.A. (1996) 'Contemporary Research: alcohol, drugs, HIV/AIDS and risk taking', *Journal of Substance Misuse* 1: 32–7.

Plant, M.A. (1997) 'Alcohol, drugs and social milieu', in Scambler, G. and Scambler, A. (eds) *Rethinking Prostitution*, London: Tavistock/Routledge, 164–79.

Plant, M.A. (1999) 'Patterns and consequences matter' (Editorial), *Addiction Research* 7: 463–8.

Plant, M.A. (2000a) 'Young people and alcohol use', in Aggleton, P., Hurry, J. and Warwick, I. (eds) *Young People and Mental Health*, London: John Wiley, 13–28.

Plant, M.A. (2000b) 'Learning by experiment', in Houghton, E. and Roche, A. (eds) *Learning about Drinking*, Philadelphia, PA: Brunner/Mazel (forthcoming).

Plant, M., Bagnall, G. and Foster, D. (1990a) 'Teenage heavy drinkers: alcohol related knowledge, beliefs, experiences, motivation and the social context of drinking', *Alcohol and Alcoholism* 25: 691–8.

Plant, M.A., Bagnall, G., Foster, J. and Sales, J. (1990b) 'Young people and drinking; results from an English national survey', *Alcohol and Alcoholism* 25: 685–90.

Plant, M.A. and Foster, J. (1991) 'Teenagers and alcohol: results of a Scottish national survey', *Drug and Alcohol Dependence* 28: 203–10.

Plant, M.A. and Miller, P. (2000) 'Drug use has declined among UK teenagers', *British Medical Journal* 320: 1536–7.

Plant, M.A. , Miller, P., Plant, M.L. and Nichol, P. (1994) 'No such thing as safe glass', *British Medical Journal*, 308: 6–7.

Plant, M.A., Orford, J. and Grant, M. (1989) 'The effects on children and adolescents of parents' excessive drinking: an international review', *Public Health Reports* 104: 433–42.

Plant, M.A., Peck, D.F. and Samuel, E. (1985) *Alcohol, Drugs and School Leavers*, London: Tavistock.

Plant, M.A., Pirie, F. and Kreitman, N. (1979) 'Evaluation of the Scottish Health Education Unit's 1976 campaign on alcoholism', *Social Psychiatry* 14: 11–24.

Plant, M.A. and Plant, M.L. (1992) *Risk Takers: Alcohol, Drugs, Sex and Youth*, London: Tavistock/Routledge.

Plant, M.A. and Plant, M.L. (1997) 'Alcohol education and harm minimisation', in Plant, M.A., Single, E. and Stockwell, T. (eds) *Alcohol: Minimising the Harm: What Works?*, London: Free Association Books, 193–210.

Plant, M.A., Plant, M.L. and Vernon, B. (1996) 'Ethics, funding and alcohol research', *Alcohol and Alcoholism* 30: 1–9.

Plant, M.A., Single, E. and Stockwell, T. (eds) (1997) *Alcohol: Minimising the Harm: What Works?*, London: Free Association Books.

Plant, M.L. (1985) *Women, Drinking and Pregnancy*, London: Tavistock.

Plant, M.L. (1997) *Women and Alcohol: Contemporary and Historical Perspectives*, London: Free Association Books.

Plant, M.L., Abel, E.L. and Guerri, C. (1999) 'Alcohol and Pregnancy', in MacDonald, I. (ed.) *Health Issues Related to Alcohol*, Oxford: Blackwell, 181–214.

Plant, M.L., Miller, P., Plant, M.A., Thornton, C. and Bloomfield, K. (2000) 'Life stage, alcohol consumption patterns, alcohol-related consequences and gender', *Substance Abuse* (forthcoming).

Plant, M.L. and Plant, M.A. (1979) 'Self-reported alcohol consumption and other characteristics of 100 patients attending a Scottish alcoholism treatment unit', *British Journal on Alcohol and Alcoholism* 14: 197–207.

Plant, M.L. and Plant, M.A. (2000) *Alcohol and Drug Problems Amongst Women in Prison: Epidemiology and Responses*, Edinburgh: Alcohol and Health Research Centre.

Plant, M.L., Plant, M.A. and Foster, J. (1991) 'Alcohol, tobacco and illicit drug use amongst nurses: a Scottish study', *Drug and Alcohol Dependence* 28: 195–202.

Plant, M.L., Plant, M.A. and Morgan Thomas, R. (1990) 'Alcohol, AIDS risks and commercial sex: results from a Scottish study', *Drug and Alcohol Dependence* 25: 51–5.

Pogue, T.F. and Sgnotz, L.G. (1989) 'Taxing to control social costs: the case of alcohol', *American Economic Review* 79: 235–43.

Poikolainen, K. (1995) 'Alcohol and mortality: a review', *Journal of Clinical Epidemiology* 48: 455–65.

Pollak, B. (1975) 'A two year study of alcoholics in general practice', *British Journal of Alcohol and Alcoholism* 13: 24–33.

Portman Group/Health Education Authority (HEA) (1992) *Alcohol Education: Promoting Good Practice*, London: Portman Group/(HEA).

Prescott-Clarke, P. and Primatesta, P. (eds) (1998) *Health Survey for England 1996*, London: Office for National Statistics.

Preusser, D.F. and Williams, A.F. (1992) 'Sales of alcohol to underage purchasers in three New York counties and Washington, DC', *Journal of Public Health Policy* 13: 306–17.

Prochaska, J.O. and DiClemente, C.C. (1986). 'Toward a comprehensive model of change for problem behaviors', in Miller, W.R. and Heather, N. (eds) *Treating Addictive Behaviours: Processes of Change*, New York: Plenum, 3–27.

Prochaska, J.O. and DiClemente, C.C. (1992) 'Stages of change in the modification of problem behaviors', in Hersen, M., Eisler, R.M. and Miller, P.M. (eds) *Progress in Behavior Modification*, Newbury Park, CA: Sage, 184–214.

Project MATCH Research Group (1993) 'Project MATCH: rationale and methods for a multisite clinical trial matching patients to alcoholism treatment', *Alcoholism: Clinical and Experimental Research* 17: 1130–45.

Project MATCH Research Group (1997a) 'Matching alcoholism treatments to client heterogeneity: Project MATCH posttreatment drinking outcomes', *Journal of Studies on Alcohol* 58: 7–29.

Project MATCH Research Group (1997b) 'Project MATCH secondary a priori hypotheses', *Addiction* 92: 1655–82.

Project MATCH Research Group (1998a) 'Matching alcoholism treatments to client heterogeneity: treatment main effects and matching effects on drinking during treatment', *Journal of Studies on Alcohol* 59: 631–9.

Project MATCH Research Group (1998b) 'Matching alcoholism treatments to client heterogeneity: Project MATCH three-year drinking outcomes', *Alcoholism: Clinical and Experimental Research* 22: 1300–11.

Puska, P., Tuomilehto, J., Nissinen, A. and Vartiainen, E. (eds) (1995) *The North Karelia Project: 20 years Results and Experiences*, Helsinki: National Public Health Institute.

Rabow, J., Schwartz, C., Stevens, S. and Watts, R. (1982) 'Social psychological dimensions of alcohol availability: the relationship of perceived social obligations, price considerations, and energy expended to the frequency, amount, and type of alcoholic beverages consumed', *International Journal of the Addictions* 17: 1259–71.

Rabow, J. and Watts, R.K. (1982) 'Alcohol availability, alcoholic beverage sales, and alcohol-related problems', *Journal of Studies on Alcohol* 43: 767–801.

Raistrick, D., Hodgson, R. and Ritson, B. (eds) (1999) *Tackling Alcohol Together: The Evidence Base for a UK Alcohol Policy*, London: Free Association Books.

Rampas, H. and Pereira, S. (1993) 'Role of Acupuncture and Alcohol Dependence and Abuse', *Acupuncture in Medicine* 11: 80–4.

Randall, D. and Wong, M.R. (1976) 'Drug education to date: a review', *Journal of Drug Education* 6: 1–21.

Rankin-Box, D. (1995) 'Competence in the clinical setting: issues in nursing practice: the responses', *Complementary Therapies in Medicine* 3: 25–7.

Raskin White, H., Hansell, S. and Brick, J. (1993) 'Alcohol use and aggression among youth', *Alcohol, Health and Research World* 17: 144–50.

Reason, P. (ed.) (1994) *Participation in Human Inquiry*, London: Sage.

Rehm, J. (1999) 'Draining the ocean to prevent shark attacks?', *Nordic Studies on Alcohol and Drugs* 16: 46–54.

Rehm, J., Ashley, M-J., Room, R., Single, E., Bondy, S., Ferrence, R. and Giesbrecht, N. (1996) 'On the emerging paradigm of drinking patterns and their social and health consequences', *Addiction* 91: 1615–21.

Reid, D. (1995) *Sustainable Development*, London: Earthscan.

Resnick, H. and Gibbs, J. (1988) 'Types of peer program approaches', in Gardner, S. (ed.) *Adolescent Peer Pressure: Theory, Correlates and Program Implications for Drug Abuse Prevention*, Rockville, MD: NIDA, 47–89.

Rhodes, T. (1996) 'Culture, drugs and unsafe sex: confusion about causation', *Addiction* 91: 753–8.

Rice, D. (1986) *Estimating the Cost of Illness*, Health Economics Series, no. 6, Rockville, MD: Department of Health, Education and Welfare, DHEW Publication No. (PHS) 947–6.

Richardson, J. and Crawley, S. (1994) 'Optimum alcohol taxation: balancing consumption and external costs', *Health Economics* 3: 73–87.

Riley, D.M., Sobell, L.C., Leo, G.I., Sobell, M.B. and Klajner, F. (1987) 'Behavioral treatment of alcohol problems: a review and a comparison of behavioral and nonbehavioral studies', in Cox W.M. (ed.) *Treatment and Prevention of Alcohol Problems: A Resource Manual*, Orlando, FL: Academic Press.

Rimmele, C.T., Howard, M.O. and Hilfrink, M.L. (1995) 'Aversion therapies', in Hester, R.K. and Miller, W.R. (eds) *Handbook of Alcoholism Treatment Approaches: Effective Alternatives*, Needham Heights, MA: Allyn and Bacon, 134–47.

Ritson, E.B. (1995) *Community and Municipal Action on Alcohol*, Copenhagen: World Health Organization Regional Publications European Series No. 63.

Robertson, I. and Heather, N. (1986) *Let's Drink to Your Health! A Self-Help Guide to Healthier Drinking*, Leicester: British Psychological Society.

Robertson, I., Heather, N., Dzialdowski, A., Crawford, J. and Winton, M. (1986) 'A comparison of minimal versus intensive controlled drinking treatment interventions for problem drinkers', *British Journal of Clinical Psychology* 25: 185–194.

Robertson, J.A. and Plant, M.A. (1988) 'Alcohol, sex and risk of HIV infection', *Drug and Alcohol Dependence*, 22: 75–8.

Robinson, D. (1979) *Talking Out of Alcoholism: The Self-Help Process of AA*, London: Croom Helm.

Robinson, D., Maynard, A. and Chester, R. (eds) (1989) *Controlling Legal Addictions*, London: Macmillan.

Roche, A., Single, E. and Heath, D. (forthcoming) 'What constitutes a beneficial pattern of alcohol consumption: a multidisciplinary review', *Alcohol and Drug Review*, forthcoming.

Rogers, C.R. (1951) *Client-Centred Therapy*, Cambridge, MA: Riverside Press.

Roman, P.M. and Trice, H.M. (1968) 'The sick role, labelling theory and the deviant drinker', *International Journal of Social Psychiatry* 14: 245–51.

Room, R. (1980) 'Concepts and strategies in the prevention of alcohol-related problems', *Contemporary Drug Problems* 9: 85–106.

Room, R. (1984) 'Alcohol control and public health', *American Review of Public Health* 5: 293–317.

Room, R. and Collins, G. (eds) (1983) *Alcohol and Disinhibition: Nature and Meaning of the Link*, Washington, DC: NIAAA, Research Monograph 12, US Department of Health and Human Sciences.

Room, R., Graves, K., Giesbrecht, N. and Greenfield, T.K. (1995) 'Trends in public opinion about alcohol policy initiatives in Ontario and the US: 1989–91', *Drug and Alcohol Review* 14: 35–47.

Rosenberg, H. and Davis, L.A. (1994) 'Acceptance of moderate drinking by alcohol treatment services in the United States', *Journal of Studies on Alcohol* 55: 167–72.

Rosenberg, H., Melville, J., Levell, D. and Hodge, J.E. (1992) 'A 10-year follow-up survey of the acceptability of controlled drinking in Britain', *Journal of Studies on Alcohol* 53: 441–6.

Rosett, H.L., Weiner, L., Lee, A. et al. (1983) 'Patterns of alcohol consumption and fetal development', *Journal of the American College of Obstetricians and Gynecologists* 61: 539–46.

Ross, H. (1992) *Confronting Drunk Driving: Social Policy for Saving Lives*, New Haven, CT: Yale University Press.

Rossi, D. and Tempesta, E. (1999a) 'Evolution of female alcohol consumption in Italy 1991–1997', Paper presented at Conference on Gender and Alcohol in Europe, Berlin, May.

Rossi, D. and Tempesta, E. (1999b) 'Alcohol in Italy', Paper presented at International Conference on Gender and Alcohol, Berlin, May.

Royal Colleges (1995) *Alcohol and the Heart in Perspective*, London: Royal Colleges of Physicians, Psychiatrists and General Practitioners.

Royal College of General Practitioners (1986) *Alcohol: A Balanced View*, Royal College of General Practitioners, London: Tavistock.

Royal College of Physicians (1987) *A Great and Growing Evil: The Medical Consequences of Alcohol Abuse*, London: Tavistock.

Royal College of Psychiatrists (1979) *Alcohol and Alcoholism*, London: Tavistock.

Royal College of Psychiatrists (1986) *Alcohol: Our Favourite Drug*, London: Tavistock.

Rush, B.R., Gliksman, L. and Brook, R. (1986) 'Alcohol availability, alcohol consumption and alcohol-related damage. II. The role of socio-demographic factors', *Journal of Studies on Alcohol* 47: 11–18.

Russ, N.W. and Geller, E.S. (1986) *Evaluation of a Server Intervention Program for Preventing Drunk Driving*, Final report no. DD-3. Blacksbury, VA: Virginia Polytechnic Institute and State University, Department of Psychology.

Russ, N.W. and Geller, E.S. (1987) 'Training bar personnel to prevent drunken driving: a field evaluation', *American Journal of Public Health* 77: 952–4.

Russell, M., Martier, S.S., Sokol, R.J. et al. (1994) 'Screening for pregnant risk taking', *Alcoholism: Clinical and Experimental Research* 18: 1156–61.

Rydon P., Stockwell T., Jenkins, E. and Syed, D. (1993) 'Blood alcohol levels of patrons leaving licensed premises in Perth, Western Australia', *Australian Journal of Public Health* 17: 339–45.

Rydon, P., Stockwell, T., Lang, E. and Beel, A. (1996) 'Pseudo-drunk patron evaluation of bar-staff compliance with Western Australian liquor law', *Australian and New Zealand Journal of Public Health* 20: 290–5.

Saffer, H. and Grossman, M. (1987) 'Beer taxes, the legal drinking age, and youth motor vehicle fatalities', *Journal of Legal Studies* 16: 351–74.

Saltz, R.F. (1985) 'Server intervention: conceptual overview and current developments', *Alcohol, Drugs, and Driving: Abstracts and Reviews* 1: 1–14.

Saltz, R.F. (1987) 'The roles of bars and restaurants in preventing alcohol-impaired driving: an evaluation of server education', *Evaluation of Health Professionals* 7: 5–27.

Saltz, R. (1997) 'Prevention where alcohol is sold and consumed', in Plant, M.A., Single, E. and Stockwell, T. (eds) *Alcohol: Minimising the Harm: What Works?*, London: Free Association Books, 72–84.

Saltz, R.F. and Hennessy, M. (1990a) *The Efficacy of 'Responsible Beverage Service' Programs in Reducing Intoxication*, Berkeley, CA: Prevention Research Center.

Saltz, R.F. and Hennessy, M. (1990b) *Reducing Intoxication in Commercial Establishments: An Evaluation of Responsible Beverage Service Practices*, Berkley, CA: Prevention Research Center.

Saltz, R.F. and Stanghetta, P. (1997) 'A community-wide responsible beverage service program in three communities: early findings', *Addiction* 92, Supplement 2: S237–S249.

Sanchez-Craig, M., Wilkinson, D.A. and Walker, K. (1987) 'Theory and methods for secondary prevention of alcohol problems: a cognitively-based approach', in Cox, W.M. (ed.) *Treatment and Prevention of Alcohol Problems: A Resource Manual*, New York: Academic Press.

San José, B., Bongers, I. and Garretsen, H. (2000) 'Drinking patterns and attitudes towards drinking in the late middle aged', personal communication.

Savitz, D.A., Schwingl P.J. and Keele M.A. (1991) 'Influence of paternal age, smoking and alcohol consumption on congenital anomalies', *Teratology* 44: 429–40.

Schaps, E., Dibartolo, R., Moskowitz, J., Balley, C.G. and Churgin, G. (1981) 'A review of 127 drug abuse prevention programme evaluations', *Journal of Drug Issues* 11: 17–43.

Schaps, E., Churgin, S., Palley, C.S., Takata, B. and Cohen, A.Y. (1980) 'Primary prevention research: a preliminary review of program outcome studies', *International Journal of the Addictions* 15: 657–76.

Schaps, E., DiBartola, R., Moskowitz, J., Palley, C.S. and Churgin, S. (1981) 'A review of 127 drug abuse program evaluations', *Journal of Drug Issues* 11: 17–43.

Schinke, S.P. and Gilchrist, L.D. (1984) *Life Skills Counselling With Adolescents*, Baltimore, MD: University Park Press.

Schinke, S.P. and Gilchrist, L.D. (1985) 'Preventing substance abuse with children and adolescents', *Journal of Consulting and Clinical Psychology* 53: 596–602.

Schuckit, M.B. (2000) *Drug and Alcohol Abuse: A Clinical Guide to Diagnosis and Treatment*, Dortdrecht, Netherlands: Kluwer Acadmic/Plenum.

Scotch Whisky Association (1996) *Statistical Report*, Edinburgh: Scotch Whisky Association.

Scottish Council on Alcohol (1997) *Alcohol Statistics*, Glasgow: Scottish Council on Alcohol.

Scottish Executive (1999) Personal communication.

Scottish Office Home and Health Department (SOHHD) (1994) *Drugs in Scotland: Meeting the Challenge*, Edinburgh: HMSO.

Secretary of State for Health (1998) *Our Healthier Nation*, London: The Stationery Office.

Shakus, M. and Smith, M. (1979) 'The use of acupuncture in the treatment of drug addiction', *American Journal of Acupuncture*, 7: 223–8.

Shapiro, D.H. (1992) 'Adverse effects of meditation: a preliminary investigation of long-term meditators', *International Journal of Psychology* 39: 62–7.

Sharma, K. and Shukla, V. (1988) 'Rehabilitation of drug-addicted persons: the experience of the Nav-Autila Centre in India', *Bulletin of Narcotics* 150: 43–9.

Sharp, C., Hurford, D.P, Allison, J., Sparks, R. and Cameron, B.P. (1997) 'Facilitation of internal locus of control in adolescent alcoholics through a brief biofeedback-assisted autogenic relaxation training procedure', *Journal of Substance Abuse Treatment* 14: 55–60.

Sharp, D. and Lowe, G. (1989) 'Adolescents and Alcohol – a review of the recent British research', *Journal of Adolescence* 12: 295–307.

Shaw, S., Cartwright, A.J.K., Spratley, T. and Harwin, J. (1978) *Responding to Drinking Problems*, London: Croom Helm.

Shepherd, J. (1994) 'Violent crime: the role of alcohol and new approaches to the prevention of injury', *Alcohol and Alcoholism* 29: 5–10.

Shepherd, J. and Brinkley, J. (1996) 'The relationship between alcohol intoxication, stressors and injury in urban violence', *British Journal of Criminology* 36: 546–66.

Shoovanasai, A. and Visuthuimak, A. (1975) 'Acupuncture in the treatment of heroine addiction', *International Criminal Police Revised* 292: 256–8.

Shulz, J., Rice, D., Parker, D., Goodman, R., Stroh, G. and Chalmers, N. (1991) 'Quantifying the disease impact of alcohol with ARDI software', *Public Health Reports* 106(4): 443–50.

Simnett, I., Perkins, E. and Wright, L. (eds) (1999) *Evidence-Based Health Promotion*, Chichester: John Wiley.

Single, E. (1993) 'Public drinking', in Galanter, M. (ed.), *Recent Developments in the Treatment of Alcoholism, Volume 11: Ten Years of Progress*, New York: Plenum Press.

Single, E. (1997) 'The concept of harm reduction and its application to alcohol: the 6th Annual Dorothy Black Lecture', *Drugs: Education, Prevention and Policy* 4: 7–22.

Single, E., Collins, D., Easton, B., Harwood, H., Lapsley, H. and Maynard, A. (1996a) *International Guidelines for Estimating the Costs of Substance Abuse*, Ottawa: Canadian Centre on Substance Abuse.

Single, E., Robson, L., Rehm, J. and Xie, X. (1999) 'Morbidity and mortality attributable to substance abuse in Canada', *American Journal of Public Health* 89(3): 385–90.

Single, E., Robson, L., Xie, X. and Rehm, J. (1996b) *The Costs of Substance Abuse in Canada* (Main Report), Toronto: Canadian Centre on Substance Abuse.

Single, E., Robson, L., Xie, X. and Rehm, J. (1998) 'The economic costs of alcohol, tobacco and illicit drugs in Canada, 1992', *Addiction* 93: 983–98.

Single, E. and Storm, T. (eds) (1985) *Public Drinking and Public Policy*, Toronto, Addiction Research Foundation.

Single, E. and Wortley, S. (1993) 'Drinking in various settings: findings from a national survey in Canada', *Journal of Studies on Alcohol* 54: 590–9.

Slade, M.E. (1998) 'Beer and the tie: did divestiture of brewer owned public houses lead to higher beer prices?', *Journal of the Royal Economic Society* 108: 569–601.

Smart, R.G. (1980) 'Availability and the prevention of alcohol-related problems', in Hartford, T.C., Parker, D.A. and Light, L. (eds) *Normative Approaches to the Prevention of Alcohol Abuse and Alcoholism*, NIAAA Research Monograph No. 3, Rockville, MD: US Department of Health, Education and Welfare.

Smart, R.G. and Liban, C.B. (1981) 'Predictors of problem drinking among elderly, middle-aged and youthful drinkers', *Journal of Psychoactive Drugs* 13: 153–63.

Smith, M.O. (1979) 'Acupuncture and natural healing in drug detoxification', *American Journal of Acupuncture*, 7: 97–107.

Smith, M. and Harding, G. (1989) *Health Education and Young People*, TCRU Occasional Paper No. 9, London: Thomas Coram Research Institute.

Sokol, R.J., Martier, S.S., Ager, J.W. et al. (1993) 'Paternal drinking may affect intrauterine growth', *American Journal of Obstetrics and Gynecology* 168: 48.

Stall, R. (1987) 'Research issues concerning alcohol consumption among ageing populations', *Drug and Alcohol Dependence* 19: 195–213.

Stall, R. and Leigh, B. (1994) 'Understanding the relationship between drug or alcohol use and high risk sexual activity for HIV transmission: where do we go from here?' *Addiction* 89: 131–4.

Stall, R., McKusick, L., Wiley, J. et al. (1986) 'Alcohol and drug use during sexual activity and compliance with safe sex guidelines for AIDS: The AIDS Behavioral Research Project', *Health Education Quarterly* 13: 359–71.

Standing Conference on Drug Abuse (SCODA) (1999a) *The Right Approach: Quality Standards in Drug Education*, London: SCODA.

Standing Conference on Drug Abuse (SCODA) (1999b) *The Right Responses: Managing and Making Policy for Drug-Related Incidents in Schools*, London: SCODA.

Steffenhagen, R. and Burns J. (1987) *The Social Dynamics of Self-Esteem*, London: Praeger.

Stein, L.I., Newton, J.R. and Bowman, R.S. (1975) 'Duration of hospitalisation for alcoholism', *Archives of General Psychiatry* 32: 247–52.

Steinglass, P., Bennett, L.A., Wolin, S.J. and Reiss, D. (1987) *The Alcoholic Family: Drinking Problems in a Family Context*, London: Hutchinson.

Stevens S.J. and Arbiter N. (1995) 'A therapeutic community for substance-abusing pregnant women and women with children: progress and outcome', *Journal of Psychoactive Drugs* 27: 49–56.

Stewart, K. and Sweedler, B.M. (1997) 'Driving under the influence of alcohol', in Plant, M.A., Single, E. and Stockwell, T. (eds) *Alcohol: Minimising the Harm: What Works?*, London: Free Association Books, 126–42.

Stinnet, J.L. (1982) 'Out-patient detoxification of the alcoholic', *International Journal of Addictions* 17: 1031–46.

Stockwell, T. (1987) 'The Exeter Home Detoxification Project', in Stockwell, T. and Clements, S. (eds) *Helping the Problem Drinkers: New Initiatives in Community Care*, London: Croom Helm.

Stockwell, T. (1992) 'On pseudo-patrons and pseudo-training for bar staff', *British Journal of Addiction* 87: 677–80.

Stockwell, T. (1993) 'Influencing the labelling of alcoholic beverage containers: informing the public', *Addiction* 88, Supplement: S53–60.

Stockwell, T. (ed.) (1994) *An Examination of the Appropriateness and Efficacy of Liquor-Licensing Laws Across Australia*, Canberra: Australian Government Publishing Service.

Stockwell, T. and Beel, A. (1994) *Public Support for the Introduction of Standard Drink Labels on Alcohol Containers*, Perth, Western Australia: Curtin University, National Centre for Research into the Prevention of Drug Abuse.

Stockwell, T., Blaze Temple, D. and Walker, C. (1991a) 'The effect of "standard drink" labelling on the ability of drinkers to pour a "standard drink"', *Australian Journal of Public Health* 15: 56–63.

Stockwell, T., Bolt, E., Milner, I., Pugh, P. and Young, I. (1990) 'Home Detoxification for problem drinkers: acceptability to clients, relatives, general practitioners and outcome after 60 days', *British Journal of Addiction* 85: 61–70.

Stockwell, T. and Honig, F. (1990) 'Labelling alcoholic drinks: percentage proof, original gravity, percentage alcohol or "standard drinks"?', *Drug and Alcohol Review* 9: 81–90.

Stockwell, T., Lang, E. and Rydon, P. (1993a) 'High risk drinking settings: the association of serving and promotional practices with harmful drinking', *Addiction* 88: 1519–26.

Stockwell, T., Murphy, D. and Hodgson, R. (1983) 'The Severity of Alcohol Dependence Questionnaire: its use, reliability and validity', *British Journal of Addiction* 78: 145–55.

Stockwell, T., Rydon, P., Gianatti, S., Jenkins, E. et al. (1992b) 'Levels of drunkenness of customers leaving premises in Perth, Western Australia: a comparison of high and low "risk" premises', *British Journal of Addiction* 87: 873–81.

Stockwell, T., Rydon, P., Lang, E. and Beel, A. (1993b) *An Evaluation of the 'Freo Respects You' responsible alcohol service project*, Perth, Western Australia: Curtin University, National Centre for Research into the Prevention of Drug Abuse.

Stockwell, T., Single, E., Hawks, D. and Rehm, J. (1997) 'Sharpening the focus of alcohol policy from aggregate consumption to harm and risk reduction', *Addiction Research* 5: 1–9.

Stockwell, T., Somerford, P. and Lang, E. (1991b) 'The measurement of harmful outcomes following drinking on licensed premises', *Drug and Alcohol Review* 10: 99–106.

Stockwell, T., Somerford, P. and Lang, E. (1992a) 'The relationship between license type and alcohol-related problems attributed to licensed premises in Perth, Western Australia', *Journal of Studies on Alcohol*, September, 495–8.

Stockwell, T. and Stirling, L. (1989) 'Estimating alcohol content of drinks: common errors in applying the unit system', *British Medical Journal* 298: 71–572.

Strang. J. and Stimson, G.V. (eds) (1990) *AIDS and Drug Misuse*, London: Tavistock/Routledge.

Streissguth, A.P., Martin, D.C. and Buffington, V.E. (1977) 'Identifying heavy drinkers: a comparison of eight alcohol scores obtained on the same sample', in Sexias, F.A. (ed.) *Currents in Alcoholism Vol. 11*, New York: Grune and Stratton.

Sulkunen, P. (1997) 'The ethics of alcohol policy in a saturated society', *Addiction* 92: 1117–22.

Sussex Police (1987) *Sussex Police Liquor Licensing Project. Brighton 86/87: A Project to Identify and Reduce Alcohol-Related Crime*, Sussex: Sussex Police.

Sutton, M. and Godfrey, C. (1995) 'A grouped data regression approach to estimating economic and social influences on individual drinking behaviour', *Health Economics* 4, 237–47.

Sutton, S. (1987) 'Social psychological approaches to understanding addictive behaviours: attitude, behaviour and decision models', *British Journal of Addiction* 82: 355–70.

Swadi, H. (1989) 'Adolescent drug education programmes: methods and age targeting', *Pastoral Care* 7: 3–6.

Sweedler, B. (1990) 'Strategies to reduce youth drinking and driving', *Alcohol Health and Research World*, 14: 76–80.

Teachers' Advisory Council on Alcohol and Drug Education (TACADE) (1991) *Skills for the Primary School Child*, Part I Foundation Programme, Salford: TACADE.

TACADE (1992) *Alcohol Education: Issues for the '90s*, Salford: TACADE.

TACADE (1994) *Skills for Life*, Salford: TACADE.

Telles, S., Nagarathina, R. and Nagundra, H.R. (1993) 'Physiological changes in sports teachers following 3 months of training in yoga', *Indian Journal of Medical Sciences* 47: 235–8.

Tether, P. and Robinson, D. (1986) *Preventing Alcohol Problems: A Guide to Local Action*, London: Tavistock.

Thom, B. (1997) *Women and Alcohol: Issues for Prevention*, London: Health Education Authority.

Thom, B. (1999) *Dealing with Drink*, London: Free Association Books.

Thomas, M., Walker, A., Wilmot, A. and Bennett, N. (1998) *Living in Britain Results from the 1996 General Household Survey*, London: HMSO.

Thoresen, C.E. and Mahoney, M.J. (1974) *Behavioral Self-Control*, New York: Holt, Rinehart and Winston.

Thorley, A. (1982) 'The effects of alcohol', in Plant, M.A. (ed.) *Drinking and Problem Drinking*, London: Junction Books, 23–64.

Tierney, J., Cohen, J. and Bates, C. (1991) *Two Pints of Lager and a Packet of Crisps Please: A Study of Young People's Use of Pubs in Tameside*, Tameside and Glossop Health Authority.

Tigerstedt, C. (1999) 'Alcohol policy, public health and Kettil Bruun', Paper presented at 25th Annual Alcohol Epidemiology Symposium, Kettil Bruun Society for Social and Epidemiological Research on Alcohol, Montreal.

Tobler, N. (1986) 'Meta-analyisis of 143 adolescent drug abuse prevention programs: quantitative outcome results of program participants compared to a control or comparison group', *Journal of Drug Issues* 16: 537–67.

Tones, K. (1987) 'Role of the health action model in preventing drug abuse', *Health Education Research, Theory and Practice* 2: 305–16.

Traeen, B. and Kvalem, I. (1996) 'Sex under the influence of alcohol among Norwegian adolescents', *Addiction* 91: 995–1006.

Traeen, B. and Lewin, B. (1992) 'Casual sex among Norwegian adolescents', *Archives of Sexual Behavior* 21: 253–69.

Trotter, T. (1813) *An Essay, Medical, Philosophical, and Chemical, on Drunkenness*, New York: Arno Press, 1981 (2nd edition).

Tuck, M. (1989) *Drinking and Disorder*, Home Office Planning Unit Report No. 108, London: HMSO.

Tupler, L.A., Hege, S. and Ellinwood, E.H. Jnr (1995) 'Alcohol pharmacodynamics in young-elderly adults contrasted with young and middle-aged subjects', *Psychopharmacology* 118: 460–70.

Turtle, J., Jones, A. and Hickman, M. (1997) *Young people and Health: The Health Behaviour of School Age Children*, London: HEA/BMRB.

Ullman, A.D. (1962) 'First drinking experience as related to age and sex', in Pittman, D. and Snyder, D. (eds) *Society, Culture and Drinking Patterns*, New York: John Wiley.

Vaillant, G.E. (1983) *The Natural History of Alcoholism*, Cambridge, MA: Harvard University Press.

Vaillant, G.E. and Milofsky, E.S. (1982) 'Natural history of male alcoholism', *Archives of General Psychiatry* 29: 237–41.

Vandamme, T.H. (1986) 'Hypnosis as an adjunctant to the treatment of a drug addict', *Australian Journal of Clinical and Experimental Hypnosis* 1: 41–8.

Van de Goor, I. (1990) *Situational Aspects of Adolescent Drinking Behavior*, Netherlands: Rijksuniversiteit Limburg, Faculuteit der Gezonheidswetenschappen.

Van de Goor, L., Knibbe, R. and Drop, M. (1990) 'Adolescent drinking behaviour: an observational study of the influence of situational factors on adolescent drinking rate', *Journal of Studies on Alcohol* 51: 548–55.

Van Oers, H., Bongers, I., van de Goor, I. and Garretsen, H. (1999) 'Alcohol consumption, alcohol-related problems, problem drinking and socio-economic status', *Alcohol and Alcoholism* 34: 78–88.

Van Oers, H. and Garretsen, H.F.L. (1993) 'The geographic relationship between alcohol use, bars, liquor shops and traffic injuries in Rotterdam', *Journal of Studies on Alcohol* 54: 739–44.

Vestal, R.E., McGuire, E.A., Tobin, J.D., Andres, R., Norris, A.H. and Mezey, E. (1977) 'Ageing and ethanol metabolism', *Clinical Pharmacology and Therapeutics* 21: 343–54.

Victorian Community Council against Violence (1990) *Inquiry into Violence in and Around Licensed Premises*, Melbourne: Victorian Community Council against Violence.

Voas, R.B., Holder, H.D. and Gruenevald, P.J. (1997) 'The effect of drinking and driving interventions on alcohol-involved traffic crashes within a comprehensive community trial', *Addiction* 92, Supplement 2: S221–36.

Vroublevsky, A. and Harwin, J. (1998) 'Russia', in Grant, M. (ed.) *Alcohol and Emerging Markets: Patterns, Problems and Responses*, International Center for Alcohol Policies Series on Alcohol in Society, Philadelphia, PA: Bruhner/Mazel, 203–22.

Wagenaar, A.C. and Holder, H.D. (1991) 'Effects of Alcoholic Beverage Server Liability on Traffic Crash Injuries', *Alcoholism: Clinical and Experimental Research* 15: 942–7.

Wagenaar, A.C. and Wolfson, M. (1994) 'Enforcement of the legal minimum drinking age in the United States', *Journal of Public Health Policy* 15: 317–53.

Wallace, P., Cutler, S. and Haines, A. (1988) 'A randomised controlled trial of general practitioner intervention in patients with excessive alcohol consumption', *British Medical Journal* 297: 663–8.

Walpole, I.R., Zubrik, S. and Pontré, J. (1989) 'Confounding variables in studying the effects of maternal alcohol consumption before and during pregnancy', *Journal of Epidemiology and Community Health* 43: 153–61.

Walsh, R.A. (1995) 'Medical education about alcohol: a review of its role and effectiveness', *Alcohol and Alcoholism* 30: 689–702.

Warner, J. (1992) 'North, South, male, female: levels of alcohol consumption in late medieval Europe', personal communication. Cited by Plant, M.A. (1995) 'The United Kingdom', in Heath, D. (ed.) *International Handbook on Alcohol and Culture*, Westport, CT: Greenwood Press, 290.

Warner, R.H. and Rosett, H.L. (1975) 'The effects of drinking on offspring: an historical survey of the American British literature', *Journal of Studies on Alcohol* 36: 1395–420.

Warrier, G. (1997) *The Complete Illustrated Guide to Ayurveda*, London: Element Books.

Watts, R. and Rabow, J. (1983) 'Alcohol availability and alcohol-related problems in 213 California cities', *Alcoholism: Clinical and Experimental Research* 17: 47–58.

Webb, D. (1999) 'Current approaches to gathering evidence', in Simnett, I., Perkins, E. and Wright, L. (eds) *Evidence-Based Health Promotion*, Chichester: John Wiley, 34–46.

Webb, M. and Unwin, A. (1988) 'The outcome of outpatient withdrawal from alcohol', *British Journal of Addiction* 83: 929–34.

Weisner, C.M. (1990) 'Coercion into alcohol treatment', Appendix D in Institute of Medicine, *Broadening the Base of Treatment for Alcohol Problems*, Washington, DC: US Government Printing Office.

Wells, S. and Graham, K. (forthcoming) 'The frequency of third party involvement in incidents of barroom aggression', *Contemporary Drug Problems*.

Wells, S., Graham, K. and West, P. (1998) 'The good, the bad, and the ugly: responses by security staff to aggressive incidents in public drinking settings', *Journal of Drug Issues* 28: 817–36.

Wells-Parker, E., Bangert-Drowns, R., McMillen, R. and Williams, M. (1995) 'Final results from a meta-analysis of remedial interventions with drink-drive offenders', *Addiction* 90: 907–26.

White, D. and Pitts, M. (1997) *Health Promotion With Young People for the Prevention of Substance Misuse*, London: HEA.

Whitehead, M. (1997) 'How useful is the "Stages of Change" model?', *Health Education Journal* 56: 111–12.

Wilks, J., Callan, V.J. and Austin, D.A. (1989) 'Parent, peer and personal determinants of adolescent drinking', *British Journal of Addiction* 84: 619–30.

Wilkins, R.H. and Hore, B.D. (1977) 'A general practitioner study of the estimated prevalence of alcoholism in the Greater Manchester area', *British Journal of Addiction* 72: 198–200.

Williams, A.F. (1992) 'The 1980s' decline in alcohol-impaired driving and crashes and why it occurred', *Alcohol, Drugs and Driving* 8: 71–6.

Williams, G.P. and Brake, G.T. (1982) *The English Public House in Transition*, London: Edsall.

Wilsnack, R.W. and Wilsnack, S.C. (1992) 'Women, work and alcohol: failures of simple theories', *Alcoholism: Clinical and Experimental Research* 16, 172–9.

Wilsnack, S.C. and Wilsnack, R. (1995) 'Drinking and problem drinking in US women', in Galanter, M. (ed.) *Recent Developments in Alcoholism, Volume 12: Women and Alcoholism*, New York: Plenum Press, 29–60.

Wilson, P. (1980) *Drinking in England and Wales*, London: HMSO.

Windham, G.C., Fenster, L., Hopkins, B. et al. (1995) 'The association of moderate maternal and paternal alcohol consumption with birth weight and gestational age', *Epidemiology* 6: 591–7.

Windham, G.C., Fenster L., Swan S.H. (1992) 'Moderate maternal and paternal alcohol consumption and the risk of spontaneous abortion', *Epidemiology* 3: 364–70.

Windle, M. (1999) *Alcohol Use among Adolescents*, Thousand Oaks, CA: Sage.

Wine and Spirit Association memoranda to HM Treasury on excise duty.

Wittman, F.D. (1981) *Zoning Ordinances, Alcohol Outlets, and Planning: Prospects of Local Control of Alcohol Problems*. Report prepared under funding provided by the National Institute on Alcohol Abuse and Alcoholism, Grant Nos AA-04868–01/ AA-05622–02. Berkeley, CA: Alcohol Research Group, December 1981.

Wittman, F.D. (1983) *Local Regulation of Alcohol Availability in Selected California Communities: Introduction and Summary of Findings*. Report prepared for the California State Health and Welfare Agency, Department of Alcohol and Drug Programs, under Contract A-0138–2. Berkeley, CA: Prevention Research Group, Institute of Epidemiology and Behavioral Medicine, Medical Research Institute of San Francisco, October.

Wittman, F.D. and Biderman, F. (1992) 'The California community planning demonstration project: experiences in planning for prevention of alcohol problems in four municipalities', in *Experiences With Community Action Projects: New Research in the Prevention of Alcohol and Other Drug Problems*, CSAP Prevention Monograph 14. Center for Substance Abuse Prevention, US Department of Health and Human Services.

Wodak, A. (1994) 'Just say "no" to alcohol abuse and misuse', (Editorial), *Addiction* 89: 787–9.

Woodham, A. (1994) *HEA Guide to Complementary Medicine and Therapies*, London: HEA.

World Health Organization (WHO) (1985) 'Health promotion: a WHO discussion document on the concept and principles', *Journal of the Institute of Health Education* 23: 5–9.

World Health Organization (WHO) (1994a) *European Alcohol Action Plan*, Copenhagen: WHO Regional Office for Europe.

World Health Organization (WHO) (1994b) *Alcohol and HIV/AIDS*, Copenhagen: WHO Regional Office for Europe.

World Health Organization (WHO) (1994c) *World Health Statistics*, Geneva: WHO.

World Health Organization (WHO) (1998) *1996 World Health Statistics*, Geneva: WHO.

World Health Organization (WHO) (1999) *Lifestyles and Behaviour Change*, Copenhagen: WHO Regional Office for Europe.

Wright, L. (1991) 'Promoting health through teacher education', in Falk, J. (ed.) *Professional Development in Health Education: A Role for Universities?*, London: Health Education Authority.

Wright, L. (1993) *More Drinking Choices: Training Materials to Promote Sensible Drinking in the 1990s*, London: Health Education Authority.

Wright, L. (1999a) 'Alcohol and Youth Work'. Unpublished PhD thesis, University of Durham.

Wright, L. (1999b) *Alcohol and Young People: What 11- to 24-Year-Olds Know, Think and Do*, London: Health Education Authority.

Wright, L. (1999c) 'Evaluation in health promotion: the proof of the pudding?', in Simnett, I., Perkins, E.R. and Wright, L. (eds) (1999) *Evidence-Based Health Promotion*, Chichester: John Wiley, 393–403.

Wright, L. and Buczkiewicz, M. (1995) *Awaaz: Asian Young Women and Alcohol*, Salford: TACADE.

Wylie, A. and Casswell, S. (1991) 'A qualitative investigation of young men's drinking in New Zealand', *Health Education Research* 6: 49–55.

Zador, P., Lund, A., Fields, M. and Weinberg, K. (1989) 'Fatal crash involvement and laws against alcohol-impaired driving', *Journal of Public Health Policy* 10: 467–85.

Zander, A. (1990) *Effective Social Action by Community Groups*, San Francisco, CA: Jossey-Bass.

Ziglio, E. (1997) 'How to move towards evidence-based health promotion interventions', *Promotion and Education* 4: 29–32.

Zinn, J.K., Massion, A.O., Kristler, J., Peterson, L.G. and Fletcluske (1992) 'Effectiveness of meditation-based stress reduction program in the treatment of anxiety disorders', *American Journal of Psychiatry* 149: 936–43.

Zollman, C. and Vickens, A. (1999) 'ABC of complementary medicine', *British Medical Journal* 319: 693–6.

Index

Compiled by Judith Lavender

NOTE: page numbers in italics refer to figures or tables